Blowing in the Wind

Drug-Resistant TB and the Poor

"MEN UNDER THE GUIDANCE OF REASON DESIRE NOTHING FOR THEMSELVES WHICH THEY DO NOT DESIRE FOR THE REST OF MANKIND."

Spinoza (1632-1677)[1]

"IT'S THE SAME THE WHOLE WORLD OVER:
IT'S THE POOR WHAT GETS THE BLAME.
IT'S THE RICH WHAT GETS THE PLEASURE;
AIN'T IT ALL A BLOOMIN' SHAME."

Anonymous English street ballad (late 19th century)

[1] Baruch Spinoza has influenced a diverse collection of intellectuals across four centuries, including Karl Marx, George Santayana, Jorge Luis Borges and Albert Einstein. He died aged 44 of lung disease – almost certainly from silicosis-triggered tuberculosis.

For my mother Gillian Young

in memoriam memoriae

Acknowledgements

Immeasurable thanks go to Jenny Craig for her insight and advice, for her generosity, collaboration and encouragement, and also for her contributions especially with the cover design.

Similarly huge appreciation goes to William Baldwin for his skills above and beyond the call of duty. Also to Lynda Bowen for support and advice, Chloe Weber for encouragement, and to Kirsten Muzeen for critical help.

Thanks also to the team at the Northern College of Acupuncture (especially Peggy Welch and Richard Blackwell) and also to John McCarthy for helping me out with the statistics. (I should add that any mistakes that exist in these tricky sections are mine and mine alone.)

Huge thanks to Donald Eadie and Bernie Arscott for their faith, their constancy and their candles… and a million thankyou's to Yuki Itaya, Ulick Burke and Kat Chu for climbing aboard the runaway train and staying on it.

My gratitude as ever to my lovely wife Jo for living through this with me.

And *arigato gozaimasu* and a deep bow to Doctor Shimetaro Hara – for providing the guiding light and for having given a damn in his own troubled times.

About the author

In 2008 Merlin Young got infected with tuberculosis - not in the sense described in the text that follows, but from a realisation of the appalling neglect that patients with this terrible disease have been and still are suffering from. He remains convinced that when the history of the 20th century is finally written by future historians the story of TB will be up there with both World Wars.

In more normal life he practises as an acupuncturist in the West Midlands in the UK. In his less normal life he is co-founder and chair of Moxafrica, a UK charity set up to investigate whether a traditional therapy might help in the desparate fight against TB where resources are the worst (which is the subject of the final appendix). In the six years since the charity was founded, he has learnt so much about tuberculosis, enough to convince him that an appalling fresh chapter of human tragedy is unravelling right under our noses. This book is written in the hope that it might help prevent some of this happening.

Table of Contents

An Introduction

I was born in 1955. This means that my life so far has almost completely coincided with the only time in human history when tuberculosis has been effectively controlled – at least in my particular part of the world. As will become clearer in the course of reading just the first 20-odd pages of this book, this amounts to some stroke of luck.

I was also born on what might be most accurately described as the 'right side of the tracks' in terms of both time and space – meaning that my lifetime has also coincided with a period of unprecedented general affluence and peace in the society in which I live – in the so-called 'developed' or 'post-industrialised' world of Western Europe. This has also massively reduced the likelihood of my even coming into contact with this disease, let alone being infected by it. So I have very good reasons to be cheerful about life and to be very grateful about the time in which I find myself to be alive.

But this book is specifically about global TB and unfortunately on many counts the subject is anything but a cheerful one. TB is often described as being man's oldest bacteriological foe, as well as being its most deadly (which it almost certainly has been). Mosquitoes may well have inoculated a bunch of diseases into human beings which have resulted in larger piles of human corpses, but as far as infectious diseases go (i.e. ones that are directly transmissible between members of our species) the TB bacillus has been at the top of the unholy league of infectious agents for a very long time.

My personal early exposure to TB was probably typical of anyone of my generation in my particular corner of the world. At the age of 15 I was made to queue up for a skin test to see whether or not I should receive the BCG vaccination against the disease. I failed the test (in my eyes) because no tiny lumps subsequently showed up on my skin which would have dictated that I didn't need the jab. Then there was a mobile X-ray van drawn up outside the Students Union at my university – it was explained that this was for TB. What was the point, I thought, and moved off without joining the short queue.

Actually, this wasn't all I knew about TB at that second instance. There had been another the previous year, one which offers up a curious retrospective co-incidence for me in connection with events that have more recently taken over my life.

I had elected to take what is now known as a gap year. On 14th September 1972 I found myself hitch-hiking out of Bury St Edmonds in Suffolk, England in order to get to an old Royal Air Force base. It was the same day that the first of an as yet unknown number of Ugandans with British passports – people of original South Asian origin – were arriving in the UK. They were being peremptorily booted out of Uganda by its then megalomaniac president Idi Amin Dada, and the camp that I was trying to get to in the Suffolk countryside had been co-opted into becoming the first reception and resettlement camp for them.

I arrived at the camp literally three hours before the first refugees, and I probably knew as much about the people who were about to arrive as anyone already on the camp, which amounted to literally nothing – neither about their language, their culture, their customs nor their religions. Amin had only notified the world of their possible expulsion a month earlier, and for weeks no-one had even known whether or not his threats were to be taken seriously.

When the first coach arrived the chaos was effectively completed as it was swarmed over by a group of over-eager journalists.

My memories of this time are now far from complete. Once we'd worked out that almost no-one who stepped off the first coach spoke Hindi (which was the provision that had been made for interpreting) but that the dominant tongue was in fact Gujerati, and once the cooks had worked out that they were going to have to cook a lot of lentils which was hardly a staple ingredient on the North Sea oil rigs from which they'd just been hastily transferred, things began to settle down a little. I know that I didn't see a bed for the first three days, so, looking back, it all must have been pretty frenetic. I certainly recall that the camp was already seriously overcrowded by the time the second one came on-stream as planned, with beds in some cases having to be shared.

Once daily patterns began to settle in the camp, however, I found myself mainly being used to help some of its members get to and from the nearest railway station on their way to attend prospective job or housing interviews. Apart from arranging their transport to and from the station (including driving them in a retired Red Cross ambulance) we also had to ensure that they were properly logged both out of and back into the camp so that their movements were appropriately monitored.

One morning I was entrusted with the task of taking a particular resident refugee to the station because he had been invited to a formal reception in Peterborough. I recall that he was (or rather had been until just a few weeks before) an eminent professor from Makerere University in Kampala, one of the oldest and most prestigious universities in Africa.

I duly obliged by taking him to the station but, on returning, I found that a balloon had gone up in my absence.

The camp had a resident nurse – in fact she was a senior registered midwife and was one of the 'old school'. She was someone I had been personally finding more than a little fearsome having attracted her wrath by accidentally cut her off on the very first night of the camp being operational when, totally untrained, I had been entrusted with manning the camp's antiquated plug-in internal telephone system through the night.

Soon after I'd left the camp with the professor, she had apparently rushed into the office – and she was still there when I got back, wanting to know if he had got on the train. "Of course!.." I proudly reported. "Damn!" she retorted, "you shouldn't have let him out of the camp – he has TB." She then phoned the police in Peterborough to ensure that he was brought back to the camp as soon as he got off the train.

All the refugees had been initially screened by X-ray for TB on arrival at Stansted airport. I assume that the results of his particular X-ray had shown signs of advanced disease which had probably been subsequently confirmed to be infectious. So, for this brief moment, I found myself exposed to the instinctive human fear that this disease had been exerting on so many generations before mine.

That then was pretty much the sum of it regarding TB for quite some time until it began to show much more frequently on my radar. The disease threw up one unexpected and curious co-incidence just over 40 years later when I found myself , along with my friend and colleague Jenny Craig, making a presentation on the subject of the same disease at the same African university's School of Health Sciences that the professor had been removed from. But by then my awareness and understanding of the dangers of this ancient disease had increased exponentially.

Back then in 1972, however, I really had known nothing about TB – but my ignorance was understandable given that the disease had pretty much disappeared from the public radar. I initially assumed that the reason for this was simply due to the discovery of a clutch of drugs in the three preceding decades which had removed the disease from being any sort of serious infectious threat in the world in which I lived. My deepening understanding of the disease, however, made me realise that even this was a gross over-simplification. As Dr Ibanda Hood, a Ugandan doctor with whom we have been collaborating has advised me, "Nothing to do with tuberculosis is straight line stuff". Over the last few years I have come to realise more and more how true this observation is.

What I also hadn't known was that the disease had essentially never gone away at all in many parts of the world, and that there were equally complex reasons for this as well.

With these anecdotes, I'm hoping that I may have set up a useful starting place from which we can take this exploration and exposition much further. My intention is to promote a much needed and far more detailed understanding of this ancient disease than I myself had back then in 1972.

The main part of this book consists of a comprehensive review of the disease itself and the state of tuberculosis in the 21st century. Without apology, I explore it whenever it is appropriate more from the perspectives of those who are most at current active risk from the disease rather than from the perspective of the world in which I live.

In the course of developing the work, I came to realise two things: one was that there is surprisingly no book in print that takes a look at the evolving state of the disease today from this point of view; the other was that almost all the current references to it in the media in our world of higher incomes and lower rates of infectious disease are troublingly misleading. They either relate exaggerated scare stories (often themselves mixed up with emotive issues of immigration), or hyped-up stories of new drugs or vaccines (some of which I tend to believe may be being spun a little more optimistically than they deserve to be). The complexities of the immense global humanitarian and social problems that this disease has been creating, along with the enormous challenges of effective programme management in the environments where the disease is causing devastating human tragedy, are almost always ignored. These issues will need to be properly confronted if we hope to seriously reduce its incidence wherever the disease is running rife.

So it seems reasonable to suggest that a book which takes on the task of discussing these issues is actually rather badly needed given that, from almost any informed perspective, TB is such a huge problem. It also seems to be a good idea to try to insert a little more realism into the public debate such as exists, even if this may be disquieting.

Doing so, unfortunately, does not make for very cheerful reading. TB is almost certainly one of the greatest public health challenges of our age – and could well prove to be the greatest – so seeing it more properly exposed should be of interest to anyone with an interest in human current affairs. Some of the more complex associated issues of ethics and human rights also deserve far wider exposure than they currently enjoy.

I personally first found myself caught in the headlights of tuberculosis whilst reading Tracy Kidder's book about Dr Paul Farmer, entitled "Mountains beyond Mountains". Dr Farmer is not just a fearless advocate of the rights of all to decent health care, but he is also an expert on TB and other infectious diseases. Although the title of the book was not intended to specifically reflect tuberculosis alone, I think that it very accurately reflects the complex layers of problems most of which need exposing, confronting and solving if we seriously hope to see TB defeated today, particularly so in respect of the emerging pandemic of drug-resistant TB disease.

I have done my best to expose some of these layers in a systematic way in the following pages. It's not been an easy task. I peer backwards into the past because I'm convinced that there are clues there concerning what may work and also what may not be working in the fight today. I also have had no alternative but to look forward rather nervously because I see humanitarian horror stories developing in some countries in the next decade, particularly in southern Africa and India. Maybe there is still time left to avoid the worst of them.

I do my best as well to unravel some of the more complex ramifications of the disease itself given my own substantially better informed understandings today. It is simply impossible to understand the scale of the current threat without also understanding some of the paradoxical complexities that co-exist within the phenomenon that is tuberculosis.

My own starting point, I am happy to admit, was an ignorant one – and I have assumed similar ignorance on the part of most readers in order to give them a better chance of understanding the disease. In order to develop such an understanding I have deliberately chosen to build up layer upon layer of detail. Such an approach necessitates some inevitable instances of repetition, and I hope that the more informed reader will be patient and forgive me for them.

I do my best to help this process, from time to time, by changing both tunes and time signatures, hoping not just to enrich understandings by doing so, but also to fire imaginations and to develop the reader's interest in the subject in anticipation of some important later parts which I readily accept may be a hard and demanding read for the less bio-scientifically minded.

The following pages also include several personal critical analyses of some of the so-called 'facts' about TB as they have been being serially presented over the past two decades – and as they are still being presented – and I choose to challenge some of them in the process. Some of my observations may on occasion seem impudent – some may even be misinformed. I am not a trained pulmonologist, nor an immunologist – neither am I an epidemiologist nor a social scientist. But my understanding of the disease has necessarily developed into one which steps tentatively into each of these fields of expertise. Given the nature and scale of the growing problem, I am happy to accept that there may be mistakes in my analyses, although I have made every effort to ensure that the official facts, estimates and statistics which I use are as up-to-date as possible. I do, however, welcome any comments or corrections from anyone generous enough to offer them in case they might be included in further editions of this book which might then benefit from them.

This much I am sure of, however: the central themes of this book are not flawed and they must somehow be addressed or history will judge us terribly for not having done so.

On 20th March 2013 a group of Health Ministers from several African countries, along with leaders of international agencies, met in Swaziland and launched a fresh offensive against tuberculosis in Africa. Swaziland is burdened with the highest national rates of TB anywhere in the world and its people also have one of the world's lowest life expectancies, so it was certainly an appropriate place for these leaders to meet. They collectively signed what has been called the "Swaziland Statement" which included a commitment to catch up on targets in the following "thousand days" – the same targets which have been massively missed in the previous 10,000 days when they were originally set out as part of the Global Targets for TB.

Amongst these targets was the goal of halving death rates from TB by 2015 in comparison to what they had been back in 1990. Currently deaths from TB in southern Africa are running at rates that are probably three times higher than they were in 1990, and some suggest even higher still, so there is an awful lot of work that still needs to be done. Benedict Xaba, the

Health Minister for Swaziland, clearly wanted to sound a hopeful note in his call-to-arms for a more intensive response to what is now an undeniable emergency. He pronounced that he and his colleagues "did not gather … to underline the problem – we know the problem very well." He is a politician, so he has to be cut a little slack for making such a statement, but, when I read his words in the context of the commitment that he and his fellow political leaders had made, I found myself wondering exactly how well either he or his colleagues really ***do*** understand the problem. Given the history to date, could they possibly really understand the problems and still commit themselves to such an incredibly ambitious target at this point of time, because there is not a chance that this target will be met.

I'd even go a little further and suggest that only a very few people really do seem to fully understand the reality of fighting this disease today where it is most rife. Certainly remarkably few individuals or NGOs seem prepared to publicly describe its true current scale and complexity, and the names of most of those prepared to do so will be appearing again and again in the following pages.

Such relative silence may even be necessarily deliberate. Richard Coker has described that:

> "The art of media relations in TB is the art of controlled hysteria… you want people to be worried enough to give you more resources, but not so worried that they make you do all sorts of stupid things."

So are we being manipulated by some kind of orchestrated "controlled hysteria" on the subject? I'm not entirely sure, but I do worry that insufficient information is being properly disseminated for wider debate. And exactly what sort of "stupid things" are those managing global health so worried that they may end up being forced to do? This I feel even more uncomfortable about, but I'm convinced that far too many lives already depend on some very difficult choices being made in this most challenging field of public health.

There is a saying that if you scrape beneath the surface of the mud you'll always find more mud. This is not an unfair summary, unfortunately, of much the main part of this book. There's an awful lot of mud that has to be scraped away to properly understand TB today, and in doing so, there's an awful lot more mud left in view. There are massive clinical issues that deserve exposure, as well as social, ethical, political and economic ones – and these economic ones may turn out to be the thorniest of all, at least from the perspective of those at most threat from the disease. TB, unfortunately, is not just a lethal disease of the poor (unfortunately, probably more so now than it ever has been) – it's also a disease which actually ***makes*** people (and even populations) poor as well.

As far as those global institutions which effectively 'manage' our world today are concerned, any solutions for such a problematic phenomenon as TB today must first and foremost be demonstrably economically justifiable. They must, of course, also be safe and it is clear that current treatment policies or options in low-income countries often only tick one or the other of these boxes. Epidemiologically-speaking at least, I'd suggest that they rarely tick both. Just as importantly, however, they must also be both environmentally and socially appropriate.

Until world bodies like the G8 the G20, the UN, and the WHO fully alert themselves to the scale of this problem and then decide to meaningfully direct an appropriate proportion of their available resources towards it, it looks like all primary point-of-care responses must, first and foremost, be safe, cheap and easy to use if they are genuinely intended to be of real benefit to any more than a tiny proportion of the host of people most at threat from the disease today. This is understandably not an idea that is popular with some of the loudest advocates for better treatment provision, some of whom see the current TB epidemic as a stain on our ability to provide adequate health care for the whole of humanity. It's impossible to disagree with them but, nevertheless, I find myself wondering how much is truly possible – at least in the shorter term.

Professor Donald Sadoway of the Massachusetts Institute of Technology has suggested that "if you want to make something dirt cheap, make it out of dirt – probably dirt that's locally sourced". This is a very interesting idea. In the final appendix of the book I will discuss a potentially useful and so-far unexplored approach to the problem – one that is based on some debatable historical evidence, on some decades-old scientific research, and on some recently emerging clinical evidence from a randomised control trial that is being completed in Kampala. It has been run under the auspices of that very same Makerere University, the one which that infectious professor had been a faculty member of before being expelled from his country in 1972. The treatment under investigation in the study is certainly cheap. It's not made out of dirt, but it ***is*** most definitely appropriate in terms of the technology required to implement it from start to finish.

I should add that I am not suggesting it as being any sort of final solution to TB, but it could at least prove be part of a solution while the world gets its act together and begins to set its strategies properly back on track.

"The Number One Enemy of the Human Race"

"WHETHER MEASURED BY PREVALENCE, COST,
SOCIAL CONSEQUENCE, SHEER MISERY OR ANY YARDSTICK,
I BELIEVE THAT ANY OBSERVER WOULD CONSIDER
THE BACILLUS OF TUBERCULOSIS AS
THE NUMBER ONE ENEMY OF THE HUMAN RACE."

H. Corwin Hinshaw[2]

The number one enemy of the human race? That's some claim. So let us familiarise ourselves a little with this supposedly mega-dangerous pathogen. Tuberculosis, in its simplest terms, is an infectious disease caused by what is known as the Tubercle Bacillus (hence the simple acronym TB) or, rather more fancifully (if we are using the Latin as is the medical custom), by the *Mycobacterium Tuberculosis* (*M. tuberculosis*). It is most frequently characterized by the formation of tubercles in the lungs but sometimes in other tissues of the body as well. In essence, a tubercle is simply a small nodule, and these tuberculous nodules often develop long after the initial infection. It is an aerobic disease, and its growth rate is highly affected by the amount of oxygen available to it – hence its favoured home in the human body is in the lungs.

This "pulmonary TB" (the most common form) is characterized by the coughing up of mucus and often blood, with fever, weight loss and chest pain. Untreated it generally kills between 50% and 70% of those showing active symptoms, often taking years to do so. This can be a long, painful and drawn out affair.

Until the 1950s no real treatment existed for it and it was a truly dreaded disease. Until the early 1990s, in fact, it was still recognised as the most lethal infectious disease known to mankind – that was until the HIV virus appeared and stole its limelight, as it is still doing in very dangerous and complex ways as we shall see. But, given the number of HIV-positive patients who actually die from this older bacteriological enemy (as many as 25% globally and almost certainly nearer 70% in Africa) and given that the diagnostics and surveillance of HIV/AIDS has more recently been rolled out far more reliably and rigorously than for TB, it is arguable that TB

[2] One of the key researchers of Streptomycin in the 1940s, Horton Corwin Hinshaw conducted the first animal and human trials of the drug.

might ***still*** be mankind's arch-enemy in the infectious disease department. I will be recycling a few statistics in the course of the following pages which will make a very strong claim that this is indeed so – not only that it is still so, but also that its viral rival is causing the scale of the threat from TB to be either obscured or dangerously underestimated while the global health authorities and NGOs continue to mount a much stouter defence against the more recently emerged pandemic of HIV/AIDS.

Whilst it may normally kill 50-70% of those left untreated, in concert with HIV/AIDS it is much more lethal if left untreated. To my knowledge, no accurate percentage statistic yet exists regarding the probability of mortality when there is untreated co-infection of the two diseases, although there has been more than one attempt to do so.[3] It may well be that it is still too much of a moving target to really get a fix on as the control of HIV continues to improve whilst similar control of TB languishes. Because of the high rates of HIV in Africa, the rates both of TB mortality and also of latent infection are the highest of any in the world, in fact they are terrifyingly so in those countries where the HIV epidemic is the most acute. This is also the case (quite logically) anywhere where the proper tools for diagnosis and appropriate treatment are most scarce, but the fact that they are also absent, or at least most unreliable, in Africa means that this is the region where the disease is now not just the hardest to confirm but also to contain – and this has been the case for some time.

Unusually for an infectious disease, tuberculosis has a highly unpredictable incubation period from the time of first contact to signs of active disease developing. This is something which can vary enormously (in most cases with the disease remaining in a latent state, thankfully never developing into an active state at all). This has huge significance not just in terms of the nature of the disease but also in respect of its management, since paradoxically most of the epidemic remains almost entirely invisible as a result. But if active disease does develop, it does so most often very slowly with a correspondingly chronic development of symptoms. As a result, the peaks of any TB epidemic are hard to predict and equally hard to follow. In fact they are invariably most easily viewed in hindsight. These peaks, like

---

[3] This has been addressed in the most recent 2013 WHO Global Tuberculosis Report on TB. It involves the application of a complex formula [*M=(I N)Fu +NFn]* which is intended to be calculated using four component factors, only one of which [*N*] is definitively measurable – the other three being based on estimated numbers. It attempts to correlate HIV-positive TB incidence rates with case fatality ratios of notified and non-notified incidence cases.

those symptoms of then afflicted, also develop in slow waves and then tend to last for far longer periods of time than those of other infectious diseases.

TB is also possibly the best example of a disease of what is rather grandly termed "complex multi-factorial causation" – and, as we shall see, some of the more successful efforts to defeat it have not only been driven by direct therapeutic interventions but have been driven by (and have in some instances even actually ***driven***) social and political change.

TB unquestionably is a disease which endemically afflicts the poor more than any other socio-economic group. It's also reasonable to suggest that this may be truer today than at any other time in humanity's long relationship with it. Such a suggestion has to offer us much speculative and challenging food for thought as to how it might best be combatted today, given that the gaps between rich and poor are still widening. The people whom it currently most particularly afflicts are those who are sometimes euphemistically referred to as the 'bottom billion' (although, with regards to TB, this might more realistically add up to the bottom two billion, those who are most likely to be latently infected). The principal reason for this is simple – they also happen to be the most endemically immune-compromised of our species, often both living and working the closest to each other in challenging conditions which inevitably foster disease.

As if all this weren't enough, TB bacteria have more recently revealed an innate propensity for lethal mutation resulting in what is known as drug-resistant TB (DR-TB). This is something which is particularly difficult to diagnose and contain in any country with poor medical resource – because when TB becomes resistant to even just two drugs, it becomes both very difficult and expensive to treat. The world has been extremely slow in waking up to the potential implications of this.

No-one knows exactly why the TB bacillus has such a deft capacity for mutation, but this capacity, along with the relatively late arrival of TB drugs in Sub-Saharan Africa (which unfortunately happened only shortly before the emergent continental epidemic of HIV/AIDS) is still adding up to what has been described as a 'perfect storm' of untreatable disease in the region. A two-step dance of disease has now exploded in virulent hotspots in southern Africa. In fact this perfect storm is not only composed of just these two diseases (TB and HIV) but it is also being fed by many other individual storms cells as well – more than are regularly recognised, and all of which together may combine to make the approaching super storm itself as powerful and lethal as any that has ever afflicted mankind.

Some key facts

The following are four facts which are widely used to describe the TB epidemic.

- Tuberculosis (TB) today is second only to HIV/AIDS as the greatest killer worldwide by a single infectious agent.
- In 2012, 8.6 million people fell ill with TB and 1.3 million died from the disease.
- Only 66% of the pandemic is getting spotted and treated
- Over 95% of TB deaths occur in low- and middle-income countries[4]

As we will see in later pages, such figures, as shocking as they may at first appear to be, fail to tell us the whole story, nor will they be seen to make as much coherent sense as might be expected. In fact, any attempt which intends to develop a more coherent picture by combining them leads only to further uncertain conjecture and questions.

So let's start with the very first statistic above – that TB is second only to HIV/AIDS as a lethally infectious pathogen. The official figures certainly suggest that this is the case: there were 1.3 million TB deaths in 2012 as opposed to 1.8 million deaths from HIV/AIDS.

There is, in fact, a current international classification for recording cause of death which dictates that, if someone is confirmed as HIV-positive and then dies, the cause of death that will be attributed to that individual will be HIV/AIDS, even though the actual illness that caused the death was another opportunistic infectious agent. (The HIV virus does not of itself kill – it promotes the condition of compromised immunity which then creates the opportunity for other pathogens to do the killing on its behalf.)

The reason for this international classification of cause of death is simple: the HIV epidemic is viewed as being so dangerous a threat to global health that the utmost importance is awarded to keeping an active eye on it, something which includes very actively monitoring its associated rates of mortality. No global survey of deaths and of causes of deaths can maintain any sort of coherent accuracy if a single death is counted twice by being attributed equally to two diseases at the same time, so the disease which is

[4] These are the most recent statistics at the time of going to print, published in 2013.

judged to be more serious (in this case HIV) takes pride of place in the register of death.

It's been estimated that (globally) the cause of around 25% of deaths of people who have been living with HIV/AIDS (often just referred to as PLWH) is actually directly attributable to TB. In Africa this percentage is much higher. It turns out to be rather important to keep this in mind when reviewing any mortality statistics relating to either disease, because the deaths of PLWH who die of TB often aren't counted as deaths from TB at all. Sometimes they are; sometimes they aren't. (They are computed in the estimated figures above, for instance, but they're not in the global targets for reducing death from tuberculosis for 2015).

But the more compelling reason for speculating that TB might still be the most lethal infectious pathogen is simply because, whilst there has been such a consistent focus on actively monitoring HIV for nearly two decades, there has been a simultaneous neglect of accurate TB surveillance for as many as five decades, something which, as we will see, is only just beginning to be properly addressed. Wherever or whenever it does get better addressed, however, a strong suspicion emerges that the rates for TB incidence may have been, for many reasons, significantly under-reported or under-estimated. What is even more unfortunate is that, just as this has begun to be addressed, the disease has also begun to mutate, diverging into different strains of drug-resistant disease which are far harder to diagnose and which require quite different responses to contain.

All of this raises a very important question to which we will return several times in the following pages: is one of the reasons that the current TB global pandemic has been dangerously under-estimated because HIV/AIDS has been taking precedence over it in terms of both focus and resource? Certainly some anecdotal reports from TB health workers would suggest this. The allocation of funding from the Global Fund (the largest source of funding for the control of HIV, Malaria and TB) would also support this view: until 2013 TB had been receiving only 15% of the allocated funds dedicated to help these three diseases (i.e. a sixth). Even now, this has only been adjusted to a quarter so it is still not being awarded what might be assessed to be an equitable or predictable third of the available pot. Given the scale of the problem, and the amount of resource that is recognised to be needed to combat it in any adequate way (particularly as drug-resistance grows), such a disproportionately smaller allocation of resource is certainly perplexing.

Now let's try the second fact – that 8.6 million caught TB and that 1.3 million died during the most recent year for which figures are available (in 2012). Since both of these global figures are now declining very slowly in similar and consistent ways, this would suggest a very rough *adhoc* annual death rate of over 15% of those who get infected with TB (though they may well not do so in the same year). So even today, with a clutch of drugs that have been widely available for 50 years and which are generally reported to be effective, a little over one in six people who get infected with TB across the world still appear to end up dead. This has to be pretty shocking. It should certainly be to anyone who is unfamiliar with the current state of the disease and accepts the commonly promoted statement that TB today is 'fully treatable' (which it almost certainly is – at least it is in countries with higher incomes and lower rates of infectious disease).

But there is another anomaly here, and it is one which feeds directly into this questionable death rate. If only 66% of cases are spotted and treated (the third of the 'facts' that are quoted above) then every third infectious case must be being missed entirely. And if this is true, then 50%-70% of these unspotted cases can be expected to die (a reasonable estimate if we accept the figures which are normally quoted for the risk of death from untreated tuberculosis). In this case, then 17%-24% of those infected with TB (or 1.5 to 2 million people) must die each year simply because they get no treatment at all. This figure doesn't include any of those who are treated but who die because of poor treatment, poor drug supply, because of HIV infection, advanced disease, non-compliance or because of drug-resistant disease. So those 1.3 million officially estimated mortalities look to be something of an under-estimation, and quite possibly TB still is mankind's most lethal infectious killer disease.

So our very first cursory unpacking of a couple of the official figures shows us that we should be cautious of treating any of them as if they are entirely reliable, and this is largely because almost all of them are subject to significant variabilities.

And so we come to the fourth fact – that 95% of deaths from TB occur in middle- or low-income countries. What this figure suggests by omission is that death from TB is, in essence, entirely avoidable – at least it is avoidable unless you happen to be very poor. The remaining 5% of deaths which occur in higher income countries still tell us the same story as well – because those that do most frequently succumb to this disease in such countries are also their poorest citizens, or the addicted, or the destitute, and almost invariably they are also the most vulnerable. To put this in perhaps better context, currently one-fifth (or 20%) of ***all*** deaths of adults in developing or low-income countries today are said to relate to TB. In many countries, in fact, it is still the most common cause of adult death. All told, it is still a ***very*** common lethal disease in the poorer quarters of our planet.

A more accurate re-evaluation of this fourth fact, therefore, might constitute the following:

- When it comes to actually dying from TB today, almost ***all*** of those who finally succumb to it are poor.

There are a lot of composite reasons for these social risk factors as well as for such statistical anomalies, and we will unpack them one by one in the hope of developing an appropriate understanding the disease. In the course of doing so we can also speculate how best the disease should be fought in those places where the battle against it is currently being so terribly lost. It is these particular battlefields which are by far the most important ones in the wider war against tuberculosis if such a war is to be meaningfully waged at all.

Unfortunately, there are currently some signs which suggest that, despite the reported positive trends, the course of this war may be about to take a worrying turn for the worse. Before we look further at them, however, we need to understand a little more about tuberculosis, not just about how it infects people today, but also how it has affected humanity itself – from the dim and distant past right up to today and tomorrow.

Some more about tuberculosis and how it develops

Tuberculosis is remarkably unusual among the major infectious diseases for three principal reasons:

- One is that it generally still lacks both accurate and rapid point-of-care diagnostic tests (ones, in other words, that can be reliably used locally to the patient).[5] We will be discussing the reasons for this (and its implications) in much more detail later, but for now it is enough to suggest that this has perhaps

[5] This (to some degree) has changed with the approval of the GeneXpert device, although, as welcome as the device is, it still doesn't have all the solutions to the problems of diagnosis of the disease today.

been the single most significant factor that has contributed to our ongoing failure to control the spread of the disease. We are still basically unable to properly detect the disease in those places where it thrives, with a consequence that infectious cases are not treated in as timely a fashion as is necessary. Such a simple equation of inadequacy means that far too often *Mycobacterium tuberculosis* is still able to survive and transmit at will, and it does this most devastatingly in any community with a poor medical infrastructure and resource.

- A further unusual anomaly is that a naturally occurring infection of TB does not appear to confer much long-term subsequent protective immunity to it in the person infected as is commonly the case with many other infectious diseases. In other words, even with the disease cured, there remains a strong possibility of re-infection – something which is much more likely in a 'high incidence' environment with lots of infection in the air, most especially amongst those who are already immune-compromised.

- The third factor is that the disease develops in stages and does so very, very slowly. Whilst this might be assumed to give advantage to those intent on hunting down and eradicating the infectious pathogen, it paradoxically gives more advantage to the hunted, to these curious mycobacteria.

Most often TB infection initially occurs as a result of the chance inhalation of air-borne droplets which contain the tiny infectious bacilli. Such droplets can be breathed in while in close-quarters to an ***infectious*** person (not just an ***infected*** one as we will see) who is coughing.

There is still a surprising deficiency of understanding from start to finish in terms of the longer processes of infection, as well as of the host response which either is or isn't ramped up to combat it. The sorry explanation that is most frequently used by immunologists for this is that, despite its being such a long-term enemy of mankind, its 'mechanisms are still poorly understood'.

No-one, in fact, has even developed a complete understanding of exactly how infectious this disease truly is. It is generally proposed that a person with active infectious disease will infect a further 10-15 people in a 12 month period if he or she remains infectious throughout it. Essentially, this adds up to pretty much one new infection during every month that an individual remains infectious.

It can, however, take years for the disease to naturally develop from first infection to active infectious disease with virtually no visible symptoms, and then it can take a few more years until death (if this finally occurs). Without effective treatment to reduce infectivity whilst these later stages of infection are occurring, on-going transmission is unfortunately almost inevitable, although this risk can be usefully reduced by very simple measures. Certainly, in comparison to a rapid viral infection like 'flu or measles, TB may not seem very infectious at all, but its insidious infectivity is feared for very good reason by all who have any sort of understanding of the consequence of infection or knowledge of the history of the disease.

To put this into perspective in the sort of environments in which the disease flourishes, HIV-negative individuals (i.e. those with uncompromised immune systems) who are infected by TB in resource-poor settings (i.e. where most of the disease exists) have been estimated to be infectious for as long as three years prior their first diagnosis. If such estimates are correct, it implies that a single person with active TB could be anticipated to infect as many as 45 other individuals before beginning their treatment.

The most acute risk of developing active disease is recognised to be highest in children under three years of age, lowest in later childhood between five and 13 (which is called the 'safe school age'), but then rising again for adolescents, young adults and then again for the very old. It is still unclear exactly why this is, although there is a theory, as we will see, which has been recently proposed to explain it.

We still know neither the minimum time of exposure to the bacillus that is required for the possibility of infection to become a probability, nor the quantity or quality of exposure that is necessary for infection to become inevitable. There is one report of an infection from a single infectious case being contracted whilst on a flight which lasted just eight hours;[6] there is another example from a school in the UK which suggested it occurred in a

[6] Ibrahim Abubakar - "Tuberculosis and Air Travel: a systematic review and analysis of policy", Lancet Infectious Diseases, 10 (2010) 176-83.

period of 130 hours of shared unventilated air.[7] Neither report, however, can be considered conclusive given that, up to the point of known contact, there must have been chances of prior infection with genetically identical strains of disease which had previously remained latent, and also because there were probably others who were equally exposed on both occasions who reported no later signs of disease.

There is also some limited evidence of natural resistance in human populations. Some close-contact investigations in the US revealed that an estimated 20–30% of the close contacts of a known infectious individual developed a latent infection, while around 1% developed active TB. This logically suggests that 70–80% of exposed individuals might not become infected at all because of some sort of natural resistance (or maybe because they were vaccinated, a whole minefield of its own which we will also review later). This data is far from conclusive, however, and would be difficult to prove, particularly since the results would almost certainly be highly variable in different environments – but such findings do suggest that a proportion of humans are probably genetically resistant to infection.

There may also be complexities involved in this, both in terms of ethnic groups who may have developed specific resistance to certain strains over many generations and also in terms of discrete genetic strains of disease. A more recently identified type of TB (known as the Beijing strain), for instance, is widely believed to be more virulent in terms of its infectivity than others, but this may be simply because of new exposure to this strain of pathogen by populations which have only recently ever been exposed to it. Such variables probably play a huge role in the way that the human immune response does or doesn't respond to the bacteria.

A small study conducted in the Gambia indicated that contacts of infectious TB patients who were definitely confirmed as having been initially latently infected with *Mycobacterium africanum* (a minority and older member of the tuberculosis family of diseases) were less likely to progress to active TB (i.e. they were more likely to remain with the disease in a dormant or latent state) than those who were confirmed to have been

[7] Ajit Lalvani et al. - "Comparison of T-cell-based assay with tuberculin skin test for diagnosis of *Mycobacterium tuberculosis* infection in a school outbreak", The Lancet, 361 (2003) 1168-73.

initially latently infected with other *M. tuberculosis* strains, including the so-called Beijing strain which we will encounter again in a later section.[8]

In another study, a different pattern of response was observed to emerge – it was found that strains of disease of a Euro-American lineage were more likely to cause pulmonary disease rather than meningeal TB (of the brain) compared with other strains.[9] In other words, the final character of the disease may differ dependent upon its discrete strain.

Such findings suggest that generations of exposure to a locally occurring strain could possibly confer a significant level of natural herd immune response in the population exposed to it. Such resistance might offer only a small evolutionary advantage because of the lengthy process in the disease's development, but it could still be significant over generations. In the particular Gambian case it might have been exactly such an inherited immune response that apparently made an individual better able to resist a similar germ's efforts to break out of latency. This trick of breaking out into active disease is one of *M. tubercolis's* trump cards, and a tiny genetic modification that could disable this could just prove to be the bug's undoing if it could be found.

But we are already moving ahead too far and too fast.

The basic risk of infection of any sort is definitely increased by several factors, the most simple being the proximity of the infectious person (and their coughing etiquette), the length of the exposure, and the degree of ventilation in the environment.

Having been exhaled by the infectious person by cough or sneeze, these tiny infectious droplet nuclei may hang around in the air and then be inhaled into a recipient's respiratory tract and then get drawn down into the lungs. Such nuclei are quite tiny, less than one micrometre in size, but within them lie the tubercle bacilli. They come to rest deep in the lungs

---

8 de Jong et al. – "Progression to active tuberculosis, but not transmission, varies by Mycobacterium tuberculosis lineage in The Gambia", Journal of Infectious Diseases, 198 (2008) 1037–43. The conclusions drawn by this study must be uncertain, however, simply because it is impossible to ascertain the strain of mycobacteria until after active disease has developed.

9 Caws, M. et al. – "The influence of host and bacterial genotype on the development of disseminated disease with *Mycobacterium tuberculosis*", PLoS Pathog. 4 (2008) e1000034.

where they soon stimulate a response from their new host's immune system once it detects their presence. This first response involves specialised macrophages (which are specialist White Blood Cells) which are programmed to recognise potentially dangerous invaders and instinctively ingest them.

Such White Blood Cells (WBCs) more often than not successfully mop up most bacterial infections after initial infection. This is to an extent also true of infection with TB except that, with this disease, the job may never get completed properly. Unfortunately, having ingested the invaders these macrophages are unable to completely finish them off allowing the TB bacilli to start to multiply very slowly within the macrophages themselves, dividing roughly once a day. This is an exceptionally slow rate for bacterial development which seems to effectively disarm the host immune response. To give an idea how relatively slow this process is, normal bacterial rates for division are measured in minutes, not days, so TB is a very slow developer by any normal bacterial standards. This is something else which has ultimately proved to be of singular advantage to the bacillus, however, because this slow progression essentially seems to allow it to slip beneath the radar of the immune system which is far better programmed to respond to speedier progressions. Finally, the macrophages themselves split open in defeat, releasing more of the bacteria, and the process gets repeated.

This initial period of infection usually continues for a period of a few weeks. Sometimes during this time the bacilli can even spread straight to places outside the lungs, to the lymph nodes near the lungs or even to other parts of the body. The likelihood of this happening, however, is limited – although it is more likely to occur in people with an immune system which is already compromised – something else we will come back to later because of its importance in connection to HIV co-infection. It also happens much more frequently in young children, again because of their inadequate immune response.

This initial response process most frequently concludes with the development of an initial 'acquired' immunity in these first two to 10 weeks – something which amounts to a final halt to this initial stage of bacterial multiplication. The WBC's, however, have still not been able to completely finish off their job, having failed to dispose of the ingested bacteria in the way they have evolved to do. The possibility that the bacilli themselves might be continuing to eat the WBCs from within and then be growing and multiplying within the cells themselves poses a very dangerous threat to the host immune system which is now finally waking up to the severity of the infection. In response, the host opts for stalemate by effectively walling all of this off and forming a fibrous shell around the infection site to contain it. These shells are called granulomas, which are tiny nodules formed by another collection of macrophages, forming in response to the presence of antigens that are resistant to 'first-responder' immune cells (neutrophils and eosinophils) which have themselves set up this state of alarm and response. A collection of dead cells then materialises in the centre of the granuloma. If viewed under a microscope a granuloma will appear as a mass of formless debris with no apparent nuclei present. These formless centres are further defined as 'caseous' or cheese-like and are regarded as being typically identifiable as the granulomas of tuberculosis.

Infection → initial immune response → 'walling off' → latent infection

All now becomes quiet, and the disease becomes latent – but the risk still remains that the bacteria might break out again at any time in the future.

Some very recent research suggests that this risk may be even more insidious than has been previously thought, and also suggests that this first phase of disease just might not even be as cut and dried as it has just been described.

It is still generally accepted that, during these early stages of the disease, the active TB bacteria do most frequently replicate inside human macrophages in the lungs (or at least in the site of primary infection), but there now appears to be less conclusive evidence than had been assumed that it is these immune cells alone that harbour the dormant TB which finally breaks out.[10] According to a study published in 2013 in Science Translational Medicine it seems that the TB bacilli can hide out, not just in the lungs, but also in stem cells deep within bone tissue, where they can effectively avoid detection completely not just by the immune system but also possibly even by any drugs which might be prescribed to cure the latent infection.

This is a new field of research, one that is exciting for microbiologists, but it may yet prove to be truly problematic for those focusing on how to address the immense human pool of latent infection which exists worldwide. Horacio Frydman, a specialist microbiologist, has commented that this apparent trick of the bacteria of "hitching a ride in [stem] cells that

---

[10] http://www.thescientist.com/?articles.view/articleNo/34286/title/Stem-Cells--Safe-Haven-For-TB/

are self-renewing" could have evolved as a very neat strategy for later re-infecting tissues in the host.

Bikul Das of Stanford University, the lead author of the study, first stumbled across this possible reservoir some 15 years ago, while working for the World Health Organization in Bhutan, a country where TB is severely endemic. He was conducting bone marrow biopsies of patients with otherwise unexplained fever, and began to wonder whether TB could possibly inhabit bone marrow. When he examined surplus biopsy material, Das detected a surprising number of patients who were harbouring TB quite literally within their bones.

Be this as it may be, the likelihood of the bacteria ever breaking out from anywhere to develop into active disease generally remains largely dependent upon the subsequent health of the host because, for 90% or more of those infected, those first symptoms (if there ever were any) never reappear and their infection can be considered, therefore, to have been effectively contained for the duration.

At such a stage the patient is defined as being 'latently infected': they are not infectious, nor do they carry any visible signs of the disease, nor will the vast majority of them ever suffer further from the infection. They remain most definitely still infected, however. While faint signs might be spotted by careful analysis of a chest X-ray, more conclusive evidence of their infection can be picked up and confirmed by a specific skin test for the detection and diagnosis of latent TB.

In a very small minority of patients who are first infected the disease continues to progress linearly without any real check, and it can reach a symptomatic level in around two years or in some cases much less. This phenomenon is known as 'primary tuberculosis'. In most others, however, if the disease activates further it will flare up at a much later date – and this is a much more common phenomenon which is technically known as 're-activation tuberculosis'.

For most, thankfully, the disease will never flare up again at all however. The following gives a rough idea of the process:

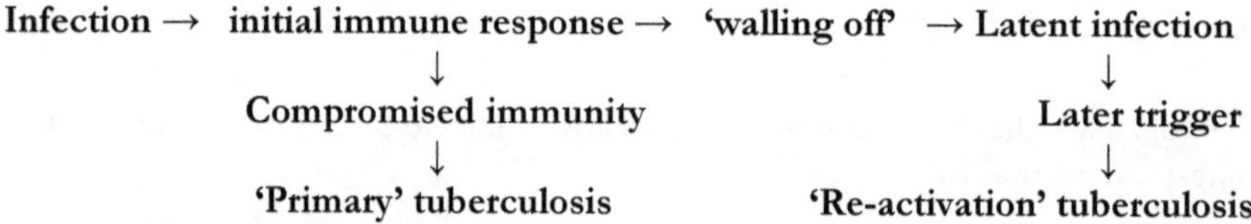

If the disease does develop into a re-activated state, it is believed that the same basic process unfolds all over again: the original tubercle breaks down and then releases still viable bacilli to cause further infection. The early symptoms of such re-activated disease include a loss of both energy and weight and (if the disease is in the lungs) a persistent cough. At this point the patient will also become infectious to others. The patient's health will also most probably continue to very slowly deteriorate, with increasing coughing – possibly even with the subsequent spitting up of bright red arterial blood. In advanced disease this might even cause a haemorrhage which can have sudden and fatal consequence. Otherwise the growing tubercular masses might finally end up destroying so much lung tissue that normal respiration can no longer supply the body with enough oxygen to allow it to survive, and at that point the patient will die. This whole process, however, may well take years to complete.

There are specific known risk factors for TB – factors which can make both the initial infection and the subsequent development of the disease into infectious tuberculosis a lot more likely:

- Alcoholism
- Certain medical conditions, such as -
    - Cancer of the head or neck
    - Diabetes mellitus
    - HIV/AIDS
    - Leukemia or Hodgkin's disease
    - Silicosis
- Certain medical treatments (such as corticosteroid treatment or organ transplants)
- Certain treatments for rheumatoid arthritis or Crohn's disease
- Crowded living conditions
- Homelessness
- Intravenous drug abuse
- Low body weight
- Malnutrition
- Poverty
- Severe kidney disease
- Smoking

These are the sorts of factors which might prompt a doctor to suspect a lingering cough to be something more insidious than a normal lung infection.

Simple malnutrition is a very important risk factor for the development of TB. Malnutrition has a negative effect on immunity to almost any disease, profoundly affecting what is known as cell-mediated immunity (CMI), and CMI is considered to be the principal host defense against TB. There are other risk factors as well, however. TB is known to be prone to re-activation during times of stress, and this factor curiously helps explain why it ***doesn't*** re-activate so often in particular age groups.

The chemical most closely associated with stress is cortisol, and cortisol itself is also well known to have a negative effect on the functions of white blood cells. But cortisol is in its turn controlled by another naturally occurring chemical, something called dehydroepiandrosterone (or, more manageably, DHEA). The relative presence and also the potency of this chemical fluctuates naturally during life, following a pattern which very closely reflects exactly those age-related comings and goings of TB incidence rates in humans. The chemical has also been shown to diminish significantly in advanced TB disease.[11] As such the presence or absence of DHEA is suspected as being a major factor in the re-activation as well as the final outcome of TB disease.

TB is not always first caught in the lungs – but because the bacillus likes oxygen in its environment a lung offers itself not only as its easiest access point, but also as its favoured home in the body. Contact with urine from a patient with TB in the bladder or kidneys could also be the pathway for infection, however. TB can be ingested through the digestive tract as well, the most common way being through the drinking of unpasteurised milk from cows that are infected with bovine TB. Animals, as we will see, can also be infected with TB although they carry a distinct mycobacterial disease which itself can have impact on any human epidemic. It is extremely similar to *M. Tuberculosis*, however, and infects human beings with tuberculosis type symptoms, and TB type disease. This certainly wasn't something which was initially fully understood – Robert Koch, the man who first identified the bacillus in 1882, originally denied this possibility. It was only a little later that it was realised that it was cows which carried a slightly different strain of disease which was contributing to the pandemic.

Before we take a look at the history of the disease, however, we need to take a slightly closer look at the nature of bacteria themselves since this also will help us better understand some of the characteristics of both the disease and the pandemic.

---

[11] Robert Baker - "Quiet Killers. The Rise and Fall of Deadly Disease", Sutton Publishing (2008).

The world of bacteria

Bacteria are micro-organisms that come in various shapes and sizes. Some are round grape-like ones like the *staphylococci* which often cause boils and abscesses. Others have bodies that are elongated and appear threaded together, like the *streptococci* which infect the throat. Then there are also tiny infectious threads (*mycelia*) which aren't bacteria at all but which are fungi or mould which themselves can also divide and breech like bacteria and which also cause disease.

TB is actually none of these. It is an elongated bacillus, but, because it visibly resembles those fungal threads (or *mycelia*) it is termed a 'mycobacterium'. There are at least 50 different species of mycobacteria, only a fraction of which cause serious disease, but those that do are not only feared but also reveal themselves invariably to be difficult to treat.

Mycobacterium tuberculosis, as it is termed, isn't even itself a single bacterial phenotype – it is just one in a group of very similar mycobacteria which are referred to most often as MBTC (or *Mycobacterium Tuberculosis* Complex). This complex comprises several other disease-causing mycobacteria, among them *M. africanum, M. microti, M. bovis*, *M. avium intracellare* and *M. canetti.*

M. microti is not known to cause disease at all in humans, whilst infection with *M. africanum* causes TB type disease but is rare globally. It is more common in West Africa, having been shown in one study conducted there to have been involved in around 40% of TB cases. *M. bovis* has a much wider host range and is the main cause of tuberculosis in cows and other animal species. Humans, as already mentioned, can become infected by *M. bovis* via milk or milk products, but infection can as easily occur as a result of eating insufficiently cooked meat from an infected animal, or even from working closely with them or through contact during slaughtering. Each type of MBTC disease can cause recognisable tuberculosis-type disease and each in turn also has its own preferred mammalian host. There are other TB-like bacteria as well (like *Mycobacterium chelonei*), which, although quite common in the environment, thankfully rarely cause illness in humans except in the old, or in those with inherited defects or in the seriously immune-compromised.

Some mycobacteria are not that dangerous at all. *Mycobacterium marinum*, for instance, causes not much more than skin eruptions. It is sometimes referred to as 'Fish Fancier's Finger' because it is most frequently seen in keepers of tropical fish who clean their fish tanks with ungloved hands.

There is another mycobacterium, however, that has been universally feared by the human race similarly to TB – which is leprosy (*M. leprae*). Leprosy is a true curiosity because, whilst it was the very first disease to have a specific causative bacterium definitively identified with it (back in 1873), there is still no agreement even today in respect of its basic means of transmission – and yet, in spite of this most fundamental lack of knowledge, this ancient and dreaded disease has completely disappeared from Europe.

Like TB, leprosy is closely associated with poverty, but more particularly also with rural residency and also barefoot walking. Interestingly, it disappeared in many countries at around the same time as they underwent industrialisation. Unlike TB, however, as many as 95% of humans are naturally immune to infection from the disease so that, even in those countries where it is still endemic there is much less risk of infection and so far less prevalence.

It has also been observed, rather intriguingly, that patients infected with leprosy only very rarely develop TB even in environments where tuberculosis is commonplace. Its infection would therefore appear to somehow confer some level of resistance to an infection from its more lethal cousin.

One of the reasons why infections with all of these mycobacteria are so difficult to treat is because the bugs themselves originally evolved to successfully survive by developing uniquely thick cell walls, helping them resist even long exposures to threatening or competing agents of any sort in their original natural environments. Such threatening agents have more recently come to include man-made antibiotics – the biochemical agents specifically developed by mankind to penetrate or destroy such protective cell coatings in more common and more vulnerable disease-forming bacteria. These structurally sturdy mycobacterial cell walls probably also explain why the TB bacterium is so slow to divide, because they also hinder its process of cell replication and thus make for the chronically slow nature of the disease and its development. The cell walls also help to explain why TB has been such a persistent slow-burning plague that has never ever completely gone away. They also explain why, unlike most other infectious diseases, tuberculosis never flares up in a sudden local epidemic and so also never burns itself out like some simpler diseases do. TB just comes and goes in endlessly slow waves, never disappearing, and during times that are less to its advantage it hunkers down in reservoir populations of latently infected cases biding its time.

This slow rhythmic phenomenon of epidemic disease, however, still fails to completely explain its particularly devastating trick of breaking out of its dormant state – as to how it somehow might chemically sense the appropriate opportune moment to do so. If this critical moment in the disease's individual development could be identified and unpacked and the process of re-activation somehow blocked, the disease could potentially remain latent until it became too late for it – when all of those it had latently infected had died through other causes. In such an event, the potentially infectious pool of latent disease would literally have dried up, and the disease and its ancient rolling epidemic would finally die out with the demise of the last surviving latently infected individual.

Given the devastation that this disease has been wreaking on mankind across so many millennia, that is a thought that's worth considering for a moment or two.

Identifying bacteria through the microscope

There is another thing which we need to understand about bacterial cell walls – and it relates to the different ways through which they have been able to be identified, since this has further classified them into different types. It can also sometimes suggest differential ways in which the diseases they create can be better treated. Unfortunately, in the case of tuberculosis, this definitive identification of active bacteria through the microscope still remains a challenging problem and adds to the many reasons why the disease has remained such a challenge to get on top of.

Generally bacteria are large enough to be identified under a microscope, but a little trick is often required to make them stand out visibly.

A small diversion into the story of the discovery of bacteria by microscope may be helpful and of interest at this point, if only because it reveals how often good timing can contribute to scientific discoveries (and bad timing can do the opposite) as much as it illustrates the brilliance of those who have made the major discoveries. The story also suggests the possibility that the discovery of the tuberculosis bacillus might have occurred many years before it did if the character of a single individual had been different.

This particular possibility relates to the commercial idiosyncrasies of one Antony van Leeuwenhoek (1632-1723), a Dutch business man. Van Leeuwenhoek is also commonly referred to today as the father of microbiology because of his contribution to the magnification capacity of microscope lenses.

While running his draper's shop business, van Leeuwenhoek developed a parallel fascination with the quite unrelated business of lens making. Up until this time, the ability to view the world of the microscopically small had been very limited. Lens grinding was, to say the least, a painstaking and highly skillful affair, and what had been developed up until van Leeuwenhoek's contribution to the field had been limited by the available technology. Quite by chance van Leeuwenhoek found that, by placing the middle of a small rod of soda lime glass in a hot flame, he could pull the red hot section of the rod apart. This created two long whiskers of glass, and he found that if he re-inserted the end of one whisker back into the flame he could create a very small, high-quality glass sphere. He then used these relatively simply created spheres as the lenses for his microscopes which he began to commercially manufacture, with the smallest spheres of all providing the highest magnifications.

He took to examining everything around him –he peered through his lenses at his dental plaque, at his semen and just about anything else he thought might offer him something interesting to look at. What he was seeing through his lenses had never been seen before by any other human being – and among the many other things he saw were tiny objects moving about mysteriously on his microscope slides. He wrote to the Royal Society in London about them, and he was even elected to the society in 1680 on the back of his revelations.

What he saw were bacteria, some of which would have been ones which cause human disease – but unfortunately no link was made by anyone at the time between these tiny "animalcules" (as he called them) and illness: it took nearly two centuries before these connections were finally and fully made. A large part of the reason for this delay was down to the slightly shady nature of the man himself. Being a canny Dutch businessman he figured that, if he revealed his simple method for creating the critically important lens to the wider world, the scientific community would adopt it whole-meal and would then almost certainly disregard or even forget his role in the development of science and microscopy because it had been essentially so simple. The price he commanded for his instruments would also immediately crash. He therefore allowed the world of science to believe that he was laboriously spending most of his nights and free time grinding these increasingly tiny lenses for use in his microscopes, even though it should have been realised that this would have been practically impossible given that he made hundreds of microscopes in his lifetime. By the end of the 17th century, van Leeuwenhoek was holding not just a global monopoly on microscopic technology, but also on its associated study and consequential discoveries.

Leeuwenhoek maintained that there were aspects of microscope construction "which I only keep for myself" – and in particular this included the crucial secret of how he created his lenses. As a result of his secrecy, for many years no-one was able to reconstruct Leeuwenhoek's design techniques and the science of microscopy effectively stagnated.

The next step forward in the identification of bacteria was made possible a century later. This time it was not because of an inventive draper, but because of technical advances in the dyeing industries. Mill owners looking for commercial advantage in the 19th century textile industry wanted new and more permanent dyes for their cloth instead of having to rely on the staple natural ones which had been used for centuries – and they particularly wanted ones that were brighter and more vivid. It fell to the chemists of the day to produce them, and what they found were new dyes that could do far more than just colour cloth – they could penetrate, stain and even adhere to living tissue as well.

The world of microscopy instantly borrowed this new technology. In 1884 Hans Christian Gram (1853-1938) invented a new way of working with the stains: he spread liquid samples on to the surfaces of his glass slides and then applied different dyes to them. Gram found that some of his samples stood out more strongly than others as a result, often appearing in deep colours under the microscope. Different methods of staining samples were then systematically developed in a general process that has become known since as 'gram staining'.

Such methods were found to differentiate bacteria in terms of both the chemical and physical properties of their cell walls. This was something which was later also found to be all-important for developing the appropriate drugs to kill them. Bacteria that could readily be identified by the basic Gram method simply became known as 'gram-positive' bacteria. They also happen to be bacteria that can generally be effectively treated with penicillin. 'Gram-negative' bacteria, on the other hand, (which are ones which couldn't be identified by the basic method) had to be counter-stained, after which they showed up as red or pink. The plague bacterium is one of these, and this bacillus also happens to be significantly resistant to any penetration of its cell walls by penicillin.

Then there were what became known as the 'acid-fast' bacteria. These were trickier still, since they couldn't be distinguished by gram staining at all, effectively resisting being decoloured by all the acids tried during the staining process. *Mycobacterium tuberculosis* is one of these, as are all of the other mycobacteria. Such acid-fast organisms contain large amounts of lipid substances within their cell walls (in the case of *M. tuberculosis* this substance is mycolic acid) which resist staining by all the ordinary methods, but the bacteria do succumb if a special reagent stain is applied to them in which case they then can show up bright red. In the case of *M. tuberculosis*, this is done by first spreading a small sample of the patient's sputum on to a slide and then applying the special stain to it.

The particular chemical stain that was finally found to reveal the elusive *M. Tuberculosis* was first developed by two Germans, and has been known since as the Ziehl Neelsen stain in their honour. It was a method that was used for over a century after its initial discovery, only recently being supplanted by auramine which is now considered a superior stain.

A diagnosis of TB which uses this method is commonly simply referred to as being 'smear-positive', which amounts to the fact that the particular patient's sputum sample has been recognised through this test to contain some acid-fast bacteria (almost certainly mycobacteria). Significantly, however, this method of diagnosis cannot actually determine which distinct strain of mycobacteria is showing itself on the surface of the glass slide – but it does almost certainly confirm the presence of some type of mycobacterial infection.

All of this may sound both over-complicated, but the terms 'acid-fast bacilli' (or 'AFB') and 'smear-positive' or 'smear-negative' will come up many times when we start looking more deeply, not only at the real practical difficulties in definitively diagnosing TB but also at the challenges of properly estimating the extent of the pandemic. They will also reappear when we look into the further challenges of diagnosing drug-resistant strains of the disease, and one time further when we review the challenges of differentiating between the different mycobacterial diseases themselves as well.

Latent TB infection – what happens exactly?

So much for identifying the bacillus – we now need to return to the disease it engenders.

Generally, as we have seen, people only show symptoms of tuberculosis if they develop the active form of the disease, and so, for most people who breathe in or ingest the tuberculosis bacteria and thus become technically infected, the disease is successfully halted by their immune system which stops the bacteria from growing further by walling the infection off.

This stand-off state is frequently termed LTBI (an acronym standing for 'Latent TB Infection'). People with latent tuberculosis show no symptoms, do not feel sick, cannot spread TB, but (importantly) they do usually show a positive TB skin test if it is given to them.

Unless the latent bacilli are destroyed (which is entirely possible with targeted drug treatment targeting the latent infection), there remains a risk for approximately 5-10% of these LTBI individuals of going on to develop active and infectious disease at a later stage of their life.

This risk is sometimes calculated more accurately as being very roughly a 5% possibility in the first two years after infection and then 0.1% per year thereafter. But this risk is unfortunately of a very different order for the immune-suppressed, whether such a condition is caused by malnutrition, ageing, by medical treatment which suppresses the immune system (such as chemotherapy), systematic steroid treatment (or immune suppressing drugs), or by an immune suppressive disease – particularly HIV/AIDS.

Under such circumstances, the bacteria are much more likely to break out and cause active or re-activated tuberculosis. They are not just likely to wreak a more devastating effect in the process but will probably also be more difficult to diagnose as well – often, unfortunately, not until it is already too late.

Active (or re-activation) tuberculosis

If the disease becomes more active, either at first infection or some time later, some early symptoms will begin to manifest. The early symptoms of active tuberculosis may be vague, however, and may even go completely unnoticed by the affected person.

The more specific symptoms of tuberculosis which might alert a doctor to the possibility of pulmonary TB disease include:

- A cough that lasts three weeks or longer
- Pain in the chest
- Low grade fever
- General malaise
- Otherwise unexplained weight loss even without loss of appetite
- Laboured breathing (dyspnea)
- Coughing up of blood (hemoptysis) or sputum.

None of these symptoms are sure signs of the disease, however, because other health problems could also cause these symptoms so, ideally, a positive definitive diagnosis is necessary before drug treatment is begun. Without it, some patients who don't have TB will receive challenging and unnecessary treatment. We will see later how comparatively infrequently such a truly definitive diagnosis is made, however, and exactly why this is so.

The lungs often begin to bleed because of the cumulative breakdown of the granulomas. Every time the granulomas split they release more tubercle bacilli along with pus and dead tissue, on each occasion creating larger and more numerous cavities on the tissue of the lungs. The more extensive the destruction caused by this process, the greater the bleeding, and the more difficult it will become for the patient to fully recover, with an increasing likelihood of a permanent reduction of functional lung tissue. All of these signs will show up on an X-ray which may therefore give a useful picture of the state of advancement of the disease.

In theory, a person with active disease is only infectious if viable bacilli are being discharged in their sputum. In practice, therefore, for most cases of infectious TB that are put on treatment, the greatest risk of the person transmitting their infection to someone else is probably during the period immediately prior to their diagnosis and just after it – simply because this is when patient will have taken him or herself to a doctor because their coughing symptoms have become acute and disabling.

Specific measurements are used to assess this risk – to suggest whether a patient is highly infectious (+++), moderately infectious (++) or only comparatively infectious (+), the measurement being made based on the amount of bacilli visible on the slide. Any sputum 'smear-positive' case is also by definition much more infectious than a case which is only recognized as being positive after subsequent culture of a sputum sample (a more sophisticated diagnostic process which is sometimes the only way the disease can be diagnosed). This is so because visual diagnosis by simple smear microscopy dictates that there must be more bacilli present than in a sputum-negative sample that is subsequently confirmed to have TB following culture. There can be no question that there is greater potential for infection from a cough from such a smear-positive patient because there is a certainty that more viable germs will be discharged in the cough.

This fundamental risk of transmitting infection is also known to significantly reduce after a few days or at least by two weeks after appropriate effective chemotherapy multi-drug treatment has been begun, by which time the load of bacilli in the sputum will have usually dropped quite dramatically.

Most often these symptoms of disease involve just the lungs, but this is not always the case. Symptoms of tuberculosis involving areas other than the lungs vary considerably depending upon the organ or area affected. TB can attack almost any part of the body including joints, bones, the urinary tract, central nervous system, meninges, kidneys, muscles, bone marrow, the lymphatic system and even the skin. All of these conditions are known as extra-pulmonary tuberculosis (or simply 'EP'). Thankfully this occurs only in 10-15% of adult TB cases - thankfully because they are far more difficult to diagnose and treat. In the immune-suppressed and in children, however, the tendency for the disease to spread outside the lungs is unfortunately a lot more common.

In fact, in individuals with HIV/AIDS, extra-pulmonary tuberculosis can even predominate in frequency, particularly with lymph node involvement, something which makes diagnosis and treatment of TB in these patients a lot more challenging. This is something else that we will take a more detailed look at later since it has such an impact on the disease today in Africa. First, however, we need to take a look at the history of the disease since doing so can massively enrich our understanding of the challenges that exist in successfully fighting it today.

The Old Enemy...

"HUMAN HISTORY AND THE TUBERCLE BACILLUS ARE SO ENMESHED THAT TO FOLLOW THE COURSE OF THE DISEASE OVER TIME IS A PREREQUISITE TO UNDERSTANDING WHAT THE WHOLE STRUGGLE TO CONTROL DISEASE MEANS TO OURSELVES AND OUR CONTEMPORARY SOCIETY."

Barbara Rosenkrantz (1987)[12]

Early history

TB has been killing humans for a very long time – to the extent that it is often described as being mankind's oldest bacteriological foe.

We can never know if this has truly been the case, but it has almost certainly been our most dangerous one. Estimates of deaths from TB in more recent centuries are simply staggering. The number of accumulated deaths from TB estimated to have occurred between 1850 and 1950, for instance, has been estimated to be nearly one billion people (more than either famine, wars, or natural disaster)[13] – and this despite the fact that, for the last 50 years of this period, effective drugs were available.

To apply a better perspective to this figure, a few estimated death tolls from other well-known epidemic diseases from recorded history are listed below, followed by some figures which relate to tuberculosis:

The Plague of Justinian: 541–542	25 million
The Black Death: 14th century	75-200 million
The Third Plague: 1882-1927	12 million
The Great 'Flu: 1918	50-100 million
HIV (since its outbreak)	36 million
SARS: 2002-4	1 thousand
Swine 'Flu: 2009	285 thousand

[12] An epidemiologist and historian, from her introductory historical essay in the 1987 reprint of the Dubos' history of TB "the White Plague".

[13] Iseman MD – "Evolution of drug resistant tuberculosis: a tale of two species", Proceedings of the National Academy of Sciences USA, 91 (1994) 2428–9.

TB: 19th & 20th centuries	1 billion
TB: during the year 2012	1.3 million
TB: 1997-2020 (projected)	Possibly 70 million[14] – at least 40 million
MDR-TB: 2000-2009	1.5 million[15]
MDR-TB & XDR-TB: by 2030	30 million…?[16]

All of these figures should be appropriately compared against the relative global populations of their times for any valid comparative or reasonable assessment to be made, but nevertheless they offer a startling insight into the scale of the rolling TB death toll, both past, present and future.

It should be noted that, even today, almost all of these estimates are far from definite or reliable,[17] but the estimated scale of the TB pandemic of the 19th and 20th centuries is well illustrated by these figures nevertheless. It should also be noted that almost all of the figures for TB, even today, remain as estimates rather than reported figures. This is because, despite the scale of the numbers and the gravity of the pandemic, sufficiently robust disease surveillance still (both paradoxically and perplexingly) is completely absent in those countries in which the disease is most rampant and where such data is most vital. The fact that no continuous surveillance data for TB exists in any low-income country anywhere means that, as a rule, the lower the national GDP the greater the likelihood exists that the estimates of disease will be unreliable since it will have been mathematically modelled on proportionately more uncertain data.

In consideration of TB's lethal persistence it has even been suggested that the discovery of the first effective drugs for TB in the middle of the 20th century was of such importance that it may have actually changed the course of human history. Whether this has been a permanent change, a

---

[14] This was a projected figure made by Dr C. Dye of the WHO in a private communication which was quoted by Ann Leung in "Pulmonary Tuberculosis: The Essentials" in Radiology, 210 (1999) 307-322.

[15] "Multidrug and extensively drug-resistant TB (M/XDR-TB): 2010 global report on surveillance and response", Geneva, World Health Organization (2010).

[16] This is a personal 'guesstimate' based on worse case scenarios assuming rates of MDR-TB to increase without check in low-income countries.

[17] The exception being those relating to SARS and Swine Flu.

temporary illusion – or (worse still) merely a flight of fantasy made by the more fortunate- will have to remain, at least for the present, an issue of conjecture.

In fact it will be something for the historians of the future to ultimately decide.

Tuberculosis turns out to be a very old disease indeed. It is believed to have been common in ancient Egypt as long as 5,500 years ago at the very dawning of human civilisation – with a famous mummy of a high priest from 1100 BC offering us ancient physical evidence of tuberculosis in signs of a track of pus which had been discharging from an abscess in the high priest's spine. This tell-tale evidence was found remarkably well preserved in the mummified tissue of the priest's psoas muscle – something that is a common sign of extra-pulmonary tuberculous spondylitis.[18]

It is also believed that both Akhenaten and his legendarily beautiful wife Nefertiti both died from tuberculosis, and other evidence suggests that hospitals for tuberculosis may even have existed in Egypt as long ago as 1500 BC – but the real origins of the disease are now acknowledged to be much earlier – at least 20,000 years earlier, and some suggest even earlier still.[19]

Given that TB-type disease is known to infect many types of mammals as well as human beings, and being as humans are (relatively speaking) the newer kids on the block, it has been logically assumed that the disease would have found its first home in animals. It was further speculated that, since the mycobacterium probably originally evolved from micro-organisms in the soil, it could most easily have infected grazing animals either by inhalation or ingestion, and then could have naturally spread to non-grazers along existing food chains – coming to humans at around 9,000 BC at the same time as agriculture and animal husbandry first developed. This theory depends on the human disease first arriving in the form of bovine TB, a disease which is strictly speaking genetically separate from human

---

[18] Morse D - "Tuberculosis" in Brothwell D, Sandison AT (as editors), "Diseases in antiquity. A survey of the diseases, injuries, and surgery of early populations", Springfield, IL: Charles C Thomas (1967).

[19] M.Christina Gutierrez et al. - "Ancient Origin of gene mosaicism of the progenitor of Mycobaterium tuberculosis", PLos Pathogens, 1/1 (2005) e5, doi: 101371/journal.ppat.0010005.

tuberculosis, with human TB then evolving from this original source as a discrete mycobacterium with a particular penchant for human beings. Some medical historians used this model to theorise that TB probably first began really taking its toll on humanity by passing from human to human only after we began to congregate in cities or city states.

There are, however, other definite signs of the disease from earlier periods of human development, though they may, of course, have been only isolated instances. One Stone Age skeleton from Liguria in Italy displays signs of the disease from over 2,000 years earlier than the earliest evidence from Egypt, for instance. This was also some time before formal civilisation and farming began in the region. Using the model of the bacterium passing up a food chain from grazing animals (which could equally well have been wild) there should be no logical reason why this could not have been how the disease occurred, although whether this ever amounted to human-to-human transmissible disease at this earlier time must remain questionable. Certainly humans would have been living and sleeping together in close quarters (including with their livestock), and food supply would have often been sporadic and seasonal which would also have led to episodes of serious malnutrition, so there would have been good opportunity for cross-infection between members of a community even with bovine TB infection on its own.

The oldest known molecular evidence of bovine TB so far detected was found in a fossil of an extinct bison (a Pleistocene bison), which was radiocarbon dated to a much earlier age, from around 17,870 years ago;[20] the oldest in human remains so far recovered is from a 9,000 year old Neolithic settlement in the Eastern Mediterranean.[21] So the idea of the human disease originally evolving from animals appears at first to be well supported by the evidence.

But there has emerged some even more ancient evidence still, which (albeit not strictly human since it is hominid) was certainly not found in the remains of any ruminant quadruped. Part of a *Homo erectus* skull found at

---

[20] Rothschild BM et al. - "*Mycobacterium tuberculosis* Complex DNA from an Extinct Bison Dated 17,000 Years before the Present", Clinical Infectious Diseases, 33 (2001) 305–11.

[21] Hershkovitz I et al. - "Detection and molecular characterization of 9000-year-old *Mycobacterium tuberculosis* from a neolithic settlement in the Eastern Mediterranean", PLoS ONE, 3 (2008) e3426.

Kocabaş in Turkey displays lesions on its inner surface which are considered to be the result of tubercular meningitis (an extra-pulmonary type of tuberculosis). The skull astonishingly dates from around 500,000 years ago setting something of an academic cat amongst the theorists' pigeons.[22] As a result, a completely new theory has been proposed which suggests that the human disease might actually be older than the bovine strain, with *M. bovis* itself evolving from a hominid-favouring ancestor of *M. africanum.* Such an idea suggests that some more human-focused mycobacterium similar to TB just might have even been afflicting our earliest hominid ancestors in East Africa at the very dawn of mankind.

Whilst this may all seem academic and of no particular importance or relevance to us today, it might offer an answer to one of the many current epidemiological puzzles associated with the disease – which is why the BCG vaccination (which is obtained from the bovine strain) is less effective in some parts of the tropics (including East Africa) than it is in temperate zones. It may even explain the so-called 'Burmese conundrum' in which the commonly encountered local mycobacteria are suspected of making the Burmese people more susceptible to TB after vaccination rather than less, with the effect of BCG increasing incidence of the disease rather than reducing it.

What is certain is that, once TB first properly established itself as a transmissible disease within our species (whenever that may have been), it appears to have never left us, continuously coming and going in slow opportunistic waves whenever living conditions, war or famine reduced host immunities in afflicted populations. There is evidence for this in some of mankind's earliest surviving literature. In a passage in the Book of Deuteronomy in the biblical Old Testament, for instance, a list of curses describes what would befall the Jewish people if they failed to properly "hearken unto the voice of the Lord thy God" after entering their promised land having escaped from their enslavement in Egypt. The seventh listed curse pointedly promised that their God would "smite thee with a consumption" if they ever failed to listen to Him.[23]

---

[22] Kappelman J et al. - "First Homo erectus from Turkey and implications for migrations into temperate Eurasia", American Journal of Physical Anthrolpology, 135 (2008), 110-16.

[23] Deuteronomy 28.22 (King James's Bible)

There is even evidence that the disease existed in pre-Columbian times in the New World. In the Caribbean, early evidence of the disease has been identified in the Arawak culture from around 1050 BC, but far more convincing South American evidence was found in the mummy of an eight to 10-year-old Nazca child from Hacienda Agua Sala. The mummy dates to around 700 AD. What makes this find so persuasive is that scientists have been able to isolate evidence of the bacillus itself in the tissues of the mummy.[24]

Prior to such findings it was being popularly suggested (as we will see) that TB was particularly afflicting indigenous 'native' populations both in Africa and the New World during the centuries of European colonisation because these peoples had never previously been exposed to the disease. This may still be partly true, of course, since it may have been that these populations had not previously been exposed to the specific newer strains of disease that came from Europe with the settlers and adventurers.

It is in fact pretty much impossible to be certain about anything much even in the written evidence right up until the actual identification of the bacterium itself in 1882, unfortunately, without good archaeological evidence to back it up – evidence which we can now genetically check so that what we assume to have been tuberculosis can now be confirmed to be TB rather than being another similar mycobacterial or wasting disease. This is because, right up until recent times, various other pulmonary and wasting diseases have been very similarly described and have inevitably been gathered together under the umbrella of consumptive disease. Given what we now know about the persistent characteristics of TB, however, it seems very probable that most of those victims described as succumbing to *phthisis* or something similar did, in fact, succumb to what we would know call pulmonary tuberculosis.

As far as the medical literature of Europe and the Eastern Mediterranean is concerned, the term *phthisis* first appeared in written form around 460 BC to describe a disease which was pretty clearly TB. Hippocrates described *phthisis* as the most common cause of illness in his time. He also identified that it typically affected individuals between 18 and 35 years of age, and that it was nearly always fatal.[25] His bleak conclusions on the matter even led

---

[24] I Prat JG, Souza SMFM - "Prehistoric tuberculosis in America: adding comments to a literature review", Memorias do Instituto Oswaldo Cruz, 98; Suppl. I (2003)151–9.

[25] Hippocrates, "Aphorisms".

him to discourage physicians from visiting victims of the disease in its later stages – not to protect themselves from the disease but simply in order to protect their reputations since the patients were so certain to die.

This Greek word *phthisis* (which literally means 'wasting') survived up until very recently in the medical vernacular, and was used to develop other associated words, such as the *phthisic* (to describe the suffering patient), and the *phthisician* (to describe the doctor who specialised in treating the disease). It was from this earliest time as well that the pervasive idea that some people were predisposed to the disease by their constitution was first proposed – often simply by their body shape if they happened to be both tall and thin.

The ways of describing the disease in other cultures were similar. In early Indian medical texts written between 800 and 1000 AD, for instance, the disease was referred to as *yaksma* (consumption), or *rajayaksman* (kingly consumption).[26]

In fact almost all historical names for TB in any early medical literature use this common defining descriptor of it being a wasting or consuming disease. The following are some of these 'wasting' names which were used by different cultures in different languages, all of which are reasonably assumed today to refer to tuberculosis:

Schachepheth – Hebrew[27]
Phthisis – Greek
Yaksma – Sanskrit
Tabey diq – Urdu
Xoy – Hindi (a term referring to the waning of the moon)
Consumptione – Latin
Chaky oncay – Incan
Nari maraz – Pathan (literally 'the thinning fever')

---

[26] An important compendium on Indian medicine from this time was the Rogaviniscaya (often also referred to as the Madhavanidana). One of a number of commentaries on this text (the 'Madhukosa') refers specifically to this disease.

[27] There are actually just two references in the Bible – in the books of Leviticus and Deuteronomy respectively. The one relates to the time that the Israelites were enslaved in Egypt, the other to just afterwards. Given the conditions that they would have endured under enforced slavery, this can hardly be coincidental.

In China, other descriptors were used which are less inclined towards wasting but which were equally, if not in some cases even more graphic:

- 'Cadaverous Infixation' (*Zhu*)
- 'Passing from Door to Door Disease' (*Chuanshi*)
- 'Lung taxation Disease' (*Feilao*)

It's still impossible to estimate in any remotely accurate fashion the typical rates of incidence or prevalence of TB in these cultures in such earlier times. All we can safely assume from what we now know is that poor living conditions, poor diet, war, famine and co-infections would all have had an impact on what would have been fluctuating continuous epidemics of disease in distinct communities, although other common diseases would also have had more acute temporary impact at certain moments – diseases like typhus in times of famine, cholera in times of natural disaster, and plague in times of epidemic outbreak. These were all diseases, however, which flared and died away in localised (or at least naturally terminating) epidemics. TB was different: it hung around.

Other lethal infectious diseases have also smouldered incessantly, of course – diseases like diphtheria, polio, smallpox, scarlet fever, and measles – but none have done so in the grand scale of slow consistency that has been achieved by TB across the centuries. Each of them, as well, has more recently been picked off to a greater or lesser degree by concerted campaigns of effective vaccination and disease control.

The same cannot yet unfortunately be said of tuberculosis.

More recent history

"I WOULD LIKE TO REMIND THOSE RESPONSIBLE FOR THE TREATMENT OF TUBERCULOSIS THAT KEATS WROTE HIS BEST POEMS WHILE DYING OF THIS DISEASE. IN MY OPINION HE WOULD NEVER HAVE DONE SO UNDER THE INFLUENCE OF MODERN CHEMOTHERAPY."

Arthur M Walker (1896-1955)

Early European monarchs took the opportunity to ascribe much of their right to rule as being a mandate from their Christian God – an idea which further developed into the pervasive philosophy of the Middle Ages of 'the

Divine Right of Kings'. As such these rulers were also sometimes seen to be quasi-religious figures as much as they were accepted as rulers, even ones with magical or curative powers. Because of such ideas, it came to be widely believed in both England and France that sovereigns could cure certain diseases by what became known as the 'Royal Touch'. Such diseases included scrofula, which was a popular term used to describe tuberculosis when it affects the lymph nodes of the neck. King Henry IV of France, for instance, usually performed his healing rites on a weekly basis, after taking communion. This practice of royal healing became so common in France (while only moderately so in England) that scrofula itself became known simply as the '*Mal du Roi*', and in England as the 'King's Evil'. The spread of tuberculosis across France and England at this time led to formal programmes for such royal touching. During the Sun King Louis XIV's reign in France placards were publicly posted indicating the days and times when the king would be available for these touchings. In England, the process became more formalised still: as late as 1633 (just a decade before the outbreak of the English Civil War put final pay to any ideas of divine right to rule in England) the Anglican Book of Common Prayer included the text for a special Royal Touch ceremony. The ceremony itself is even described in Shakespeare's *Macbeth*:

> "Strangely visited people,
> All swol'n and ulcerous, pitiful to the eye
> The mere despair of surgery, he cures,
> Hanging a golden stamp about their necks,
> Put on with holy prayers: and 'tis spoken,
> To the succeeding royalty he leaves
> The healing benediction."[28]

We know from London's Bills of Mortality, first introduced in the 17th century, that consumption was accounting for around 20% of deaths at the time. A rate of one in five of all deaths is extremely high, although we can be far from certain that all of them were actually down to TB. The understandable fear that was caused by such perceived death rates, however, is well reflected in one of the names for the disease which appeared in the literature of the time – coined by John Bunyan who famously described the disease as being the 'captain of all these men of death'. Such fear of disease must also surely have been driving some of the emigration to the New World.

---

[28] William Shakespeare –"Macbeth", Act 4, Scene 3, 171-7.

In English literature two centuries later the master novelist Charles Dickens described his character Smike as dying from what, in starker words than Bunyan's, he called simply the 'Dread Disease'. It was far from Dickens' only reference to the devastation caused by consumption in the squalid cities he provided commentary upon, but the passage that followed the two words he chose to call it by remains chilling to this day.

> "There is a dread disease which so prepares its victim, as it were, for death; which so refines it of its grosser aspect, and throws around familiar looks unearthly indications of the coming change; a dread disease, in which the struggle between soul and body is so gradual, quiet, and solemn, and the result so sure, that day by day, and grain by grain, the mortal part wastes and withers away, so that the spirit grows light and sanguine with its lightening load, and, feeling immortality at hand, deems it but a new term of mortal life; a disease in which death and life are so strangely blended, that death takes the glow and hue of life, and life the gaunt and grisly form of death; a disease which medicine never cured, wealth never warded off, or poverty could boast exemption from; which sometimes moves in giant strides, and sometimes at a tardy sluggish pace, but, slow or quick, is ever sure and certain."[29]

Both Bunyan and Dickens offer us graphic descriptions which capture something of the ever present contemporary fear of this disease in their respective times.

The prevalence of tuberculosis had been growing progressively in Britain during the late Middle Ages and Renaissance, finally peaking in the 18th and 19th centuries as agricultural field workers moved to the cities looking for work, especially once the Industrial Revolution truly flowered, bringing with it both poverty and squalour in the burgeoning new cities. By the start of the 19th Century the death rate from consumption in London was running at just over one in four recorded deaths. Of the 1,571 deaths in the city of Bristol between 1790 and 1796, 683 (or 43%) were recorded as being due to consumption.[30]

Between the 17th and 19th centuries, TB was referred to as both the 'White Death' and the 'White Plague' in Europe. It was also referred to as the *Mal de Vivir*, and the *Mal de Siècle*, as if the disease had finally found its own special era. It should be born in mind that, until only recently, this

---

[29] Charles Dickens - "Nicholas Nickleby" (1848).

[30] Chalke HD - "Some historical aspects of tuberculosis", Public Health 74, 3 (1959) 83–95.

constantly attritional European epidemic comprised at least two discrete mycobacterial diseases working together, both of which would have been recognised and described at the time as being consumption or *phthisis* – one was the airborne infectious *M. tuberculosis*, and the other was *M. bovis* which was most often being ingested in milk from infected cows. It has been estimated that *M. bovis* (from milk and meat) was responsible for about 6-7% of tuberculosis deaths in humans in the pre-antibiotic era. On this basis we can still reasonably assume that at least 90% of the fluctuating epidemic was caused by *M. tuberculosis* itself.

The disease at different times has also played an especially intimate and influential part in the development of medicine. Its treatment and diagnosis has a direct connection with the common medical use of the stethoscope, for instance, a device which was originally developed by René Laennec (1781-1826) in order to listen to his consumptive patients' chests. Laennec himself actually died from the disease at the age of 45, having probably been infected while studying his contagious patients or the still infectious tissue from their dead bodies. By listening through his stethoscope to the sounds his patients made while breathing he began to identify a correspondence between the pulmonary lesions found on the lungs of his autopsied tuberculosis patients and the respiratory symptoms he was hearing in his living patients. His most important written work is regarded today as being his *Traité de l'Auscultación Mediate* which specifically detailed his discoveries on the use of pulmonary auscultation in diagnosing tuberculosis.

Later the use of guinea pigs as animal subjects in medical research (and therefore also the colloquial adoption of the term 'guinea pig' for any experimental subject) was developed not just because they are small and manageable mammals for both experiment and dissection, but also because they have absolutely no resistance at all to the tuberculosis bacillus. They could thus be infected with the bacillus with a 100% guarantee of their rapidly developing primary disease, and were therefore perfect subjects on which to develop experimental treatments to compare treatment effects. The principle was simple: infect a group of guinea pigs and then subject them to the experimental treatment. Because of guinea pigs' innate natural vulnerability to the disease, if any animals survived such treatment it had to warrant further investigation.

In the 20th century as we will see, the very first modern large scale randomised medical trial was designed and developed to research the use of one of the first new drugs for the treatment of tuberculosis. In earlier centuries, however, TB treatments had not been based on drugs at all and they varied dramatically. For a time in Europe, for instance, copious amounts of horse riding was seen as being the best answer. Simpler, less strenuous and more accessible walking was also advocated in some instances, as were (rather bizarrely) driving in a carriage, sailing and even cold sea bathing.

One of the more famous historical victims of this disease was John Keats (1795-1821). Before dedicating himself to poetry he had studied medicine, and then nursed his younger brother Tom in the final stages of his own consumptive disease. The probability exists that both brothers had caught the disease years before from other family members since both their mother and uncle had almost certainly died of TB as well. A full two years before his own death Keats had been ill and coughed up some blood. He took a careful look at it and then dramatically announced to his brother:

> "I know the colour of that blood – it is arterial blood … that drop of blood is my death warrant – I must die."

He was far from being the only famous literary figure of the time who spectacularly fell victim to the disease. TB truly decimated the Brontë family, causing the death of the young sisters Maria and Elizabeth in 1825, and then their dissolute brother Branwell in September 1848, Emily in December the same year, then Anne five months later in 1849, and finally Charlotte in 1855.

This is an astonishing death toll for a single family at any time, and was an extreme example of something which suggested two ideas which persisted and still persist in some cultures even today. One is that TB tends to run in families, and therefore such families should be shunned and stigmatised. The other is that it is somehow a fashionable or romantic disease of the dissolute and/or artistically bohemian, as a result of which the ailing '*phthisic*' developed a peculiar and perverse cachet, perhaps a little like the appeal that the drug-addicted artist or musician has sometimes held in more recent times. The visible decline which accompanied tuberculosis was being believed to bestow upon the sufferer some type of heightened sensitivity, resulting in a perverse fashion for young and more upper-class women to purposefully pale their skin in order to achieve the look of the consumptive. The British poet Lord Byron even quite bizarrely wrote on one occasion, "I should like to die from consumption," helping to further popularize the idea that TB was somehow the disease of the artist or of the creative spirit.[31]

---

[31] Diane Yancey - "Tuberculosis", Twenty-First Century Books (2007).

This phenomenon was not confined to England. In France, at least six novels were published reflecting some of these same fashionable ideals of tuberculosis – Dumas's *La Dame aux Camélias*, Murger's *Scènes de la vie de Bohème*, Hugo's *Les Misérables*, the Goncourt brothers' *Madame Gervaisais* and *Germinie Lacerteux*, and Rostand's *L'Aiglon*. The romantic character of Mimi, in Puccini's opera *La Boheme* was also a consumptive. *La Traviata,* another Puccini opera, was also based on Dumas's *La Dame aux Camélias.*[32]

Better understandings are attempted

Thankfully there had also been developments taking place which promised better medical understandings of the disease, really beginning in the 17th century. In his "Opera Medica" of 1679, Sylvius was the first to identify the distinctive nodules as a consistent and characteristic change in the lungs of consumptive patients. Then, in 1689 the British doctor Richard Morton[33] coined the word "tubercles" to describe these small rounded nodular masses. Because of the variety of its symptoms, however, TB was not identified as a single distinct disease until the 1820s and not finally named as 'tuberculosis' until 1839 by the German professor of medicine Johann Lukas Schönlein (1793-1864) in Berlin.

At the same time as Sylvius, however, the first references to the infectious nature of the disease began to appear in the western medical literature. An edict issued by the Italian Republic of Lucca in 1699 stated that:

> "Henceforth, human health should no longer be endangered by objects remaining after the death of a consumptive. The names of the deceased should be reported to the authorities, and measures undertaken for disinfection."

Soon after, in 1720, the English physician Benjamin Marten published "A New Theory of Consumption". In it he suggested that TB could be caused

---

[32] This was further adapted in the 21st century as "Moulin Rouge".

[33] Consumption was so common in Morton's time that he is quoted as saying, "I cannot sufficiently admire that anyone, at least after he comes to the flower of his youth, can dye without a touch of consumption."

by "wonderfully minute living creatures," ones which, having gained a foothold in the body, would then generate the symptoms of the disease. He went on to state that:

> "It may be therefore very likely that by an habitual lying in the same bed with a consumptive patient, constantly eating and drinking with him, or by very frequently conversing so nearly as to draw in part of the breath he emits from the lungs, a consumption may be caught by a sound person...I imagine that slightly conversing with consumptive patients is seldom or never sufficient to catch the disease."

It has rightly been observed that, as far as understandings of infectious disease in the early 18th century were concerned, Dr Marten's writings display a great degree of epidemiological insight.

For a long time it was still being accepted that there was no hope that an effective treatment for this consumptive disease would ever be found. There were still those who were experimenting on the possibility, however, putting their ideas to the test with the full co-operation of their ever-hopeful patients.

One such innovative idea developed in America. In 1842 Dr John Croghan bought the so-called Mammoth Cave in Central Kentucky, a part of the largest known cave system in the world. Later that year, he took 15 of his tuberculosis patients into the cave in the hope of curing their disease with the help of the cave's constant temperature and the purity of its air. The patients were lodged in separate stone huts, each one individually supplied with a black slave servant to bring them their meals. One patient wrote rather enthusiastically at the time of his cave experience:

> "Some of the invalids eat at their pavilions while others in better health attend regularly the *table d'hote* which is very good indeed, having a considerable variety and being almost daily …. graced with a saddle of venison or other game."

Things all seemed to be looking rather promising. In early 1843, however, two patients died and the rest then left. All of the departing patients apparently then rapidly died as well, between three days and three weeks after resurfacing. John Croghan sadly succumbed to tuberculosis himself six years later in 1849.

In 1840, two years earlier than the Mammoth Cave experiment, George Bodington (1799-1882) an English doctor on the other side of the Atlantic, had published an essay entitled "On the Treatment and Cure of Pulmonary

Consumption". He had been noticing that country folk seemed to be generally much less prone to TB than those living in the city, something he concluded to be simply because they were less likely to be living and working in crowded conditions. In this he was certainly correct. In the absence of any other available treatment, Bodington proposed what appeared to him to be the only possible logical solution for the city-dweller: he simply advocated a retreat to what he termed a "pure atmosphere". By this he meant as much exposure as possible to dry frosty air, to a healthy diet and to a regime of gentle exercise.

Bodington was roundly attacked by his contemporaries for his ideas, and rather sadly retired completely from the world of TB and internal medicine to spend the remainder of his life caring for the mentally ill. His insightful idea survived, however, having been picked up on, and more successfully developed, by Hermann Brehner a German doctor. Brehner used the idea as the core principle of his sanatorium movement which became widely adopted during the following decades. In 1859 Brehner built the world's first small TB sanatorium, the *Brehmerschen Heilanstalt für Lungenkranke* in what was Görbersdorf (which is now Sokołowsko), in Silesia (which is now part of Poland). The sanatorium's basic regimen was quite simple and looked very much like what Dr Bodington had less successfully been recommending: bed rest, fresh air and good food.

Brehner's own story is an interesting one. As a botany student Brehner had developed tuberculosis and had been advised by his doctor to seek out a healthier climate. He had travelled to the Himalayas where he continued to pursue his botanical studies and effectively rid himself of the symptoms of the disease. On his return he took up the study of medicine and, in 1854, he presented his doctoral dissertation. It bore the radical title "Tuberculosis is a Curable Disease". In that same year, he began building the institution in Görbersdorf where, in the midst of fir trees, and with good nutrition, patients were exposed on their balconies to the same sort of continuous fresh air that he had experienced himself in the Himalayas.

Many sanatoria followed his, the most famous one of its time being built in Davos, Switzerland – where the invalid or hypochondriac elite of Europe retreated, often simply if they became struck with the idea that they might be wasting away. Robert Louis Stevenson, the Scottish novelist, spent two winters there while fighting consumption, recovering to die of other causes in Samoa in 1894.[34]

Effectively, Brehner's own ideas had developed from Bodington's including the theory that clean mountain air was particularly efficacious to the consumptive.

As such the sanatorium became the most widely accepted treatment for tuberculosis for nearly a century, although its actual efficacy was not subjected to any proper scientific scrutiny until much later.

Social changes

"THE DISEASE IS DYING A NATURAL DEATH WITH IMPROVED CONDITIONS OF THE WORKING CLASSES, AND IT IS BY FURTHER DEVELOPMENTS ON SUCH LINES, AND NOT OTHERWISE, THAT ITS EXTERMINATION WILL BE ATTAINED."

Dr T. D. Lister (1890's)[35]

By the mid-19th century TB was effectively on the rampage. A quarter oif a century later and global death rates have been estimated to have been running at around seven million a year, with London and New York being particularly badly affected. It was now being seen to be reaching epidemic proportions in the cities of literally every country which had embarked on the process of industrialisation and urbanisation, developing discrete individual national tides of disease as each country sociologically and industrially transformed itself. In this way TB remained the leading cause of death well into the 20th century although, it is important to note that some of these tides of disease were already reducing by the turn of the century in some of the countries which had been at the original forefront of

[34] There were other fascinating examples situated in the Alps. A massive 3,500 bed sanatorium was built in Italy at Sondalo in the mountains north of Milan. Another was built at St Hilaire in the French Alps, situated 600 metres above the valley floor and originally only accessible either by foot or by mule – but with a special funicular railway then purpose-built for access.

[35] Dr Lister was a doctor at Mount Vernon Hospital for Consumption, which was situated in Hampstead, London between 1864 and 1904.

industrialisation, particularly wherever living and/or working conditions were beginning to improve.

In some parts of the world an annual migration of the sick had also become a commonplace for the better off – with a seasonal stream of invalids travelling from the smog of the north in search of the sun further south. The Mediterranean coast was described at the time as being "the last ditch of the consumptive". But others were resorting to more distant shores.

Cecil Rhodes, possibly the most successful, and also (in retrospect) perhaps also the most notorious of all British imperialists, arrived in Natal in South Africa in 1869 at the age of 16. He had travelled there, journeying to his older brother's farm, in the hope of a cure for his consumption, all the way from the family home in Oxford, England. Whilst recovering (which he succeeded in doing) he began looking around the neighbouring area of Kimberly and came across significant signs of diamond deposits. Not much more than ten years later and at only 27 years of age, Rhodes had already established himself as a multi-millionaire, and the history of South Africa had been changed forever. Ironically, his recovery and mineral discoveries soon began to have devastating repercussions for the tuberculosis of others, repercussions which persist to this day as we will see.

For Americans it was the states of Florida, Arizona, California, Colorado or New Mexico that lured the sick and the sickening, again because of their cleaner air and warmer climates. The city of Los Angeles may be popularly believed to have grown up around its incipient film industry, but in its earliest days it had developed primarily as a therapeutic resort, most specifically as a place to which consumptives travelled, especially from the east of the continent. Thousands were taking themselves westward to escape the disease-promoting conditions of the eastern cities – many of them already infected with disease, all desperately hoping to find a healthy environment in which to recover and live. Not surprisingly, they were often not made that welcome in those places where they chose to settle, being pejoratively referred to simply as 'lungers'. Emily Abel chillingly described this migratory phenomenon in the first chapter of her book on the subject which she enigmatically entitled "Pestilence in a Promised Land".[36] In it she describes the mass migration westwards of thousands of people in search of both healthier climates and more therapeutic environments. She suggests that the number of people arriving in Los Angeles who were already

[36] Emily K Abel - "Tuberculosis and the Politics of Exclusion: A History of Public Health and Migration to Los Angeles (Critical Issues in Health and Medicine)", Rutgers University Press (2007).

infected with TB began to literally reshape the nature of its existing population. Unsurprisingly, there were negative consequences to this: because of the impoverishing nature of the disease, many of the newly arrived simply ended up destitute, without work, without homes, and without support. In response the city developed a series of strategies, not just to try to exclude the poor generally (including attempts to repatriate already-resident Mexican immigrants), but also to screen out and limit these 'lungers' by restricting the number of infected people entering both city and county. This characteristic stigma associated with tuberculosis can thus be seen to have indelibly marked, not just the local social fabric of the time, but also the disposition of the community, something which perhaps still shows its signs in the character of the city of angels to this day.

This particular migration to Los Angeles was reflective of a much more general drift of population westwards in the USA between 1840 and 1890 in pursuit of healthier environments in which to convalesce, recover or merely in which to live and prosper. It was a migratory phenomenon which was far from unique to North America, however. Economic migration within Britain in the early 19th century had begun by being from the country to the burgeoning cities in search of jobs, but for those who had settled in the new cities but now wanted to escape its disease and squalour, there was no going back to the impoverished and jobless country villages. Many with the means to do so looked for other ways to escape, and a trickle of migration to Britain's antipodean colonies began as a result. It was for exactly the same health-seeking reasons that were fuelling the migration westwards in the United States. None of these journeys was without substantial risk, and they can hardly have been undertaken lightly. Many of the hopeful emigrants must have spent much of the long voyages coughing or sweating at night in crowded cabins. More than a few must never have made it to their intended destinations and many more must have become infected in the cramped cabins in the course of these long voyages.

The 20th century itself witnessed many diverse and profound influences on (and innovations within) the varying social fabrics across the world and some of these can be recognised to have been directly stimulated by the ubiquitous persistence of TB. Some of them were of significant social benefit, but others proved to be particularly perverse and pernicious.

Conditions in the burgeoning industrial cities in Britain in the 19th centuryhad become almost unimaginably terrible. The average life expectancy was said to be as little as 26 in Liverpool and only 37 in London in 1841.[37] This was far from purely being down to consumptive TB, but TB was now being recognised not just as being a leading cause of death, but also as being directly linked to the dreadful urban living conditions which were still feeding it. It was in this social context that the rising death rates from TB in the industrialising nations prompted encouraging responses in some countries, taking the form of innovative social welfare legislation, legislation which both recognised and attempted to redress some of the root causes of these tides of socially-promoted disease.

Water and sewage systems began to be designed and developed in these chaotic and rapidly growing larger British towns to help counter such desperately low life expectancy rates. A series of acts of parliament then began to address the problems in an attempt to enforce further improvements. The first was the 1871 Local Government Act. This was followed by the 1872 Public Act and the 1875 Public Health Act, the 1878 Public Health (Water) Act, the Adulteration of Food Acts of the 1870's, the Weights and Measures Acts of 1878 and 1889, and the Sale of Food and Drugs Act of 1899. All contributed generally to public health, although none specifically related to TB. In 1890, however, the Housing Act offered the first concerted effort to specifically improve general living conditions amongst the poor.

Cleaner air, however, still played no part in any of any of these legislative agendas, and the ubiquitous polluted atmospheric environments were clearly seen to be affecting the rates of TB. The toxic factory atmospheres in the textile, pottery and metal-grinding industries in particular were still counterbalancing many of the benefits from improved nutrition and better sanitation and housing, particularly in relation to respiratory diseases.

The benevolent hand of tuberculosis management revealed itself particularly strikingly in the next wave of emerging social welfare reform. In the UK, Germany and also in Australia the endemic nature of TB was being properly recognised to be devastating the productive and reproductive capacities of each country's working populace during its most productive years. Such a realisation forced governments to consider adopting legislative responsibility for the care and cure of TB patients in a way that had never been considered previously and which has almost certainly never been attempted at such a scale since for any other group suffering from any other chronic infectious disease.

---

[37] "5th Annual Report of the Registrar General", Her Majesty's Stationary Office (1843).

It was the newly emergent unified Germany which led the way. The proud new nation was intensively playing rapid and competitive industrial and colonial catch up with Britain but was suffering a virulent explosion of TB in the process. In 1884 Otto von Bismarck added a clause to a legislative bill which had been passed the previous year which specifically promoted mandatory sickness insurance to cover TB. At the same time, the German concept of the *Kurhaus* developed, and it developed directly out of the TB sanatorium movement. *Kurhausen* survive to some degree right up until the present day in the German countryside and remain part of the German social welfare system for the more elderly, although cases of tuberculosis are now never seen in them.

The story in Britain was a little different. This country's military authorities had been unexpectedly shocked by the general unfitness of the soldiers who had been conscripted to fight in the two Boer Wars that had been fought in South Africa on either side of the turn of the century. Since it potentially affected national security, questions began to be asked about what should be done about this for the benefit of future campaigns with no good answers arising. Then, in 1908, David Lloyd George believed he found the answer. That year he visited Germany and found himself to be so impressed by what he encountered with the country's developing policies in public health that he formally announced in his next budget that the United Kingdom should be aiming to be "putting ourselves in this field on a level with Germany". He added a telling rider to this – one which offers salty food for thought given what was to follow in Europe in the next few years. He suggested to his fellow members of parliament that, "We should not emulate them only in armaments."

The UK's National Insurance Act followed in 1911. Today it is regarded as one of the foundation stones of Britain's modern social welfare system because it gave the British working classes their first contributory system of insurance against illness and unemployment. An estimated 13 million British workers came to be compulsorily covered under the scheme, with those suffering from TB being especially singled out for specialist provision which included not just sanatorium benefit but also specific support for their dependents. These were ideas which directly reflected Bismarck's scheme in Germany begun a full 25 years earlier. The Act was of profound social importance because it removed the need for unemployed workers, who were also automatically insured under the scheme, to rely on the stigmatising social welfare provisions of the long detested Poor Law which was finally abolished in 1926.

It's almost certain that this 40 year period between 1870 and 1911 witnessed events which provided the most critical factors for reducing mortality rates generally in both Britain and Germany, with clear reductions in the prevalence rates as well in the same period. This, it should be noted, was well before the introduction of a vaccine, the pasteurisation of milk or the first discovery of the first drug.

Medicine, meanwhile, was changing as well, and many of these changes were also linked to better understandings of tuberculosis. The British Medical Research Committee and Advisory Council (later becoming known as the Medical Research Council) was founded in 1913, with its prime role being the distribution of medical research funds under the terms of the 1911 National Insurance Act. Its immediate focus was on TB, directed by the Royal Commission on Tuberculosis which had formally recommended the creation of a permanent medical research body to investigate the disease. The Council's mandate was far from being confined solely to tuberculosis, but its major focus on the disease from its very outset is a clear indication of the gravity with which the disease was being considered at the time.

It is easy to assume that technical advances in medicine have always been the primary causes of improved health and life expectancy, but actually this is not necessarily the case. Thomas McKeown (1912-1988), a professor of Social Medicine at Birmingham University, England, made a general attack on this idea in the 1950s. He developed an alternative hypothesis suggesting that it was nutrition that had been as much or more responsible for the varying 19th and 20th century mortality rates as much any other contributory factors. Available figures suggest that he may well have been right. Between 1848 and 1854 death rates from TB were apparently running at 13.3% of all deaths in Britain at the time. By 1901, not only had there been around a 30% recorded reduction in general death rates, but about two-sevenths of this was being attributed to reductions in the prevalence of TB. McKeown thus argued that, decades before Streptomycin (the first drug) had been discovered, tuberculosis in Britain had already lost something approaching 75% of its lethal potential from its earlier highest point in the middle of the 18th century.

McKeown's case may well not be quite that easy to close, however. Other infectious diseases, including bronchial pneumonia and bronchitis (which, when totalled together, comprised the second most common cause of death in 1854 at 10.5%) actually ***rose*** in this same period, coming to represent over 16% of all deaths by 1901 (a higher percentage in fact than TB had been in 1854). This apparent anomaly might just simply have been down to fluctuating trends in diagnosis – with doctors entering bronchitis on death certificates for symptoms which they would have been previously deciding to be down to consumption.

Considering such troublesome variables retrospectively offers us a useful window through which to consider some of the complexities that bedevil the comprehensive accurate measurement of the true scale of the disease today – especially where diagnostics are known to be both insufficient in quantity and deficient in quality, much as they were in fact in these earlier times. It is certainly the case that global malnutrition has to be massively reduced if TB is seriously intended to be eradicated. But other economic and social factors which align with the McKeown thesis cry out for consideration as well – the frequent incidence of other infectious diseases, overcrowding, poor working conditions, inadequate air ventilation and certain occupational hazards are just some of them if the lessons from this period of history are to be properly learnt.

Nutritional improvements were unquestionably significant during this period, but relieving overcrowded living and working conditions may well have been even more so and it was these which were being serially and systematically addressed by the Factories and Workshop Acts, the Crowding Acts, and the Housing Acts.

Nevertheless, a London survey conducted as late as 1930 identified that an astonishing 82% of 14-15 year olds in the city had evidence of exposure to TB.[38] If this figure is in any way generally reflective of the pre-antibiotic era, it would suggest that almost all adults in the 19th and early 20th century were still being regularly exposed to active disease, with some of them (logically, as many as 18%) even possibly being naturally resistant to the disease. The actual death rates at this later time were also still tending to occur in the 15-35 age range, a phenomenon which rarely changes at any place or in any era. This in turn suggests that such deaths must have been being mainly precipitated by re-activation of latent disease and not from primary infection, and that the initial infections must have been occurring 20 or more years earlier in childhood.

One important conclusion that we can draw from McKeown's work is that a country may not necessarily need advanced medical technology nor even a

[38] Gillian Cronje - "Tuberculosis and mortality decline in England and Wales, 1851-1900" (1930), in R I Woods and J Woodward (eds), "Urban disease and mortality", Batsford (1984).

universally free health service for formidable improvements in life expectancy to be seen.[39] It does, however, suggest that, in the absence of such medical advances, there may well have to be a committed political will for social change and accompanying economic opportunity – one driven by the expectation of slow and consistent improvements in general social welfare. Given the current state of the pandemic in resource-poor environments where some life expectancies are still so shockingly low, it would certainly be foolish to completely dismiss such ideas.

Meanwhile, well into the 20th century, however much these death rates may have been reducing, a diagnosis of tuberculosis was still synonymous with death, and this was particularly so in many, if not most, of the sanatoria:

> "However much the sanatorium resembled other institutions, it had one unique feature – the omnipresence of the shadow of death. Apart from it, nothing can be understood about sanatorium life, whether it was staff enforcing rules or patients seeking sexual pleasure. Staff tried to brush it off with aphorisms about being strong and determined. But in countless ways, some personal, others collective, the sanatorium experience was at its core an encounter with mortality."[40]

Despite all of this, the sanatorium movement was still spreading worldwide. In India, for instance, the first open air sanatorium for treatment and isolation of TB patients was founded in 1906 in Tilonia, near Ajmer city of Rajasthan.[41] This was a sanatorium for 'consumptive girls' and it was opened by the American Methodist Episcopal Church, particularly intended for girls from the boarding schools and orphanages that were connected with their mission in Northern India. Cases of advanced consumption were also said to be welcomed, however, though they were segregated. Such was not the case in the other Indian sanatoria which followed where it was commonly reported that such cases would generally be turned away.

---

[39] John C Caldwell - "Routes to Low Mortality in Poor Countries", Population Council (1986).

[40] Richard Sucre - "The Great White Plague: The Culture of Death and the Tuberculosis Sanatorium". http://www.faculty.virginia.edu/blueridgesanatorium/death.htm

[41] These buildings have been more recently used (since 1972) by the extraordinary Barefoot College which is dedicated to improving the lives of the rural poor by education and improved social and ecological awareness.

A variety of other institutions were also set up around this time for the open air treatment of TB in India, but in general only those people who could pay for their stay were admitted, and by around 1920 there were still less than 500 beds available in all of South Asia in such institutions. A number of special wards were also being set up in civil hospitals, but they could do little more than provide segregation along with the questionable benefit of open air 'treatment'. The numbers that could be accommodated, however, were always tiny compared to the massive need.[42]

In 1911 the first real challenge to the dogma of bed rest in sanatoria began to emerge. William Camac Wilkinson (1858-1946), an Australian, reviewed follow-up studies of patients who had attended 31 sanatoria in the very home of the sanatoria movement itself, in Germany. Four years after discharge, he could identify that 80% of such patients had either died or reverted to becoming invalids. A similar report from Cumbria in the UK suggested the same thing but even worse – within six years 80% could be confirmed as being dead.

The days of the primacy of the sanatorium were now being seen to be numbered. In fact they turned out to be pretty much completely finished off by the opening volleys of the Second World War – as many as 15,000 British TB patients were peremptorily turned out of their sanatoria at its very outbreak, as the institutions were peremptorily requisitioned for other purposes.

Tuberculosis and race

Wherever or whenever a sanatorium may have been located in the world the emphasis for recovery was almost invariably being primarily placed on the patient, in particular on how he or she could better influence their cure by adhering to the stringent sanatorium rules.

Such regimes were tough. Patients were often as not out in the fresh air in their beds even in the coldest of weathers, and they were as frequently deliberately physically restricted to almost no activity at all. The basic idea behind their treatment always included exposure to as much fresh air as possible, even in extreme cold – and even sometimes ***especially*** in the cold and frost. Whether or not such outdoor regimes were of ultimate benefit to such patients is highly questionable, but it may well have been very usefully

[42] Lankester A - "Tuberculosis in India", London, Butterworth, 1920.

protective for the staff attending them who would themselves, by such extreme measures, have been substantially less exposed to infectious pathogens.

The 'Daily Schedule' for patients of Catawba Sanatorium, in Virginia USA, for instance, was as follows:

7:15 - Rising Bell
8:00 to 8:30 - Breakfast
8:30 to 11:00 - Rest or Exercise as Ordered
11:00 to 12:45 - Rest on Bed
1:00 to 1:30 - Dinner
1:45 to 4:00 - Rest on Bed, Reading but no talking allowed. Quiet hour.
4:00 to 5:45 - Rest or Exercise as Ordered
6:00 - Supper
8:00 - Nourishment if ordered
9:00 - All patients in pavilions
9:30 - All lights out

Catawba was Virginia's first sanatorium. In 1918, the state's second state-sponsored sanatorium, Piedmont Sanatorium, had opened in Burkeville – but this one was strictly for Negro consumptives. Up until then the best treatment facilities that black TB patients could hope for had been in state mental institutions where the hygiene levels and the quality of treatment were both extremely poor. Piedmont's own "Rules and Information for Patients" spelt it out loud and clear for its negro patients, however, in a way which differed rather ominously from what was being dictated in sanatoria more generally elsewhere: "If you expect to get well you must work for it" was the command. It somehow has the ring of "*Arbeit macht frei*" and the German concentration camp about it.

A report from H.G. Carter, the director at Piedmont, reveals the dominant views of the time:

> "It is up to the white man who controls his destiny to see that he [the Negro] gets the proper treatment when sick; for the sake of humanity first, from an economic point of view second and for his own sake and that of his family if he sees no other reason."

Tuberculosis was certainly a big problem within the black community in America and black tuberculosis mortality rates were generally substantially higher than the mortality rates of the white population. Of the total of deaths in Virginia in 1920, for example, 61% were white and 39% black – a generally accurate reflection of the state's racial mix; of all of the deaths that were specified as being tubercular, however, only 37% were white and 63% were black.

The state's growing concern for the black tuberculosis problem was largely arising because so many Negroes were working intimately as servants within white households. The disease was thus being defined by colour and was being viewed as providing a racially-defined reservoir of potentially infectious disease. The devastation being caused by the disease in the black communities themselves could just as easily spread to the white population, however, and so something had to be done about it. Unfortunately, given some of the ideas concerning race which were pervading medical thought across the world at the time, what efforts that were made were often far from what would be considered acceptable today.

South Africa contains its own special early story concerning race and TB – one that was far from insignificant, and which is still having impact not just on the African epidemic but also on the wider global pandemic. The story was especially influenced by Lyle Cummins (1873-1949), a British doctor who was regarded as an expert on TB at the time. Cummins believed that Africans exhibited a "biological dissimilarity in their average response to tuberculous infection". This idea reflected the contemporary 'seed and soil' theory of disease – the seed being the disease itself, and the soil being the particular ethnic population which it might infect. It was widely believed that there were racial differences which left some populations considerably more susceptible to certain diseases than others.

Cummins's ideas had immediate influence on those managing the rapidly developing highly profitable mining industry in South Africa. They directly promoted the concept of racial segregation but, in doing so, they also engendered almost perfect conditions, not just for the disease to flourish, but also for particularly insidious political ideas to develop alongside them. In retrospect, TB historian Helen Bynum suggests that:

> "Cummins's new ideas.. helped condemn the mine workers and black South Africans more generally and [subsequently] fed into the prejudices of the apartheid state after the Second World War. Using Cummins's ideas as their defining logical premise, mine owners considered that the costly benefits from improving conditions in the mines and townships could only be of limited consequence in the short term, so why bother? There were lots of miners and vast sums of money to be made from the variety of minerals. The best plan was segregation, to keep the miners and their disease in labour camps and the black population generally away from the urban areas

> unless they were required to work there, in which case even then they should be better isolated in townships."[43]

Thus were the seeds of apartheid sown.

The architects of this proto-apartheid were creating a system in which hundreds of thousands of workers were forced to live in over-crowded and poorly ventilated single-sex city hostels served by commercial sex workers (euphemistically referred to as 'town-wives'). This system of what has been since described as 'oscillatory migration' meant that a large proportion of black workers were only being employed temporarily or episodically in cities or towns, or were working in the mines. They were then only periodically visiting their wives and families back in their rural homelands. They were also living in desperately poor conditions in separated townships. This was ideal, not just for the spread of TB but also for other sexually transmitted infections (which much more recently has included HIV/AIDS).

It became a standard pattern of employment which persisted across southern Africa throughout the 20th century, consisting of overcrowded squatter settlements, a migrant labour force and deliberately under-developed health services for blacks, all creating the perfect environment for TB to flourish.

These same social, economic and environmental conditions were finally and deliberately brought together and formalised with the legal adoption of apartheid in 1948. The mining industry and its system of segregation were actually begun well before apartheid, but the same system continued throughout it, reaching its peak with the creation of the *bantustans*. What is not so widely realised is that the conditions within the mining industry have shamefully persisted almost unchecked since apartheid was dismantled in 1993, and they survive right up until today as a direct consequence of the ANC dropping its promises contained in its Freedom Charter relating to the country's mineral resources "belonging to the people". These conditions survive because the promises were dropped as a compromise in the face of international and multi-national pressures and because of the estimated US$2.5 trillion dollars' worth of mineral reserves which still lie waiting to be mined in the country with the profits remaining in the hands of the wealthy few.

Incidence rates of TB among South African mine workers today are among the highest in the world, running at over 3,000 per 100,000 (some suggest as

[43] Helen Bynum - "Spitting Blood", Oxford University Press (2012).

high as 9,000 per 100,000). When miners sicken, as they have done regularly for over a century, they are sent home as they always have been, effectively to infect their families and communities before they almost inevitably die. So the African epidemic doesn't just continue, but it still continues to grow, now rocket-fuelled by HIV/AIDS.

In Canada in the first half of the 20th century the treatment of infectious disease among native Canadian aboriginal people was also being influenced by ideas of race, and some of these ideas also condensed around the problems of tuberculosis. The story in Canada, however, played out somewhat differently. After the indigenous tribes had been forced to give up their hunting lifestyles and adopt sedentary ways of life, the incidence rate of infectious diseases in native populations in the Western Provinces was said to be running as high as 9,000 per 100,000, and this included high rates of TB. The response to the problem in Canada, however, was different from that in South Africa, and was one which was quite literally not so black and white. It was still murkily grey, however, given that it was also heavily influenced by ideas of racial eugenics. The consequence for native Canadians was that they were expediently enforced into racial assimilation rather than politically enforced into racial segregation.

In the 1920s R. George Ferguson, the physician and superintendent of the Fort Qu'Appelle Sanatorium in southern Saskatchewan, began to review what he called the "tuberculosis epidemic" among Canadian aboriginal people. Ferguson was himself a leading expert on TB being one of the world's pioneers in promoting the practice of BCG vaccination. He not only worked at the sanatorium, but was living there along with his family, and he was becoming increasingly conscious of the dangers from the levels of untreated tuberculosis circulating on the adjacent reserves. Native Canadian people were rarely treated in the sanatorium itself, however, only being admitted to a special ward in the sanatorium if or when space was available. Ferguson chose to apply the same 'seed and soil' analogy of the day to his own assessments of the situation, (similarly to Lyle Cummins and the other race theorists of the time) choosing to see aboriginal and indigenous peoples as comparative 'primitives' with correspondingly primitive responses to unfamiliar disease. Ferguson theorized that Native Canadians carried little or no inherited resistance to tuberculosis, as a result of which, having been restricted from their traditional lifestyles by being confined to reservations, they quickly sickened and died. He described that witnessing this phenomenon was like watching "wild birds confined in cages". But, extrapolating from the common basic soil-and-seed idea, he began to conclude that 'primitives' who intermarried with non-natives should be much more likely to be able to resist the disease and survive. He concluded that:

> "[The] introduction of white blood is not only a potent factor in civilizing primitive people, altering habits of living, appetites, and desires, but [it] also has a noticeable effect on increasing their resistance to tuberculosis."

Ferguson's work in the 1920s provided a medical and quasi-scientific rationale for concerted government efforts to assimilate Aboriginal people.[44] Whatever may be thought about such ideas today, it has to be said that it contributed to the growing global understanding of tuberculosis at that time. It was even being said that:

> "The Aboriginal populations have made substantial contributions to much of our knowledge of the prevention and control of TB."[45]

But it was not just such questionable efforts at social engineering that was apparently contributing to the reduction of TB among native populations in North America. It was also just as often down to the efforts of the indigenous peoples themselves. Death rates in reservations across the continent generally were running at horrific levels in the early 20th century. As these First Nation peoples learnt more from doctors, nurses and teachers, however, non-indigenous health care providers were increasingly being allowed to help fight the dreaded disease of TB. Across the United States, Native American or First Nation peoples were allowing non-native medical practitioners to handle what they were calling the 'travelling disease' because, just like the medical doctors of the time, they too saw it as originating among the non-indigenous. Even powerful and highly regarded medicine men and women had begun to encourage their people to seek medicine for this disease from the white people – with undoubted positive consequences. Tuberculosis deaths among many tribal peoples in California and Washington, for instance, were recorded to be declining right into the

---

[44]Maureen Lux -"White blood: race, tuberculosis and Canadian plains aboriginal people, 1920-1945", History Dept, University of Saskatchewan.

[45] Kue Young - "Tuberculosis prevention and control: the contributions of aboriginal populations", Department of Public Health Sciences, University of Toronto.

1940s, in large measure on account of these concerted efforts of both Indians and non-Indians alike.[46]

But this story is also sadly still far from over. Rates of TB among First Nation peoples in both countries in North America are still today of a different order to that of the continent overall, as indeed they are amongst aboriginal populations almost everywhere

Tuberculosis and the unfit-to-breed

The tawdry influence of eugenics on social and medical thought in the United States in the late 19th and early 20th centuries is something that most Americans today remain either unaware of or would rather see forgotten, but its influence at the time was unquestionably substantial. In fact, for a critical time it could even have had a terrible and far larger influence on the history of the rest of the last century.

In 1911 the Carnegie-supported and terrifyingly entitled "Preliminary Report of the Committee of the Eugenic Section of the American Breeder's Association to Study and to Report on the Best Practical Means for Cutting off the Defective Germ-Plasm in the Human Population" candidly recorded the options that the committee had been exploring in order to purify the country's breeding pool.[47] Proposal number 8 of a total of 11 ideas contained within the report consisted quite simply of common-or-garden euthanasia, a proposal which even included the idea of using gas chambers. In 1918, Paul Popenoe (1888-1979) whose reputation (and qualifications) mainly lay in his being a horticulturalist, along with some previous experience as an Army venereal disease specialist in World War I, co-authored a popular medical textbook entitled "Applied Eugenics". It

[46] Clifford E Trafzer - "Traveling medicine: tuberculosis among first nations in California and Washington", Department of History, University of California, Riverside.

[47] This report was presented at the First International Congress of Eugenics in London in 1912 by Bleecker van Wagenen who declared that people of "defective inheritance" should be "eliminated from the human stock". Included among the "socially unfit" were the feebleminded, paupers, criminals, epileptics, the insane, the congenitally weak, people predisposed to specific diseases, the deformed, the blind, and the deaf.

became a widely studied text. In it he suggested that, because of various defects, between five and ten million Americans were unfit to reproduce and should therefore be sterilised. Such ideas were far from extreme – in fact they were already being fostered by existing individual state legislation. Compulsory strerilisation had first been enabled by Indiana's Compulsory Sterilisation Law of 1907 which allowed for involuntary sterilisation of the mentally ill and the mentally retarded in the state's psychiatric hospitals – as well as for the sterilisation of criminals and of "idiots". It was a law which had already been copied by as many as 30 other states.

But sterilising the unfit-to-breed was at the milder end of the views expressed by Popenoe. The book unashamedly advocated that:

> "From an historical point of view, the first method which presents itself is execution...Its value in keeping up the standard of the race should not be underestimated."[48]

The grand plan of the eugenicists was to wipe out in one way or another the reproductive capacity of those who were deemed weak and inferior – the so-called "unfit-to-breed".

Fortunately there seems to be little evidence of the ultimate ideas behind such a policy ever having been implemented on American soil, but a shocking exception relates both tuberculosis and the mentally ill. It occurred in a mental institution in Lincoln, Illinois, where incoming patients were deliberately fed milk from tubercular cows on the assumption that eugenically stronger individuals would be immune to the disease, whilst the weaker would naturally succumb.

The policy resulted in an annual death rate of the institution's inmates that ran at over 30%.

Tuberculosis in Japan

Japan, meanwhile, had been fast emerging from its two centuries of self-imposed isolation and at the same time was culturally and socially exploding

[48] Popenoe comfortably redefined himself as an expert in marriage guidance counselling after World War II (and after the realities of what the eugenics movement had ultimately perpetrated were properly revealed).

in a process of frenetic industrialisation. Quite predictably, despite its physical isolation, a rapid rise in rates of tuberculosis accompanied this process, just as had happened elsewhere. Between 1850 and the end of the Second World War, TB was so pervasive in the country that it has been said that few Japanese families remained untouched by the disease. It was an epidemic which was being driven yet again by concerted industrialization, by urbanization and by the intensive barracking of its migratory workforce.

The epidemic in Japan has been divided by historians into five separate phases of disease.

In phase 1 (between 1899 and 1918) TB mortality was seen to increase alongside the initial industrialization with a high concentration of deaths within the weaving industry. During this period as well, TB mortality amongst women was much higher than among men and, quite unusually, the majority of victims were young girls. Death rates were rising more quickly in the industrialised areas than in the poverty-stricken rural areas from which the workforce was being recruited, but it was rising most noticeably amongst the proportion of the migrant workforce who were women and young girls. Peasant girls had come to the city to work and were frequently seen to sicken and then slow down at their labours. As a result, in a frighteningly similar fashion to what happened (and continues to happen) with miners in South Africa, they were dismissed and returned to their villages where they then continued to sicken and die.

These workers were mostly young (12-20 years of age) and unmarried. Most were the *dekasegi* migrant workers, working at silk or cotton mills for short periods, generally for a year or two, and living in mill dormitories throughout their period of employment. The devastating effect of tuberculosis on this particular group has led some Japanese historians to conclude that these Japanese textile workers were victims of particularly inhuman exploitation, and that their experiences were powerful evidence of the iniquities of the emerging Japanese system of capitalism.

In phase 2 (between 1918 and 1930) TB mortality actually decreased as those already suffering from the disease (or those most vulnerable to it) succumbed instead to the virulent influenza pandemic of 1918.

This decline reversed again during phase 3 (1930-1945) mainly due to a second major wave of industrialization with its primary focus this time being in heavy industry. This third phase of the epidemic was further exacerbated by the social impact of the war in Manchuria and then in China and, finally, by the wider war in the Pacific.

The all-too-familiar phenomena of ignoring consumption as well as either blaming or stigmatising consumptives characterized much of this period. In similar fashion to what had happened in Europe, it was still widely believed that TB was essentially a hereditary disease, or else that it was one that was caused by constitutional weakness caused by excessive lifestyles in relation to eating, drinking or sexual habits. Because of this the disease was often concealed within families or else deliberately misdiagnosed in order to protect its victims. Protective industrial legislation had been begun in Japan in the 1920s but the rate of registered deaths from TB continued to increase throughout this third phase in spite of this. In this period TB was recognised as being the leading single cause of natural death in the country accounting for 12-14% of all deaths, something which has been considered quite possibly an underestimation. By 1942, right at the height of Japan's Pacific War, the situation was seen as being so bad that the Japanese cabinet officially declared tuberculosis to be such an urgent issue that the very "rise or fall of the Japanese race" could directly be affected by it.[49]

In phase 4 (from 1945 until the mid-1970s) TB declined rapidly, partly due to the excessive death rates during World War II which reduced the pool of latent disease, but mainly because of the initiation of a modern programme of TB control which started in the early 1950s. In phase 5 (from the mid-1970s until today), the decline in the rate of TB has slowed down, stabilised to a large degree by the significant increasing average age of the population.[50]

The historian William Johnson has suggested that between 1900 and 1950 at least six million Japanese died of the disease – but even this may be an underestimation.[51]

[49] Janet Hunter - "Textile factories, tuberculosis and the quality of life in industrialising Japan", Economic History Department, London School of Economic (1992) http://eprints.lse.ac.uk/22459/1/04_92.pdf.

[50] Shimao T – "Tuberculosis and its control – lessons from the past and future prospect", Kekkaku, 80; 6 (2005) 481-9. [Article in Japanese]

[51] William Johnson - "The Modern Epidemic: a History of Tuberculosis in Japan", Harvard University Press (1995).

The particular European experience

In many ways, these experiences in North America, Japan, Europe and South Africa all echo each other. In Austria, however, the disease struck in one single instance in a way which had its own special impact on the wider world, one which lasted for over half of the 20th century.

On the 3rd January 1903 an otherwise insignificant Austrian civil servant died of TB. He had gone to his local inn, the Gasthaus Wiesinger in the little village of Leonding, to drink his customary morning glass of wine. On arrival, he had been offered the day's newspaper but then collapsed on the floor before he had even opened it. Taken into an adjoining room, a doctor was summoned, but he died almost immediately as a result of hemorrhaging from his lungs. The leather couch on which he died can, in fact, still be seen in the inn today.

This single otherwise unremarkable death would have remained that way had it not had a huge secondary impact on the whole world in the ensuing half century, because the man who died that day at the inn was Adolf Hitler's father, Alois.

At the time of his father's death the young Adolf was an impressionable and intemperate teenager of 13 years of age. Hitler's own revealing description of the episode was recorded in his memoirs in "*Mein Kampf*". It was not entirely accurate. He elected to write only that:

> "A stroke of apoplexy felled the old gentleman who was otherwise so hale, thus painlessly ending his earthly pilgrimage."

Very tellingly he chose to omit informing his readers that the cause had been tuberculosis. This was for reasons which, not that much later, began to reveal themselves a lot more clearly.

The young Adolf had been clashing with his father at the time. Alois, who has never been portrayed by anyone as being in any way a kindly man, was insistent that Adolf should become a civil servant like himself. The young Hitler, however, had other ideas, harbouring dreams of becoming a great artist. With his father dead, at least there was now no more arguing with his father, especially over his career choice, but nevertheless it was still being expected that Adolf should follow in his father's footsteps. He was about to be granted more freedom still in the matter, however, and once again this was courtesy of tuberculosis. Two years later, at the age of 15, Adolf himself fell ill with TB himself, but he recovered. Again he was not exactly honest in his later account of the episode in his memoirs, writing:

> "Then suddenly an illness came to my help and in a few weeks decided my future… As a result of my serious lung ailment, a physician advised my mother in most urgent terms never to send me into an office."

He got as far this time as describing a "serious lung ailment" but refrained from any further detail. What was important was the consequence of his doctor's advice because he insisted that Hitler should not work in any office environment. It meant that he would now never turn into the civil servant that he dreaded becoming and that his father had been so determined that he should become. That mysterious "serious lung ailment" had intervened on his behalf and had decided his future. It also, therefore, decided the future of millions of others as well, particularly as ever more extreme connections began to be made within Hitler's disturbed psyche, especially between tuberculosis and the Jews.

In fact many European physicians in the late 1800s and early 1900s had already been characterizing 'the Jew' as being particularly physically vulnerable to tuberculosis so that, by extension, this had been the reason for the spread of the disease throughout the world. Hitler readily subscribed to these ideas. The following is a speech he delivered in Salzburg on August 7, 1930:

> "This is not a problem you can turn a blind eye to – one to be solved by many concessions. For us, it is a problem of whether our nation can ever recover its health, whether the Jewish spirit can ever really be eradicated. Don't be misled into thinking you can fight a disease without killing the carrier, without destroying the bacillus. Don't think you can fight racial tuberculosis without taking care to rid the nation of the carrier of that racial tuberculosis. This Jewish contamination will not subside. This poisoning of the nation will not end until the carrier himself, the Jew, has been banished from our midst."

In this terrifyingly prescient diatribe a full nine years before the outbreak of war in Europe he was already describing Jews as being "carriers" of disease. He was also discussing eradicating not just the Jewish spirit along with the disease but also the disease's carriers themselves. Since Jews were neither the carriers nor the seeds of tuberculosis dissemination, this single speech stands as terrible testimony as to how the 30 year-old Hitler was beginning to twist both logic and terminology, in this case using the scourge of TB to promote and justify the idea of exterminating the Jewish people.

The rest of this story, as they say, is history.

But we must now take a look at what had been happening in the same period in the world of medicine in relation to the disease.

The Bug is identified, Tests developed, and a Vaccine found

"IF THE IMPORTANCE OF A DISEASE.. IS MEASURED BY THE NUMBER OF FATALITIES IT CAUSES, THEN TUBERCULOSIS MUST BE CONSIDERED MUCH MORE IMPORTANT THAN THOSE [OTHER] MOST FEARED INFECTIOUS DISEASES, PLAGUE, CHOLERA AND THE LIKE. ONE IN SEVEN HUMAN BEINGS DIES OF TUBERCULOSIS."

Robert Koch (1882)

At the end of the 19th century, the first signs of a turning tide in the struggle against the disease had finally begun to reveal themselves. On 24th March 1882 Robert Koch addressed the Physiological Society in Berlin with a presentation which he entitled "*Über Tuberculose*", or "About Tuberculosis".

The previous year, Koch had been experimenting by staining tuberculous material with a methylene blue dye. Viewing the results through his microscope he could just make out groups of vague oblong structures. To improve the contrast, he decided to add Bismarck Brown, and after this he could see the oblong structures a little more clearly still. He then further improved the technique by varying the concentration of alkali in the staining solution until, as far as he could determine, he had achieved the ideal conditions for viewing the bacilli. Once they were fully visible he realised that he had probably identified the causative agents of tuberculosis.

His next step was to figure out a way of establishing beyond doubt that these tiny structures were truly part of the disease process.

To do this, he employed what has since become known as the Koch-Henle postulate – a devastatingly foolproof method for linking cause and effect in any infectious disease. The basic principle for the postulate assumed that the organism under suspicion would be present in every case of the disease. With this in mind, Koch proposed that the organism should be isolated from its host and then grown independently in pure culture; then samples of the organism could be taken from this pure culture and might be seen to cause the same disease when inoculated into a healthy susceptible experimental animal in the laboratory. Finally, to clinch the case, this same organism could in turn be isolated from the newly inoculated infected animal and would then be identified as being the same as the original organism that had been first isolated from the originally diseased host.

After numerous attempts he found that he was able to successfully incubate some of the tuberculosis bacteria which he had taken from a human consumptive. He then inoculated a group of guinea pigs with these bacilli, comparing the consequences of the inoculated (and rapidly sickening) group of animals to a separate control group of non-inoculated guinea pigs. Unsurprisingly the entire inoculated group sickened. Having swiftly despatched all of the animals, both healthy and sick, he proceeded to examine each group in turn and found no sign of either the disease or the organism in the control group, but in every single one of the inoculated animals he found the characteristic tubercles and could also identify the same tell-tale bacteria from samples from them which he examined under his microscope.

With this act of conclusive systematic research he proved that this newly identified bacillus, which he now named the *tuberculosis bacillus*, was the cause of tuberculosis. Besides announcing that he had successfully identified and isolated the pathogen which caused consumptive disease, Koch also added that the "tubercle bacillus is surrounded by a special wall of unusual properties".

He summarized his findings in the *Berliner Klinische Wochenschrift* shortly after. In an article which he entitled *Die Ätiologie der Tuberculose*. He wrote:

> "In the future the fight against this terrible plague of mankind will deal no longer with an undetermined something, but with a tangible parasite, whose living conditions are for the most part known and can be investigated further."

In 1905 Koch received the Nobel Prize in honour of this discovery, one which is still regarded today as a landmark moment in immunology. Since 2000 March 24th, the anniversary of his original presentation in Berlin, has been annually marked as World TB Day.

It was Koch, as well, who first coined the term "TB", applying it as an acronym for the tuberculosis bacillus. Koch's work was just one part of a wider shift in understandings of disease, but it is widely recognised as being a primary way-marker at the very opening moments of modern immunology. It offered a new understanding of the phenomenon of disease-causing germs, one that made a massive subsequent difference to the management of health and infectious disease in the subsequent decades.

For Koch, the disease was all about the germ, and had little or nothing to do with the infected host. This was an understandable perspective given the guinea pig's inherent lack of resistance to the disease, but the scientific community was still not all of an entirely single mind on the matter. Some of his contemporaries were more inclined to stick to the more traditional ideas of family heredity and predisposition, and, even as the infectious nature of the disease was emerging more and more strongly, attention was also still being given to the environments in which it flourished.

Koch himself reckoned that one in seven deaths in Europe at the time was down to TB. His estimation can be strongly supported by contemporary records in England which suggested that in the second half of the 19th century 13% of deaths were down to consumption or TB (around 80% of which were recorded as being pulmonary).

Incidence rates almost everywhere were now directly pointing to the link with the processes of industrialisation, however. By the end of the 19th century TB rates were actually declining in London, for instance, while they were simultaneously now rising in Russia, in the Austrian-Hungarian Empire and in Japan – in fact they were rising in every country where industrialisation was playing competitive catch-up. This wasn't something that was just being noticed by physicians and epidemiologists either – it was being noted by political theorists as well. In the 1860's Karl Marx and Friedrich Engels had turned their focus on the disease, arguing in their political writing that "consumption and other lung diseases among the working people are necessary conditions to the existence of capital".[52]

The skin test

Koch's next step was to look for a treatment. In 1890 he developed tuberculin, a glycerine extract of the bacteria itself and conducted the world's first attempt at researchinga drug to fight the disease. Initially there were reports of success, but there were also rapid reports of severe allergic responses, as a result of which the idea of tuberculin being the hoped-for miracle cure was swiftly dropped.

Tuberculin did offer up the first opportunity to positively identify infection, however. The drug was picked up by Clemens von Pirquet, (1874-1929) a

[52] "*Das Kapital*", Chapter 15. If Marx and Engels were alive and still publishing they might be concluding that their views were being comprehensively confirmed 150 years later given what is happening today in the South African mining industry.

Viennese paediatrician. Von Pirquet was also one of the founders of the field of allergy research (he actually coined the word), but his discoveries respect of TB arose directly from his work with smallpox vaccines. His contributions to tuberculosis research were prompted by what he had seen happen in patients suffering from severe reactions to repeated smallpox vaccinations.

The procedure he developed to diagnose previous infection from TB was almost too simple to be true but still forms the basis for the tests that remain the most commonly used today: he scrubbed the subject's forearm, then scratched it twice with a needle and popped a drop of tuberculin on each scratch. If there had been any previous interaction between *M. tuberculosis* and the patient's immune system he expected it to show within 48 hours when a tell-tale sign of reactive inflammation would become evident at the site of scratch. Such a response was correctly assumed to be evidence of sufficient prior exposure to the bacillus for an immune system to mobilise antibodies at the site of the scratch in response to the antigenic proteins in the tuberculin.

His findings were of immense importance to the developing understanding of the disease. They began to reveal for the first time both the existence and scale of latent disease. After performing his test on 1,400 children who were previously believed to be disease free he found that 80% of them reacted positively. The only logical conclusion that could be drawn was that they had already been exposed to the bacillus sufficiently for them to have been infected by it without symptoms. It's hard to imagine what a devastating realisation this must have been for von Pirquet at the time when he began to realise what it implied. It was another massively important milestone in the developing understanding the disease, since it offered the world its first glimpse at the underlying ocean of latent infection which still continues to underpin and feed the visible epidemic of active disease.

Other variant tuberculin tests were soon being developed as well, each one looking for more reliable methods. Albert Calmette, for instance, who was soon to become famous in the field for other reasons, chose to drop his tuberculin directly into the eyes of his subjects. Unsurprisingly, it wasn't a method that was widelyt adopted.

Charles Mantoux (1877-1947), another French doctor, next began expanding on von Pirquet's ideas, injecting tuberculin intradermally just beneath the skin surface and, as a result, in 1907 his eponymous Mantoux test became today's standard diagnostic test for the disease.

The vaccine

Meanwhile Calmette, having given up on dropping tuberculin into the eyes of his potential patients, turned his attentions to the possibilities of preventing the disease in the first place. His reputation today relates to his part in the development of the first (and so far only) vaccine, in pursuit of which he collaborated with a vet, Camille Guérin (1872-1961). Their work was appropriately informed by that of Louis Pasteur with cholera and anthrax. Exactly as Pasteur had done, they set about attenuating the pathogen to the extent that it could only produce a mild infection that would be sufficient to provide subsequent immunity, and yet be of no serious consequence to the vaccinated host in the process. Both men worked under the aegis of France's famous Pasteur Institute. Using Guérin's veterinary expertise, they used bovine bacteria rather than the human strain, and in 1906 began experimenting with cattle, but they hit immediate problems in culturing the best possible candidate.

By selecting a bovine strain they were emulating the success of the Englishman Edward Jenner who had developed the vaccination technique for smallpox using a bovine variant of the disease. Jenner held claim to being the true father of modern vaccination methods, long before Pasteur himself. Jenner had lived and worked in rural Gloucestershire in England at the end of the 18th century, and had become aware of a common belief amongst local villagers that anyone infected with cowpox were then rendered immune from the far more dangerous smallpox infection. In 1796 he put the hypothesis to the test by inoculating two small scratches in a young boy's forearm with cowpox. Jenner recovered the fluid for the inoculation from the pustule of a local milkmaid who already had cowpox. The boy he vaccinated, called James Phipps, was the son of a local landless labourer who had been working for Jenner as a gardener at his residence in the village of Berkeley. Jenner later wrote that he had needed "a healthy boy, about eight years old for the purpose of inoculation for the Cow Pox", and little James fitted the bill.[53] Young James was observed to suffer a mild illness lasting for about a week after which he fully recovered. Jenner then waited another six weeks before deliberately infecting the boy with smallpox – and, given that James remained well, the result is positively recorded as a major event in the history of medicine. We remain ignorant as to how the original agreement had been struck on the matter with James's

[53] Reid, Robert - "Microbes and men", London: British Broadcasting Corporation (1974), page 7.

father and also of exactly how much Jenner had explained to him about the risks involved. Nor, unfortunately, do we have any record of how James himself felt about the episode, but Jenner did leave James and his subsequent family a cottage. Jenner's name, however, has been written indelibly into the history book of man's long battle against infectious disease, the event being regarded as being another one of the true milestones in medicine.[54]

For Calmette and Guérin a bovine strain was never going to be the end of the matter like it had been for Jenner because, unlike cowpox and smallpox, bovine TB is just as serious as TB itself. Their own quest turned out to be a far longer and more painstaking affair than Jenner's, or indeed than Pasteur's. They first realised that they needed to create some sort of ideal environment for the bacteria to grow so that it might in time decline in virulence whilst still able to provoke enough of its antigenic response in humans. Both men knew from the outset that this might take many regenerations of the bacteria to accomplish, but their first challenge of was to find this ideal environment in which they could breed the bugs. After some experimentation they finally found it in a compost of potatoes after first cooking it in ox bile which in turn was then treated with glycerine.

Calmette set to work painstakingly regenerating the bacilli in this mixture every three weeks for a total of 13 years, constantly checking and rechecking it for its slowly depleting pathogenic power throughout the period. By 1913 they dared to believe that they were making a break-through, but then war broke out in Europe and everything was put on hold. After the war, they picked up the research again and in 1921 they finally conducted the first test on a human subject, using the weakened germ – which has since become known as the BCG vaccine (or the "Bacille

[54] This is not the only extraordinary story concerning children in the story of smallpox vaccinations. In 1803, Charles IV, then king of Spain, had been convinced of the benefits of the cowpox vaccine after his daughter had been stricken with smallpox, and ordered his personal physician, Francis Xavier de Balmis, to deliver it to his Spanish dominions in North and South America. To maintain the vaccine in an available viable state during the voyage, the physician "recruited" 22 young boys from Spanish orphanages. The boys were aged between three and nine, and were known to have never had cowpox or smallpox before. During the trip across the Atlantic, de Balmis serially vaccinated the orphans in a living chain: two children were vaccinated immediately before departure, and when cowpox pustules had appeared on their arms, material from these lesions was used to vaccinate two more children, etc. etc.

Calmette-Guérin"). They first tested it out on a new born baby whose mother had died immediately after giving birth. The vaccine was given orally in three stages, at three, five and seven days, and the baby was then cared for by her grandmother who had been demonstrated to be sputum-positive therefore infectious to the new born child. At six months of age the baby showed no signs at all of disease.

It seemed to have worked.

Of course, this extraordinary finding couldn't be supported or proved now by the standard tuberculin skin test since it would now show that the infant's immune system had been triggered by the attenuated bacillus in the vaccine in exactly the same way as if she had been directly infected with TB by her grandmother. This problem remains the major challenge in measuring rates of latent infection in any immunised population to this day and so continues to hamper efforts at comprehensive disease surveillance. But at least a vaccine was now available for the world to use to try to stem the tide of disease.

The wider adoption of the vaccine, however, tells us yet another story with twists of its own. It was embraced in Scandinavia, for instance, as part of the adoption of its nascent welfare states, and stayed that way. Britain, with TB rates already recognised to be declining, was reluctant to embrace the vaccine at all, only taking it up in any general sense in the 1950s. The USA and the Netherlands have never used the vaccine routinely at any time. The authorities in the USA were resistant to the idea partly because of distrust of the French research which was suspected as being selective in its recruitment of subjects. The general preservation of health was also seen as being a matter of individual responsibility in the country as much or more as it might have been a wider social one. As a result it was being promoted that the adoption of BCG in the country might "lead to a false sense of security which could result in failure to observe other precautions that would otherwise be taken".[55] Despite this, it was intriguingly still seen fit to conduct trials of the vaccine in 1935 on various tribes of Native Americans. The results of the trials were recorded as being successful, but rates in the US and in the Netherlands declined anyway so neither country ever adopted the vaccine.

---

[55] Quoted in Linda Bryder - '"We shall not find salvation in inoculation": BCG vaccination in Scandinavia, Britain and the USA, 1921-19602', Social Science & Medicine, 1999 49; 9 (1999) page 1163.

In Germany the vaccine was initially embraced and widely adopted but, despite the extraordinary heyday of the *kurhaus*, ideas about human health and disease were now beginning to change – and they were changing ominously as the ideas of racial eugenics inexorably took stronger hold. TB had also developed special meaning in post-Great War Germany. When the French took control of the industrial Rhineland after the First World War, their troops were rumoured to be spreading the disease in the occupied population as a way of diluting the strength of the German race. The vaccine itself was finally and famously completely banned from being used in Germany in 1931, partly because of this French connection, but principally because of a batch of vaccine which had been improperly prepared and which caused of the death of 71 children in Lübeck. The true cause of their deaths was very promptly confirmed to have been down to nothing more than a production problem, but the event had a terminal effect nevertheless on the reputation of the vaccine. TB was already being described as a "racial poison" and anything associated with it was seen to be similarly tainted.

Under-reporting – and further complexities

There is also good evidence of wide-spread under-reporting of the disease from this same period.

Around the turn of the 20th century patients in the US who were insured by smaller insurance companies would find themselves losing all their insurance benefits if their disease was ever identified as being tuberculosis – and as a result the disease was often being deliberately mis-recorded either as being either pneumonia or bronchitis.

Linda Bryder published an informative study relating to the same phenomenon in the UK. She concluded that, despite there being a requirement for a formal registration of death by a doctor introduced in Britain in 1874, any statistics from this time and after regarding both prevalence rates and deaths from TB should be treated with caution.[56] She identified two main reasons for this, specifically a frequent failure in proper

[56] Linda Bryder - "Not always one and the same thing, the Registration of Tuberculosis Deaths in Britain 1900-1950", the Society for the Social History of Medicine (1996).

diagnosis, but also a ubiquitous and worrying reluctance to officially admit its presence.

Until Koch's announcement in 1882, the diagnosis of TB (whether called tuberculosis, *phthisis* or consumption) was based entirely on symptoms. The symptoms of pulmonary TB were fairly clear cut, but the symptoms of extra-pulmonary TB were far from being as easy to spot. After 1882, however, the sputum test became the most widely used confirmer of disease, although it still only offered diagnosis of pulmonary disease and would miss it completely in less infectious cases. In 1912 Dr Hyslop Thomson, the Medical Superintendent at Liverpool Sanatorium, described what was needed:

> "A good microscope fitted with a sub-stage condenser and a 1/12 inch coil immersion lens, a pair of Cornet's spring forceps, a pair of needles in wooden holders, two or three long glass pipettes, a spirit lamp and some slides which should be kept free from dust and the various solutions for staining."[57]

Then, in 1931, a German physician, Dr E.Stolkind, identified something else – a striking anomaly in the figures. He noticed that exceptionally high rates of bronchitis were being identified as the prime cause of death in Britain – as much as ten times what was occurring in other European countries – and he attributed it to simple under-diagnosis of TB. This should have been no real surprise. In 1927 Sir John Robertson, Professor of Public Health at Birmingham University, had already suggested that:

> "Long ago it was said that we doctors and statisticians juggled with the figures relating to tuberculosis by attributing deaths to bronchitis and pneumonia which ought to have been attributed to tuberculosis in order to spare the feelings of the relatives of the patient."

There were several reasons for this. One was that people known to have contracted the disease or who were known to have been in contact with it were often ostracised – as were their families. Victims could also lose both jobs and friendships. A patient's home would more often than not be officially investigated by officials as well. The consequence was predictable. Patients avoided doctors who were known to be keen notifiers, and favoured going to those who weren't.

---

[57] H Hyslop Thomson – "Consumption in General Practice", Oxford (1912) page 62.

The development of radiography provided the next important further improvement in diagnosis as well as an impetus for more proactive disease control, and this developed in the 1940s. But even X-rays were subject to variation in diagnosis and neither X-rays nor sputum tests could reliably identify extra-pulmonary disease.

Official 'notification' of TB had been established in England and Wales in 1912 but on account of all of this as late as 1929 there were still far too many uncertainties in diagnosis for the system to be seen to be reliable. To try to address this, two different degrees of diagnosis were now suggested by the Joint Tuberculosis Council – the disease could be notified either as being "beyond all doubt" or as "probably tuberculous". This could have been a useful approach, and is one which could still be usefully applied today, but the suggestion was very tellingly not adopted. The decision was made for possibly the worst of reasons – it may have been as much to protect the individual reputations of the members of the profession who were constantly being faced with such uncertainty as it was to protect the public profile of the profession itself. So this challenging dilemma perpetuated and, as a result, all of the reported figures remained uncertain across much of the world – and, as we will see, they remain so right up until today.

There was also a consensus that TB was being under-reported in the elderly with the only possible diagnostic decider being by post-mortem examination. Since TB was still so common and was also a chronic disease, whenever multiple causes of death were being considered it should have been being recorded as a possible contributor to death if there was the faintest reason to do so. A multiple cause of death, with TB (if it was at all suspected) at the very least being entered on the death certificate somewhere, should really never have posed any problem at all for the certifying doctor. But even this was not happening. A random sampling in 1949 of 1,332 sudden or unexpected deaths in Kent had post mortems performed which revealed that TB was evident in 61 of them, but only 13 had any mention at all of TB on their death certificates. It was becoming clearer and clearer that the surviving prevalence of TB was much higher than officially estimated.

Those persistent implicit pressures on a doctor not to identify TB on a death certificate still lingered as well - particularly if he or she was in any doubt about it. There were good reasons for doctors being reluctant to diagnose TB generally. As late as 1960 problems existed for obtaining life assurance in the UK if there was any evidence at all of a history of tuberculosis. Add to this the general accompanying stigma, ones which even included associations with mental illness, and many doctors were reluctant to write those telling two letters "TB" on any official pieces of paper unless there were the clearest of reasons to do so.

The enduring association of TB with poverty was also a major factor. This negative link (in terms of increasing stigmatisation) was even ironically being stoked by the authorities' intentions to finally stamp out that poetic glamour that was still associated with the disease from the century before. In a summary which was deliberate in its intent but which would shock if used in a public health awareness campaign today, one doctor stated that:

> "Tubercle is in truth a coarse common disease, bred in foul breath, in dirt, in squalor."

What followed, however, must have beent less helpful than intended in that it ultimately only served to strengthen the stigma of the disease.

> "The beautiful and rich receive it from the unbeautiful poor... Tubercle attacks failures."[58]

Before concluding this section, this perverse association of the disease with poetic and/or artistic glamour deserves final illumination. A cursory and far from exhaustive list of individuals from the artistic worlds offers an idea of how such beliefs must have developed. The following creative luminaries either died or suffered badly from TB (in alphabetical order):

> Honoré de Balzac, Manuel Bandeira, Aubrey Beardsley, the Brontë family, Charles Farrar Browne, Elizabeth Barrett Browning, Robert Burns, Albert Camus, Anton Chekhov, Frédéric Chopin, Stephen Crane, Eugène Delacroix, Fyodor Dostoyevsky, Ralph Waldo Emerson, Stephen Foster, Paul Gauguin, Maxim Gorky, Dashiell Hammett, Robert A. Heinlein, Washington Irving, Samuel Johnson, Franz Kafka, John Keats, Charles Kingsley, D. H. Lawrence, Katherine Mansfield, William Somerset Maugham, Guy de Maupassant, Amedeo Modigliani, Molière, Novalis, Eugene O'Neill, George Orwell, Niccolò Paganini, Alexander Pope, Henry Purcell, Jean-Jacques Rousseau, John Ruskin, Friedrich Schiller, Sir Walter Scott, Elizabeth Siddal, Alan Sillitoe, Tobias Smollett, Spinoza, Laurence Sterne, Robert Louis Stevenson, Dylan Thomas, Henry David Thoreau, Voltaire, Chick Webb, and Thomas Wolfe.

---

[58] H De Carle Woodcock - "The Doctor and the People", London (1912), page 184.

So despite TB being identified as an infectious disease back in 1882, it was still being regarded as hereditary by many in Europe as late as in 1950 (55% then surveyed still believed that it ran in families). Meanwhile there was still no treatment available beyond bed rest, clean air and good food.

Nevertheless, enforced isolation, patient rest, improved living conditions, surgical operations, better nutrition and a reduction in milk-borne disease all saw a remarkable lowering of incidence of TB in Britain. One other factor also played a part – the global influenza pandemic of 1918. Effectively, this strain of 'flu picked off many of those who were either already in the process of succumbing to tuberculosis or were destined to do so with their pulmonary health already compromised.

Neither should it be forgotten that while the prevalence of the disease was reducing, it was definitely not doing so consistently across all social classes – the poor were suffering and dying from TB far more than the wealthy, and this was happening more so now than ever. In 1936 a further visionary Act of Parliament attempted to address even this – dictating that any TB sufferer living in what was judged to be an 'unsanitary house' could obtain help either for renovation or for re-housing.

Despite all of this, however, in the 1930s TB was still accounting for nearly half of all deaths of 25-35 year olds in Britain, of both men and women in their productive and reproductive prime. The reductions that had been achieved, however, had not just been substantial, they were to prove critical to the success of the next phase of the fight against the bacteria – in the quest for effective drugs and their ultimate application.

In 1941 "Sick Heart River", a novel by John Buchan, was published posthumously. A passage within it stands as testimony to the terrible suffering that tuberculosis was still causing at that time. The book's protagonist, Sir Edward Leithen, ends up dying from re-activated tuberculosis triggered by the effects of a gas attack suffered in the First World War. Buchan's description of the dying aristocrat stands as one of the most terrifying literary depictions of the last throes of this disease:

> "His difficult breathing became almost suffocation. The business of filling the lungs with air, to a healthy man an unconscious function, had become for him a desperate enterprise where every moment brought the terror of failure. He felt every part of his decrepit frame involved, not lungs and larynx only, but every muscle from his feet to his brain."

The First Drugs are discovered

"WE CANNOT STEP ASIDE AND SAY THAT WE HAVE ACHIEVED OUR GOAL BY INVENTING A NEW DRUG ... TILL THE WAY HAS BEEN FOUND, WITH OUR HELP, TO BRING OUR FINEST ACHIEVEMENT TO EVERYONE."

George Wilhelm Merck (1950)[59]

In the 1930s and 40s a desperate search was being conducted across the world to see whether any natural or synthetic antibiotic could be safely used on humans infected with TB. One by one new candidates emerged, each heralded by a fanfare of hope, each one followed by disappointment.

The basic pattern of research was the same each time. First, identify a likely candidate as a possible drug. Next, apply it to the bacillus *in vitro* (literally in a test tube or on a petri dish). Then, if things looked promising, apply it to an animal which had been infected with TB *in vivo.* Finally, apply it to a human, and then another, and then another in some form of controlled trial.

Progress was pock-marked with failure and frustration – with several early candidates looking promising enough to be taken through to human testing, but then either failing to provide the same results as with animals or else producing terrible side effects. The research was also highly dangerous for those conducting it. Constant care had to be taken to avoid infection.

The first convincing reports of positive effects using drugs on guinea pigs infected with tuberculosis were published in the 1930s – first with sulfonimide and then with diamino-diphenyl-sulfone. Unfortunately both drugs subsequently proved useless in the treatment of human tuberculosis, but the demonstration of their effectiveness in animals kept the torch alight for further research.

It was turning out to be far as easy as hoped. Some years later, the Swede Jorgen Lehmann recalled that by 1940 the outlook for finding a drug to treat TB was one of "complete defeatism. People had given up on a cure". Lehmann himself was not much later one of the key players in the development of PAS, one of the first TB drug which is still used as a second line drug for resistant disease today.

---

[59] In an address to the Medical College of Virginia.

The wind finally changed, courtesy of a Russian born scientist called Selman Waksman while working in the USA. Waksman (1888-1973) was first and foremost a soil biologist, and he was convinced that it was in the soil that there were the best candidate bacteria to play around with. Louis Pasteur had realised that there had to be substances in soil which could control or destroy other bacteria, because without them the soil would have become a mass of teaming bacteria millions of years ago with one bacteria becoming totally dominant. It was dawning on soil biologists that it was most probably other different types of soil bacteria that were synergistically managing this ecological balancing trick, with each one having unique properties which would have necessarily evolved over millions of years enabling them to destroy or constrain other competitive types of bacteria. The fundamental question now became whether one could be found or adapted that could not only control *M. tuberculosis* (the easier bit) but not damage any part of a normal healthy human being in the process.

Waksman had all the right skills for the search, having begun to systematically screen soil bacteria and fungi from as early as 1914. By 1935, Waksman knew that tuberculous germs could happily survive in sterile soil, but he also had observed that they slowly died out in soil that was contaminated by other organisms. By 1939 he was discovering fungi that had inhibitory effects on the bacterium's growth. The following year he and his team at Rutgers University in New Jersey isolated the first effective anti-TB antibiotic, actinomycin. Unfortunately it proved to be far too toxic for use in either animals or humans.

Then in 1944 he announced the discovery of a second new drug which he called Streptomycin. It was another chemical that had been derived from one of the bacteria-controlling soil microbes – this one originally purified from *Streptomyces griseus*,. After testing it on animals his team had found that the drug combined maximal inhibition of *M. tuberculosis* with relatively low toxicity in the animals themselves.

On November 20, 1944, the antibiotic was administered for the very first time to a human – to a critically ill TB patient – and the effect was observed to be almost immediate. His advanced disease was arrested, the bacteria disappeared from his sputum, and a rapid recovery followed. The new drug still had sid-effects, particularly to the inner ear, but *M. tuberculosis* was now no longer the bacteriological exception for which no drug could be found. It began to look like there really might be a pharmaceutical answer to the disease. In every sense this constituted an immense moment for medicine, and its discovery led to Waksman being awarded a Nobel prize in 1952. By 1952 as well, over 10,000 studies had been published on the drug.

Streptomycin is still regarded as being 'essential' in the current armoury of drugs being used to treat the disease, although, because it is not easy to tolerate and is also difficult to administer (needing to be done by daily injection in the buttocks), it is not used as one of the standard first line drugs.

There was also a bitter twist to the triumphal story of its discovery. Waksman's award was subsequently publicly challenged by Albert Schatz, a member of his team. Schatz (1922-2005) had been working under the direction of Waksman at Rutgers, and he was convinced that it had been his own painstaking work that had been crucial to the drug's discovery. He cuts us an interesting figure, one that must have made his claim a more believable one, both working and sleeping in his basement laboratory. After marrying, he even moved his wife into his tiny working space. And it had indeed been Schatz himself who had first isolated Streptomycin back in 1943. Because of this he sued Waksman for a share of the royalties and won an out-of-court settlement whereby the royalties were henceforward split – 3% to Schatz and 10% to Waksman.

The story of Streptomycin was far from being all about professional disagreement or dishonour, however. By 1945 George Merck and Co were manufacturing Streptomycin under Waksman's direction and with his support. The company was being overwhelmed by the demand for the drug, however, and consequently decided to cancel all prior claims to it in a historic gesture of public benevolence over and above commercial self-interest. In an action which was rare even then in the pharmaceutical industry the company gave its exclusive patent rights for the drug to the Rutgers Foundation freeing up its license to any other interested pharmaceutical companies in order to maximise global manufacturing capacity.[60] Not only did this mean that much more of the new drug became

---

[60] In fact, this is not the only instance of Merck showing a striking streak of benevolence, having more recently developed a drug, Invermectin, for treating River Blindness (onchocerciasis), the most common cause of blindness in the developing world. An anti-parasitic chemical found in the *Streptomyces avermitilis* fungus, had been first found on a golf course in Japan. It was then passed by the Japanese Ktasato Corporation to Merck who added simple modifications to its molecular structure and patented it as a drug. Merck could recognise that the drug would not be affordable, however, and the company then approached the WHO, USAID and the US Department of State to find a solution, all to no avail. Finally, in 1987, Merck's then Chairman Dr Roy Vagelos decided that Merck would donate Ivermectin to the world free of charge for perpetuity. This act stands in stark contrast to the more recent

available but it also allowed for fully competitive manufacture of the drug which forced its cost down.

In 1950 George Merck himself offered a postscript to this decision in an address which he made to the Medical College of Virginia:

> "We try never to forget that medicine is for the people. It is not for the profits. The profits follow, and if we have remembered that, they have never failed to appear. The better we have remembered it, the larger they have been."

This company's decision along with the content Merck's personal address offers us an idea of how the pharmaceutical industry viewed itself half a century ago in comparison to how it does so today. It is difficult to believe that something similar could possibly be voluntarily done on such a scale today with any new blockbuster drug. Companies now see themselves as being primarily answerable to their shareholders. The shareholders are themselves perceived by the companies' CEOs as being more interested in absolute profitable dividend return to their investments than in the defeat of any pervasive pathogen. Drugs today amount to nothing more than a profitable commodity. And meanwhile both politicians and those entrusted with the management of global health have become sensitised to these same supposed shareholder pressures as well.

As a result of Merck's decision six American companies were manufacturing the new drug within a year and it was being widely marketed throughout the US. Post-war Britain, however, was still too poor to buy sufficient supplies, and out of necessity the British authorities were urging caution on the public's anticipation of the drug.

George Orwell, one of the most famous British victims of the disease of this time, managed to secure a personal supply of his own through his connection with David Astor, the editor and owner of the Observer newspaper. He bought it with the proceeds of his new novel "Animal Farm". In so doing he also ironically proved the point that, when it comes to accessing medication, some are most definitely more equal than others, not just in terms of wealth and purchasing power but also in terms of

---

shameful record of the company with its Vioxx drug which, until its recall in 2004, may have contributed to as many as 500,000 premature deaths, with Merck already knowing of some potentially lethal side-effects of the drug before its launch of the drug five years earlier.

connections. His own story unfortunately shortly afterwards ended as unhappily as those of some of the animal characters in the book – in 1949 he wrote a sorry letter from the sanatorium at Cranham in Gloucestershire, UK:

> "I have been horribly ill the last few weeks. I had a bit of a relapse, then they had another go with the Streptomycin, which previously did me a lot of good, at least temporarily. This time only one dose of it had ghastly results."

He had suffered a severe reaction to the re-administration of the drug. Streptomycin, it was turning out, was proving just too difficult to tolerate, not just for Orwell, but for many others too.

A second drug followed close on the heels of the first. PAS (or para-aminosalycic acid) was developed in Sweden by Jörgen Lehmann and Karl Rosdahl, with its discovery announced in the Lancet in 1946. Lehmann, however, is recognised as the leading discoverer of the drug, deservedly so because he tried it first on himself as a human guinea pig in order to prove its safety.

Orwell's doctors tried this new drug too but it proved unsuccessful in containing his disease. On 21st January 1950, at the age of 46, Orwell died by drowning in his own blood, blood that had haemorrhaged from his lungs as had happened to so many before him.

The first sign of drug-resistance

"THE EQUILIBRIUM BETWEEN MAN AND THE TUBERCLE BACILLUS IS VERY PRECARIOUS."

René Dubos (1952)

Both of these newly developed drugs were proved to be effective, but unfortunately they were not found to be as effective for many as first hoped, particularly with more advanced cases. They were also drugs which were difficult to tolerate and which needed to be taken for a long time.

But then, in 1948, the first signs of something far more worrying began to emerge. That year Waksman received a letter saying that one of two children who had made a complete recovery from TB with Streptomycin had subsequently relapsed and died despite further treatment – and it looked probable that the child's germs had become resistant to his drug.

This should not have been an unexpected event. Alexander Fleming, in his Nobel acceptance speech in December 1945, had already rung the bell loud and clear concerning what could easily happen with the new antibiotic wonder drug which he himself had developed:

> "I would like to sound one note of warning. It is not difficult to make microbes resistant to penicillin in the laboratory by exposing them to concentrations not sufficient to kill them, and the same thing has occasionally happened in the body."

His message was clear: fail to properly kill the bacteria and the disease inevitably strikes back as strongly as ever.

Fleming's reasons for offering his warning deserve developing a little further at this point because they suggest how readily bacteria can develop resistance by developing strategies to combat any new threat to them. Penicillin itself is produced from a naturally occurring substance which in turn is produced by a naturally occurring fungus – so it was reasonable to suspect that a resistant pressure to the new antibiotic agent would also be a naturally occurring phenomenon within the microscopic world of bacteria once the bug was regularly exposed to it. In fact this amounted to an inevitability which was proportionately predicated by nothing more than the size of the windows of opportunity that were opened for it. So with Streptomycin, and with any of the other new antibiotics, it was really only a matter of how long this might take to happen.

By 1948 there was rapidly emerging evidence of this inevitability already occurring with the new TB drugs. That same year, the British Medical Research Council (BMRC) conducted the first large-scale clinical trial of Streptomycin. This study is said to be the world's first published drug trial that involved the randomization of participants, something which has since become the basic methodological standard for all modern controlled trials of new drugs and medical procedures. Although many patients enrolled in this trial were shown to be cured as expected, a substantial proportion of the cohort were shown to relapse, something which strongly suggested a resistance.

In response this threat, the idea was promoted of combining both of the two new drugs. It was thought that this might be enough to combat the tendency of the bacillus to mutate and so resist the effects of any drug when prescribed on its own. The first ever attempt at a TB drug combination therefore used these first two drugs together – PAS and Streptomycin.

The BMRC immediately developed a three-pronged trial to test this theory. It involved two arms each testing either Streptomycin or PAS on its own, with a third one testing the two drugs in combination. It became clear from the trial's results that the risk of the development of resistance to one of the drugs was significantly reduced if they were prescribed in combination with each other.

Random mutations in TB bacilli leading to resistance to a single drug are estimated to occur around once in every million to ten million replications. The chance of such resistance to two drugs happening when they were being prescribed together was therefore estimated to be around a further ten million times less likely. This seemed to make it an extremely unlikely event. Unfortunately things didn't pan out quite the way that they were being predicted. First of all the side effects from the new combination therapy proved to be severe, but also, even with such seemingly unlikely odds, it turned out that further strains of combined drug-resistance were not that far away either.

Meanwhile, the research on other new drugs that might be better tolerated continued. The same story, however, was repeated again and again. Even the safest and strongest of candidates showed the same consistently worrying weakness: given the smallest of opportunities, the TB bacilli would develop resistance to the new agent rendering it useless if it was administered on its own.

Isoniazid (isonicotinic acid hydrazide) was the next major drug to be announced. It was revealed as an effective new TB drug in New York in 1951 – and was also demonstrated to be more effective than any drug so far discovered. Quite astonishingly, it then became evident that this 'new' compound had been originally synthesised by two Czech scientists nearly 50 years earlier, though its effect on tuberculosis had never been tested. The good news was that this rendered it technically unpatentable from its very outset, although three companies simultaneously made attempts to do so.[61]

---

[61] There is a fascinating possibility to consider here. If Isoniazid had, in fact, been identified as an agent against TB so many years earlier, it would have possibly remained the sole active pharmaceutical anti-TB drug until 1946. Given the mechanisms of drug resistance, it would then have been a certainty

The drug was first tested in a Navajo community in the USA, one which had a severe TB problem but whose members who suffered from TB had never been exposed to Streptomycin.

Pyrazinamide followed in 1952, then cycloserine also in 1952, and ethionamide in 1956.

There were always two simultaneous aims to any drug programme: the first was to get patients bacteria-free and therefore non-infectious as fast as possible; the second was to fully cure patients by eradicating the bacteria completely from their systems. In 1957 a new and far more effective combination therapy was developed by a group of doctors in Edinburgh, this time consisting of, not two, but three drugs – Streptomycin, PAS and Isoniazid. Once again, things were looking positive: the Scottish team claimed that they were able to cure every patient they treated with the combination as long as he or she was infected for the first time. Developing such a combination was never as easy as it might forst sound, however – a careful balance having to be found between the relative effective dosages of each drug used and their side effects.

The final 'team' of first line drugs is formed.

Despite global death rates from TB being estimated to have reduced by around 30% from the highs of the previous century, as late as 1954, the global death rate from the disease was still running at five million each year. There was still a mountain to climb to bring this death rate down much further. TB, in fact, was one of the three global disease priorities on which the WHO was originally founded in 1948, the other two being malaria and venereal disease. As such an effective campaign was now being launched to defeat the disease with an international body created in order to manage it.

Treatment was still generally being seen at this time to be best carried out within the isolation of the sanatoria, but even this had changed a decade before the discovery of Rifampicin. The British Medical Research Council

---

that the bacillus would have developed resistance to this drug within a decade which might have become almost comprehensive by the 1940s. If this were the case, the Isoniazid would almost certainly not be a first line drug today, nor would it be the drug of choice for treating latent infection. Fate, in this instance, may just have been kind to humanity.

had teamed up with the Indian Council for Medical Research to see how community treatment might be best developed in a society with a self-evident deficiency of in-patient health facilities. Something else other than sanatoria had to be considered as a practical alternative for the country.

This collaborative research, known as "the Madras Study", was published in the Bulletin of the WHO in 1956. It compared two distinct treatment regimens – one performed within the sanatoria and the other carried out by ambulatory community care. Both used the same drug combinations in order that the results of the two approaches could be properly compared. What was also particularly appealing was the fact that, being as it was being conducted out in India, almost all of the patients enrolled would be 'TB drug-naïve' – not having had any prior exposure to any of them. The results therefore could not be affected by any pre-acquired resistances.

There were unexpected and interesting surprises in store for the researchers. The first was that the patients whose treatment was being administered at home were seen to be sticking to their treatment regimens better than those in sanatoria. This was not at all what had been expected. Also, in spite of efforts at randomisation it was evident that more of those with severe disease had ended up in the home treatment group – and yet, despite this, there were no corresponding difference in cure rates as would have been logically expected. Furthermore, it was found that those enrolled on the self-administering home treatment proved to be no more liable to relapse in the follow up period of two years than those treated in the sanatoria.

For the majority of cases, therefore, there was now seen to be no need for the sanatoria at all. What was also being identified, however, was an absolute need to replace the sanatorium with a fully equipped and well-run supportive service, one with good case finding, with a reliable drug supply and with good facilities both for examining sputum and for culturing bacilli. There was also an identified prerequisite for a well-trained and supportive staff of sufficient strength to manage such programmes.

This was back in 1956. Nearly 60 years later, with these same drugs still in use, these self-same prerequisites exist.

Much that is still of immense importance for successful treatment of TB in the wider world today is there in this study for us to reflect upon. In fact what got left behind from this first trial has not just proved fundamental to the disease's survival in South Asia, but it also informs us of both best and worst practices for containing TB today. It even shows us embarrassingly clearly the best way to sow the seeds for a drug-resistant pandemic. The highly motivated specialist staff that had been initially used so successfully in the trial moved on with local staff with less training and lower morale replacing them. Patient monitoring swiftly suffered. A secondary sociological study was carried out in Bangalore and it described this phenomenon of subsequent loss of morale as being "the slippery slope of sloppy treatment organisation". It can be argued that inadequate treatment programme management is the single most significant boon for the bacillus. It creates the perfect breeding ground for drug-resistant disease, a development which, since 1956, can thus be defined as having been inexcusably generated from inadequately managed and resourced treatment programmes.

This study also highlighted another significant risk factor for new programmes as they were being further rolled out. It stated that the rate of case-finding should never exceed any country's capacity to treat the disease. If it did so it would inevitably lead to disillusionment in the treatment by both patients and health workers. This is yet another factor which deserves consideration today as new diagnostics finally come on stream as hoped.

Last of all it taught the lesson that any effective treatment programme absolutely depends upon the maintenance of a reliable supply of effective drugs.

Almost all of these conclusions may seem obvious to us in retrospect but they were merely emerging realities at that time. They all remain of the most acute importance today. Each of them will be further explored in later chapters as the current challenges of containing the disease begin to be systematically further unpacked.

By 1959, and after several years of concerted case detection, the WHO was estimating that "between 0.5 and 1% of the world's population are coughing up tubercle bacilli" (i.e. had active infectious TB). This amounted to 12 to 15 million prevalent cases worldwide, with around 10% in India.[62]

The research for more and better new drugs, meanwhile, was continuing. Ethambutol was the next drug to arrive in 1961, replacing PAS in the early drug combinations. Finally in 1966 the current standard team of four first line drugs was made possible with the discovery of Rifampicin (or Rifampin as it is known in the US), the star striker. Three years earlier the drug company Lepetit had discovered a new drug which it called Rifamycin B.

[62] The prevalence estimate 54 years later is still 12 million.

This drug had in turn been further manipulated by the pharmaceutical company CIBAS to develop Rifampicin. It was far less toxic than Streptomycin (which it replaced in the newer combinations) but was also stronger still than Isoniazid. Like all of these drugs, however, it was still not without side effects, although one of them (turning both urine and tears to orange) turned out to be a rather useful one since it offered a simple way of monitoring treatment compliance.

The discovery of Rifampicin is still considered to be one of the greatest achievements in the story of the development of anti-TB drugs since no drug has yet been discovered that is more efficiently effective. One further advantage was that it replaced those painful intra-muscular injections of Streptomycin which posed such problems for patient and physician. It also was strong enough in effect to bring down the treatment time from two years to just six months. As such, it was (and still is) the star of the team. This wonder drug, incidentally, was named after "Rififi", the title of a French gangster novel and subsequent 1955 acclaimed film adaptation – clearly seen by its discoverers to be a little different to the drugs that preceded it.[63]

A new series of multi-country clinical trials led by the BMRC finally confirmed the four-drug regimen that is still recommended for use in patients with newly diagnosed tuberculosis today. Whilst at first two drugs had been used together, and then three, now four were being used in a combination. This was found to be effective in almost all cases and simultaneously minimised the risks of drug-resistance if the treatment was properly completed. Together these were now called the 'First Line Drugs' (Isoniazid, Rifampicin, Ethambutol and Pyrazinamide), often referred to simply as the 'FLDs'.

The backbone of this empirical regimen, however, was the combination of Isoniazid and Rifampicin, the two most effective and reasonably well-tolerated oral agents yet found. Because the total treatment was now only six to eight months instead of the previous two years, the relative term 'short-course chemotherapy' (SCC) was also born.

It was also now being recognised that TB was much easier to treat the earlier it was picked up. Alongside the wider implementation of these new

---

[63] The film, made in France and directed by Jules Dessin (an ameican who had been blacklisted in his country for his political opnions) contained a classic *heist* scene which was described by the Los Angeles Times as "a master class in breaking and entering".

drugs public health programmes were being developed in many countries looking to pick up earlier infections by using mass X-ray programmes. With radiography the tiniest of signs of re-activated disease could be spotted in otherwise asymptomatic patients. Such programmes, when administered in concert with treatment with the new drugs, looked to augur the final decline in rates of TB in many countries, particularly those where a significant decline had already occurred. By focusing intensely on locally defined black spot areas the incidence of infectious disease was being driven downwards even further.

In Britain, X-ray machines were being installed in converted furniture removal lorries with generators towed along behind them. They were then driven into the heart of some of the hotspots of disease in the bigger cities. Massive efforts were made to encourage local populations to engage with these campaigns, with focused publicity campaigns used to support them. Localities were systematically leafleted, incentives were offered and the recalcitrant were identified and then followed up.

At a certain tipping point, with the incidence numbers already reducing to more manageable levels, such a method of active case finding of early disease (and co-ordinated treatment following behind) becomes not just possible but also both effective and efficient. The alternative to this is 'passive case finding' (when patients present themselves for treatment only after becoming ill) followed by tracking down all known close contacts of such infectious cases if it is either practical or possible. It is probable that this particular type of active case-finding campaign was as important in some countries as any other part of the concerted efforts that were being made to finally control the disease in the post-war years.

Unfortunately it was far too long before it was realised that the same thing was not being done, and could not possibly be done, in developing counties with less resource and a denser and more widespread epidemic. Nor was it realised that there would be inevitable consequences from this. The epidemics in such countries were continuing pretty much as before, infact largely as they had been doing in the pre-industrialised era in Europe before the implementation of any social welfare legislation or the discoveries of any drugs. The only difference was that some of these new drugs were becoming available in such countries, but often their supply was intermittent and their application was being inadequately managed. Both of these phenomena were destined to have inevitable consequences.

The only pragmatic approach in these environments was, wherever possible, to use the newly developed drugs to try to drive down the incidence of disease as best it could be done, as if this was the only answer to the disease. There were no efforts being made towards improving living and working conditions, towards reducing in concert with the new drugs. All of these together had set the foundations for the final reductions of disease in the industrialised world. Nor, most importantly of all perhaps, was anyone rushing to close the gaps in the general medical infrastructural resources.

In the developed industrialised world, with the new combination therapy, with an increasingly affluent society, with pasteurisation of milk, with aggressive case finding and with a better administration of BCG vaccinations, TB began to be managed far better – to the extent that it began to fade in an almost unnoticed fashion from public consciousness. Incidence rates fell, mortality rates dropped and the last sanatoria closed. By 1960 death rates had fallen in England and Wales to below 10/100,000 – they had been running at around 125/100,000 around 60 years earlier.

One estimate suggests that in more developed countries national rates of infection dropped by around 50% every five to seven years, even in countries which weren't using BCG.

It really looked like it could be the beginning of the end for TB, but the bacillus had other ideas. What was now developing elsewhere were the first faint signs of the new problem.

Multi Drug-Resistance appears for the first time

"THE GREATEST DISASTER THAT CAN HAPPEN TO A PATIENT WITH TUBERCULOSIS IS THAT HIS ORGANISMS BECOME RESISTANT TO TWO OR MORE OF THE STANDARD DRUGS. THE DEVELOPMENT OF DRUG-RESISTANCE MAY BE A TRAGEDY NOT ONLY FOR THE PATIENT HIMSELF BUT ALSO FOR OTHERS, FOR HE CAN INFECT OTHER PEOPLE WITH HIS DRUG-RESISTANT ORGANISMS."

Sir John Crofton (1959)[64]

Signs of single drug-resistance, first seen at least as early as 1948, were soon being supplemented by the first signs of strains of disease that were resistant to two or even more drugs. There had been every reason to

[64] Crofton J – "Chemotherapy of pulmonary tuberculosis", British Medical Journal, 1 (1959) 1610–4. (Crofton was one of the pioneers of combination drug therapy.)

predict this but, as the disease started slipping out of the spotlight in the developed world, too few eyes were remaining focused upon it. As a result, when multi drug-resistance first really arrived, it seemed to appear from nowhere – being seen as being both unprecedented and unanticipated.

In fact the world's first national drug-resistance survey had been conducted between 1955 and 1956 in Britain. It turned up evidence of discrete strains that were separately resistant to one or another of the three early drugs. A total of 974 clinical isolates cultured from newly diagnosed cases showed strains that were resistant to Streptomycin (2.5%), PAS (2.6%), and Isoniazid (1.3%). Similarly, data from the United States showed a pattern of increasing rates of Isoniazid resistance, from 6.3% in 1964 to 9.7% in 1968.

Between 1970 and 1990, a series of individual outbreaks of drug-resistant tuberculosis involving strains which were simultaneously resistant to two or more drugs occurred. One particular an outbreak in 1970 in New York City involved a highly virulent strain which was shown to be resistant to multiple drugs, proving from the outset that resistance did not necessarily reduce the microbe's fitness as had been initially supposed and presumed. A startling 23 of the outbreak's index patient's 28 close contacts showed evidence of newly acquired latent infection and, worse still, active drug-resistant disease was seen to develop quickly in six of these 23 contacts, five of whom were children.

Then, in 1985 a 25 year-old Korean arrived in the USA. She had originally been treated for TB in Korea, but fell ill again soon after her arrival in the US. She was first treated with Isoniazid, Rifampicin and Ethambutol but continued to deteriorate. The Ethambutol was taken out of the combination and a further four drugs added (now making a combination of six drugs). These included ethionamide, cycloserine and streptomyicin, but still she continued to worsen. Culturing of her bacilli showed resistance to seven of the available drugs, leaving only PAS, Ethambutol, capreomycin, kanamycin, and ofloxacin as available options.

Dr Michael Iseman, the physician who treated the patient, was thus the first person to properly identify what he called the "chilling possibility" of a super-TB-bug. It seems, however, that his warning was not nearly well enough heeded at the time.

Russia became the first country to reveal the problem of multi drug-resistance on a grander scale – or, more correctly, it was seen to be emerging, not just in Russia, but in all of what had been the oblasts of the former Soviet Union as it began to politically disintegrate in the 1980s. As the system began to collapse under *glasnost*, a parallel collapse of the former Soviet judicial system began to occur within it. A simultaneous crime wave, largely fuelled by spiralling economic conditions, resulted in widespread overcrowding of prisons right across the former Soviet territories with prisoners being held for long periods while awaiting trial. An accompanying collapse of existing medical infrastructures along with an intermittent supply of TB drugs meant that the drugs' administration became both limited and sporadic. The standard first line drugs were being administered in the prisons in good faith whenever they were available but they were also being administered inadequately and therefore also inappropriately.

Prisons have been providing perfect incubators for *M. tuberculosis* at least since the time of Dostoyevsky. TB expert Dr Paul Farmer, who co-founded Partners in Health, described this particular situation graphically – relating how a young man picked up on suspicion of a petty crime could spend months in an overcrowded cell awaiting his right to a fair trial, and then finally find himself released guiltless and free months later. During his time inside, however, he might have developed an annoyingly consistent cough – and it could well be one which would prove to be a death sentence of untreatable disease if it was reflecting the early signs of drug-resistant TB which was increasing in frequency in Russian prisons.[65] And this might not just be a death sentence for him – it might also be one for members f his family.

Before we take a proper look at drug-resistant TB and some of its implications, however, we need to take another small step back, and develop a better picture as to how the disease in its various states can be identified and properly diagnosed. Not only that, but we need to take a look at the drugs used to treat it, as well as the vaccine, and then take a look at the further complexities of extra-pulmonary disease.

[65] Paul Farmer - "Pathologies of Power, Health, Human Rights, and the New War on the Poor", University of California Press (2005). See Chapter 4 - "A Plague on all your Houses".

Diagnosing Tuberculosis

"WE ARE COMBATING A DISEASE
THAT KILLS SOMEONE EVERY 20 SECONDS,
WITH A 125-YEAR-OLD DIAGNOSTIC TEST THAT FAILS TO DIAGNOSE HALF THE NUMBER OF CASES,
WITH AN 85-YEAR-OLD VACCINE THAT DOES NOT PROTECT ADULTS
AND WITH 40-YEAR-OLD DRUG REGIMENS."

Dr Peter Small[66]

Spotting tuberculosis

Given the different manifestations and stages of the disease, spotting TB is far from simple. Nor, unfortunately, is any reliable method readily available to help the process, even today.

There are several problematic aspects of the disease to be considered in this respect, which include:

- Spotting latent infection
- Spotting pulmonary disease
- Spotting extra-pulmonary disease
- Spotting disease in the presence of HIV/AIDS
- Spotting the disease in children
- Spotting drug-resistance.

Each of these aspects presents its own individual challenge; but when gathered together into a pandemic they present a picture of a disease which, from any angle you care to look from, is extremely difficult to get to grips with.

---

[66] Senior Programme Officer for TB for the Bill and Melinda Gates Foundation.

Spotting latent infection with tuberculin skin testing (TST)

The first level of diagnosis concerns identifying those who may have been exposed to tuberculosis and may therefore be infected by it. Such infections need not imply active or infectious disease – they are much more likely to be indicative of latent infections, but nevertheless the procedure is a vital component in the accumulative process of differential diagnosis.

To diagnose evidence of infection, tuberculin (the chemical which was originally developed by Koch himself as a potential drug to treat the disease) is injected under the skin of the forearm. If a red welt forms around the injection site within 72 hours, it suggests that the person may have been infected with *M. tuberculosis* or *M. bovis*. Unfortunately, however, if the person tested has been previously vaccinated with BCG it doesn't clinch the matter. If the person hasn't been vaccinated a positive skin test does add up to being a very reliable sign. It could, however, also just indicate previous exposure to another less dangerous mycobacterium.

Crudely speaking, tuberculin (which is also called a purified protein derivative or PPD) is a standardised dead extract of cultured TB. When injected into the skin the size of the reaction indicates a measure of the person's acquired immune response to an earlier exposure to the disease, which in turn is interpreted to help decide appropriate treatment.

Historically, there have been three methods for tuberculin testing on the skin: the Mantoux test, the Heaf test, and the Tine test. All have been shown to become positive around six weeks following an infection.

The Heaf test was first developed in 1951. Its particular advantage was that it was a simple test to apply. The test itself comprises a mechanical 'gun' with disposable single-use heads, each head having six needles arranged in a circle. There are standard heads and smaller heads for paediatric use. For the standard head, the needles protrude 2mm when the gun is actuated; for the paediatric heads, the needles protrude 1mm. The skin is first cleaned with alcohol, then some tuberculin (at 100,000 units/ml) is smeared on the skin (about 0.1 ml is used). The gun is then applied to the skin and fired. Any excess solution is wiped off and a mark drawn in waterproof ink around the injection site. The result is then read two to seven days later with the numbers of visible indurations reflecting the level of infection. The likely responses range between no signs at all, a few visible puncture points, some measurable indurations and actual ulceration.

The general UK guidelines formerly diagnosed positive latent TB if the Heaf test was seen to be grade 3 or 4 (with indurations of 5-10mm) and if there were also no signs or symptoms of active TB. In patients who had definitely not had BCG vaccination previously, however, latent TB was diagnosed if the Heaf test resulted in six visible puncture points in a circle (grade 2) with no signs or symptoms of active TB. Repeat testing was never considered worth carrying out on patients who were known to have had BCG, however, because of a recognised phenomenon of 'boosting' which risked creating false positive results.

The Heaf test was unfortunately discontinued in 2005 because the manufacturer deemed its production to be financially unsustainable. This was largely because the frequency of skin testing had reduced in parallel with fewer vaccination programmes in more developed countries. Until its withdrawal, the Heaf test had been preferred in the UK mainly because it required less training to administer but also because there was little variation seen in its interpretation. This cessation in its manufacture may yet be shown to have a negative impact on the disease in the developing world where ease of administration and reliability are such key issues.

The Tine test is a disposable variant of the Heaf test but it is one which is less reliable so has generally been much less used.

The Mantoux test is now the only test that is approved and standardised by the WHO. A dose of 0.1 ml of tuberculin (at 100 units/ml, and therefore at a concentration that is a thousand times weaker than that used in the Heaf test) is given by intradermal injection into the surface of the forearm (i.e. injected between the skin layers). If it is injected any more deeply than this it is known to give false negative results, so the depth of injection is critical to the result. A waterproof ink mark is then drawn around the injection site.

The result of the test is, similarly to the Heaf test, assessed between two and seven days later. The width of any induration is measured across the forearm and is then recorded to the nearest millimetre.

According to the current US guidelines, there are varying thresholds for declaring a positive result of latent tuberculosis from this test: for those from a high risk group, such as those who are also HIV-positive, the threshold cut-off is a 5mm width of induration; for medium risk groups it is 10mm; for low risk groups it is 15mm. The US guidelines also recommend that any history of previous BCG vaccination be ignored.

Previous BCG vaccination is known to give false positive results, however – especially if the Mantoux test is being repeated as this is known to boost an immune response in those who have previously been vaccinated. This can easily lead to unnecessary treatment with possible adverse reactions in store for those who receive it. Since the BCG vaccine (as we will see) is known to be far from 100%, there is also a very clear risk from ***not*** treating such patients. As a result the current US policy errs on the side of safety for the general public rather than for the individual: positive diagnoses tend to get treated regardless.

The US guidelines also allow for tuberculin skin testing in immunosuppressed patients (those who might be living with HIV or who might be on immunosuppressive drugs), whereas the UK Mantoux guidelines recommend that tuberculin skin tests should not be used for such patients because it is believed to be unreliable. Experts are not in complete agreement with each other on the matter, even in low-incidence/high-income countries like the UK and the USA.

The main issue which clouds diagnosis, however, is this fact that the result are deemed to be unreliable if there is any history at all of BCG vaccination. This deficiency is now being addressed, however, by a new alternative method of diagnosing latent infection – the so called IGRA (the 'interference gamma release assay') which is now approved to be used in place of (but not in addition to) TST. Put in the simplest of terms, IGRAs are blood tests which are potentially more useful for diagnosis of LTBI.

Interference Gamma Release Assays (IGRAs)

Importantly, IGRAs detect the immune response to specific *M. tuberculosis* antigens, in other words ones which are not present in BCG or in other non-tuberculous mycobacteria. They are whole-blood tests that aid in diagnosing *M. tuberculosis* infection but unfortunately they still can't differentiate latent tuberculosis infection from active disease – nor can they identify latent infection with *M. bovis* which, in some parts of the world may compose a significant part of a regional epidemic.

Two IGRA tests are currently commercially available; one is British, and the other Australian. Both are based on the principle that the T cells of an individual who has acquired TB infection will respond by secreting the interferon-gamma cytokine (IFN-γ) when re-stimulated with *M. tuberculosis* antigens and, as such, are believed to measure an individual's immune response to *M. tuberculosis*. For anyone who has never been infected with TB no release of IFN-γ should be detectable.

There are specific advantages to this newer test. One is that the results can be available within 24 hours; another is that they do not boost responses carried out in subsequent tests. Most importantly of all is that, unlike TST, prior BCG vaccination cannot cause a false-positive result in these tests.

As with practically everything connected to this disease, however, there are limitations and some of them are unfortunately also more specific to middle and low-income settings. The blood samples must be processed quickly while the white blood cells (WBCs) are still viable; there is also some uncertainty about its applicability for children, for individuals who have been more recently exposed to TB, and also for immune-compromised individuals. For these reasons in 2012 the WHO issued a caution against using IGRAs as a public health intervention for detecting latent TB infection in both low- and middle-income settings (which is unfortunate because these are exactly where most latent infection exists).

The more significant limitation, however, relates to their expense – which dictates that, like so much of the more effective resource for fighting TB, they are not affordable as an option in most high burden situations where they might be most needed and best put to use.

As with the tuberculin skin tests, IGRAs are also considered to be used as no more than an aid in diagnosing infection with *M. tuberculosis* – as a diagnosis, in other words, of variable certainty. A positive test result suggests that *M. tuberculosis* infection is likely; a negative result suggests that infection is unlikely; an indeterminate result indicates an uncertain likelihood of *M. tuberculosis* infection.

Much more important than simply identifying individuals with LTBI, however, is the challenge of identifying which ones are most likely to progress to active disease. Normally this is expected to be around 10% of latently infected individuals in their lifetimes, although this percentage will be higher in populations that are already immune-compromised. Being able to individually identify those who are most at risk of developing re-activated disease would be an important step forwards – it would mean that they could be targeted with Isoniazid preventive therapy (IPT) and this could deplete the potency of the huge pool of LTBI. In turn this would be expected to cumulatively reduce rates of incident cases of infectious disease. Unfortunately so far IGRAs have been shown to have nothing more than a low predictive ability for individual progression from LTBI to active disease. There is, however, a very small statistical indication that those with positive IGRA results do actually appear to have a slightly higher risk in this respect than those with positive TST results.

An intriguing extra layer of epidemiological complexity has been exposed by the IGRA test as well – one which has served to upset the classic dogma that stated that TB exists strictly as either active disease or latent infection without any overlap. There is now growing evidence that, similarly to how TB can manifest on a continuum of severity in its active state, there may also be a range of inactivity in latent infection. A review of IGRA results showed, quite predictably, that the overall mean of IFN-γ production is greater in active disease (i.e. much more than in those with LTBI). But there is also a tremendous degree of variability within both types of disease – something which has uncertain implications. It may even further impair the hoped-for predictive value of the assay itself.[67] With the benefit of further studies it might also shed new and challenging light on the way the disease progresses.

Another challenge relates to the evidence of efficacy of the standard treatment for LTBI. So far the only clinical evidence that Isoniazid preventive therapy (the standard treatment) reduces the risk for progression to active disease has been produced by testing the treatment on subjects diagnosed by the tuberculin skin test, and not on those with LTBI confirmed by IGRA testing. In other words it is possible that the false TST results from prior vaccinations may have skewed these studies' base measurements of latent infection which could in turn have produced invalid positive data from the IPT interventions.

Unfortunately, the final evaluation of the accuracy of any of these types of tests to diagnose LTBI is hamstrung by the fact that there is still no gold standard reliable diagnosis for latency anyway. Evaluation of both old and new techniques rely for comparative measurement on the use of proxies for LTBI such as active TB, on TB exposure gradients, on rates of TB incidence in untreated cohorts and on results of randomized clinical trials comparing the benefit of preventive treatment in patients who test positive

67 Chee CB et al. - "Quantitative T-cell interferon-gamma responses to Mycobacterium tuberculosis-specific antigens in active and latent tuberculosis", European Journal of Clinical and Microbiological Infectious Disease, 28 (2009) 667–70.

or negative. As such it remains a complex field of study. Most of the studies on the assay's sensitivity, in fact, have been performed in patients with active TB, working on the safe assumption that patients with confirmed active TB must necessarily already have been infected with the disease. There is an unfortunate drawback, however, to even this obvious and logical assumption: patients with active TB usually also have immune suppression caused either by the tuberculosis itself or by pre-existing factors which provoked the re-activation. Such immune suppression almost certainly restricts the predicted immune response either to any tuberculin injected into the skin or to the specific *M. tuberculosis* antigens introduced to a sample of the patient's blood in the IGRA tests. As a result it is very reasonably assumed that the sensitivities to both TST and IGRA tests for LTBI may well be underestimated scientifically.

Confirming active disease

Once the disease fully re-activates things unfortunately begin to become a little trickier because, unfortunately, some of the associated issues begin to become more complex as well.

First of all it is a fundamental fact that there is only one gold standard way of definitively confirming a diagnosis of tuberculosis. This is done by 'culturing' the *Mycobacterium tuberculosis* organisms from a specimen taken from the patient, a process which takes several weeks and which requires both expensive laboratory equipment and highly skilled staff. This culture will not only diagnose active disease by revealing the presence of the specific bacilli, but can also be adapted and used to determine the bacilli's sensitivity to specific drugs. Most often the requisite specimen is cultured from sputum, but the culture might also be developed from pus, from cerebro-spinal fluid, or even from biopsied tissue. It is not, however, normally recommended that a specimen should ever be cultured from a sample of blood.

A diagnosis made by any other method than this, however widely used, can only ever technically be classified as being either 'probable' or 'presumed'.

In practice, and in what amounts to global reality, things are somewhat different to this. Until very recently, in literally ***all*** of those environments where TB most thrives, diagnosis has been conducted almost entirely by sputum testing – a process which does not include the vital culturing of the bacilli. In other words, in all of those countries where the disease is most active and lethal, the best diagnosis that can be made in the vast majority of cases is one of either 'probable' or 'presumed' infection, the likelihood of which is confirmed as far as is possible by a combination of signs, symptoms, X-rays (if available) and from what is an intrinsically unreliable diagnostic method.

In such instances the patient's sputum sample will have been spread on to a glass slide, stained, and then examined under a microscope. It is a process which is relatively simple, speedy and cheap. The current preferred method for this is known as 'led microscopy', though it is still not being used at any scale. The best default uses fluorescence microscopy (with auramine-rhodamine staining), which is more sensitive than the older conventional Ziehl-Neelsen staining method, though both are still used.

In a high-income country, however, a positive smear microscopy test is usually subsequently confirmed by culture as part of automatic diagnostic practice for the proper identification of the specific active MTBC strain, and this in turn may be followed by drug-susceptibility testing (DST) if there is any reason at all to do so. These secondary assays require extended incubation times and are also significantly more expensive than the simple smear tests. They also require specialized equipment and a reliable supply of water and electricity – and they are not without risk either. Currently, TB culture laboratories in resource-poor countries too frequently lack the adequate infrastructure to provide all of this, and/or also have inadequate or outdated equipment with poor bio-safety measures in place without appropriate external quality assurance to ensure accuracy and reliability. Even if they exist there is also almost always an accompanying shortage of both human and financial resources to run and maintain them.

The sad and shocking fact of the matter therefore is that almost all of the resource-poor regions of the world which carry the highest burdens of TB still have few (if any) reference laboratories capable of reliably performing the accepted definitive diagnosis of the disease.

Blood tests for TB

Testing blood is not a good way of diagnosing tuberculosis but, for reasons that remaine far from clear, the testing of blood (rather than of sputum) as a way of identifying active TB has been being used extensively. The process is well recognised as being highly inaccurate and has never been approved by the WHO at all – a careful review by the WHO itself confirmed that they may give false results in as many as one out of every two cases. Nevertheless, they have been being used widely, almost entirely in the private sector of the health services of the countries concerned. When used, they have cost individual patients what has been estimated to have been between US$10 and US$30 each time for what amounts to being nothing of any acceptable value with a 50-50 chance of an inaccurate diagnosis.

In 2011 the WHO reported that that over a million of such blood tests were being used annually in India alone.[68] But that was not all - even more worrying was that report stated that they were being used, not just in India, but in 17 of the 22 so-called high burden countries (HBCs).

This list of 22 countries will be reviewed in much more detail in a later section. For now it is enough to identify that they are the countries on a special list because they are estimated to be collectively carrying an estimated 80% of the overall burden of global TB. They are therefore also the countries which are supposed to be being given special attention and support in their struggle to reduce this burden. That such a simple and obvious example of bad practice has been allowed to take place at any significant or visible scale within any of them for a period of nearly 20 years during an official global medical emergency must be a matter of significant concern. That it has apparently happened in over three quarters of them and that there appears to have been so little accountability on the matter is more worrying still because of what it suggests. There are therefore implications for patient welfare in these 22 countries (let alone in other ones where attention to good practice may be less) which are disconcerting given that these countries carry the focus of the world's and the WHO's attention. Many patients will have received treatment (and paid for it) when it was not required, but, worse still, many patients in these countries will not have received treatment when they should have with possible tragic consequences.

In July 2011, the WHO went a step further than simply not approving the technique by taking the decision to officially ban the practice of sero-diagnosis for TB. This ban included an appeal to those companies which make them to stop doing so, but the WHO was disquietingly cautious in

[68] WHO Press Release -"WHO warns against the use of inaccurate blood tests for active tuberculosis" (July 20, 2011), also:
Rebecca Kennedy and Karuna Luthra – "Diagnosing inaccuracy: new WHO policy shift to end ineffective TB practices - an interview with Dr. Mario Raviglione", the National Bureau of Asian Research (2011)
http://www.nbr.org/downloads/pdfs/CHA/NBR_Raviglione_interview.pdf

not inferring any direct criticism of the biological and diagnostics research industry (which irt so relies upon) in making their appeal. This initiative hardly amounted, therefore, to a vigorously implementable ban as the word might be believed to imply. Is this of significance in relation to the complex web of conflicts of interest which are inherent within such a vast organisation, conflicts which at times may be actually putting the most vulnerable at risk? It has to be suggested that it might be. And does it also reflect the amount of power and control (or lack of it) that the WHO can exert on the industries it ultimately depends upon? These give us a tatse of the challenging issues which will be explored in more detail in later sections.

A year later, in June 2012, the Indian government responded to the WHO ban and itself officially "banned the import, manufacture, distribution and sale of commercial serodiagnostic tests for TB",[69] these self-same ones which had been being so profligately misused in the country's private sector to diagnose TB. The 2013 WHO Global Tuberculosis Report hailed this Indian ban as being an "unprecedented" step as if it was some sort of triumph. Certainly both bans were unprecedented in that they hadn't been done before, but they leave an inconvenient question in the air behind them – exactly why ***hadn't*** they happened before and why had it taken everyone so long to realsie that they had to make them?

The secondary issue relates to where these tests have been being manufactured – in Australia, France, Germany, UK and US (as well as in India and China), because they are not approved for use for TB within these countries themselves. Despite this, such companies appear to be free and willing to export them to vulnerable countries in full knowledge of this fact. This anomaly begs some searching questions about the ethics, at least of the sales divisions, of these parts of the medical industry.

The announcement of the Indian ban was also accompanied by a rather sorry postscript. "Unfortunately," the report related, "this ban [has] created a gap in the private market that allowed other suboptimal tests to gain market share, especially since TB diagnostics recommended by the WHO were considered too expensive and well beyond the reach of the typical TB patient." Since the standard sputum test is both used and approved by the WHO and is comparatively cheap, it's hard to fully understand the import of this last statement. It suggests, unfortunately, that parts of the private health sector in India is still happy to exploit its patients at any opportunity. The 'Initiative for Promoting Affordable Quality TB Tests' (IPAQT) was

[69] WHO - "Global Tuberculosis Report 2013".

launched in India in 2013 in order to attempt to address this problem. We must hope that it will have some effect.

X-rays and Radiography

A further indicative confirmation of disease can be obtained from X-rays. Abnormalities on chest radiographs can strongly suggest TB, but they still cannot be definitively diagnostic of it. They can, however, very usefully support other findings. A chest X-ray can also be used (particularly in a case with an absence of signs of disease) to rule out the possibility of active pulmonary TB in a person who has a positive reaction to the tuberculin skin test.

In active pulmonary TB 'consolidations' and/or 'cavities' are most often seen in the upper lungs, although such lesions may actually appear anywhere in the lobes. In disseminated TB it's not uncommon to see a pattern of many tiny nodules appearing throughout the lungs – something which indicates what is known as 'miliary' TB. In HIV and other immune-suppressed persons any X-ray abnormality at all may indicate TB. In some such cases, unfortunately, the chest X-ray may also appear to be entirely normal.

All of this presents no simple task for the radiographer and the diagnostician, and the final result is often subject to professional and debatable interpretation. Overall, therefore, the process is recognised to be less than 100% reliable. What radiographic analysis has achieved many, many times, however, is the identification of early disease, often even before any signs of symptoms have appeared. Early disease is far easier to cure, as was witnessed by the rapid drop on incidence rates as a result of the mobile X-ray campaigns in the industrialised countries in the 1950s and 60s.

The traditional methods – smear microscopy and culture testing

In essence then, up until very recently there has been a set of generally complementary diagnostic methods to work with, all or any of which may help to contribute to a final clinical diagnosis, but only one of which has any actual definitive confirmatory capacity. To recap, these are:

- Presenting symptoms – which indicate possible disease;
- TST – which confirms possible infection which may or may not be active;
- Microscopic sputum analysis – which is not entirely reliable;
- Radiological assessment – which is also not entirely reliable; and
- Culture testing (if it's available) – which is definitive.

It is worth repeating, simply because it is so important, that only the last of these can provide a definitive diagnosis, and only the last as well can provide a clinical differentiation in the case of drug-resistance.[70]

In both high incidence and high burden countries today, TB control relies first and foremost on passive case finding. Such passive case finding consists of patients self-presenting to health care facilities with a set of symptoms who are then diagnosed either on the basis of clinical symptoms or by basic laboratory diagnosis using sputum smear microscopy. Often in these high incidence settings such patients are already in advanced stages of disease at this point, coming to a clinic because of being unable to work with some of them so weakened by disease that they are barely able to walk all.

This is in complete contrast to the way the disease was being successfully finished off in the industrialised developed world in the 1950s and 60s with teams in the community actively identifying early disease in otherwise healthy individuals as well following up all contacts of confirmed infectious cases. The contrast between these two approaches remains one that is stunningly profound.

The key symptoms which indicate pulmonary TB, as we have identified already, include a productive, prolonged cough of three or more weeks, chest pain, and hemoptysis. More systemic symptoms which could indicate either pulmonary or extra-pulmonary disease in the absence of these primary symptoms of lung disease might include low grade remittent fever, chills, night sweats, appetite loss, weight loss, easy fatigability, and production of sputum that might become purulent. Without any definitive bacteriological diagnosis, there are several further factors in a medical history which could significantly add to a probability of active tuberculosis

[70] It should be noted that this final statement should be qualified – the GeneXpert can now provide a confirmation of resistance to a single drug. This new device will be discussed further in later sections.

(and therefore which might weigh a clinician's judgement on the matter). These include prior TB exposure or infection, past TB treatment, a demographic risk factors for TB, and one or more other medical conditions that might increase the risk of re-activated TB developing. Today, of course, this includes HIV/AIDS. Depending on the patient population surveyed, it has been suggested that anywhere between as few as 20% and as many as 75% of pulmonary tuberculosis cases may be without any presenting symptoms at all. This constitutes a massive range of possibilities that would understandably challenge a physician in any age.

Sputum testing properly requires two serial sputum specimens (meaning one taken 'on the spot' and the second brought in the following morning having been expectorated first thing after rising). This means that the patient has to make a repeat visit to the health centre the very next day after his first visit for specimen delivery, and then a further one for the collection of results. It needs to be understood that for a large proportion of TB patients in high incident countries both the costs and the simple physical challenge of these two repeated visits to health care facilities (which may be quite distant) will prove prohibitive. The risk of immediate patient dropout thus becomes an immediate and significant problem in combatting and controlling the disease in these environments.

To make this situation even more challenging, the actual sensitivity of sputum smear microscopy has been reported to vary quite dramatically (it is said to be between 20% and 80% reliable – and having less than 10% reliability with children). Such sensitivity as might exist often depends on the diligence with which the specimens are collected, how the smears are prepared, and how carefully the stained smears are finally examined. The bottom line is that the sputum smear test, unfortunately, is and always has been far from desirably reliable.

To have a 50% chance of finding acid-fast bacilli on a smear it normally requires the presence of approximately 1,000 bacilli per millilitre of sputum. In contrast, a carefully performed culture can detect disease from as few as 10 to 100 cultivable bacilli per millilitre of sputum.[71] The essential part of the problem, therefore, is self-evident: even in developed countries culture testing will only be carried out if there is clear evidence of likelihood of disease; if the first step of the process fails to identify this (because it is unreliable), then the second will only confirm it one way or the other if it is

[71] Hans L Rieder et al. – "Priorities for Tuberculosis Bacteriology Services in Low Income Countries", International Union against Tuberculosis and Lung Disease (2007).

ever actually carried out. If the first part of the process fails to produce evidence of disease, the likelihood exists that the definitive second part won't be conducted even if it an affordable option. This is something which amounts to a devastating diagnostic Catch-22, meaning that as half of the global disease may be being treated on the basis of clinical judgement, and that only a tiny proportion of the pandemic is ever being definitively diagnosed.

Unfortunately the microscopic examination of sputum for acid-fast bacilli is even more unreliable with samples taken from HIV-positive individuals as well, since TB presents differently in such cases. As a result, even if the sputum smear is negative in such a case, tuberculosis still has to be considered a very strong possibility and treatment will often be begun purely on the grounds of such clinical judgement.

Some weakened patients also struggle to expectorate and produce any sputum at all, but options are still available for them. Sometimes a sample can be induced, usually by the nebulized inhalation of a saline. Some more invasive and unpleasant options exist as well, however, ones which include gastric washings, laryngeal swabs, bronchoscopies (with broncho-alveolar lavage, bronchial washings, and/or transbronchial biopsies), and also fine needle aspiration (trans-tracheal or trans-bronchial). In some cases, even more invasive techniques may be necessary, including a tissue biopsy during either a mediastinoscopy or a thoracoscopy.

Other mycobacteria are also acid-fast which means that a positive AFB smear, even if one is successfully carried out, is not necessarily infected with *M. tuberculosis*. A subsequent examination of the culture of these acid-fast bacilli can distinguish between these various forms of mycobacteria, however, although results from this may take too long. (We will be reviewing the possible wider epidemiological significances of this a little later).

The 2013 WHO Global TB Report offers us a very sobering statistical summary of all of this. Among the 5.4 million people who were notified as being diagnosed with TB in 2012 for the very first time (i.e. new cases, not recurrent ones, nor ones whose treatment regimen were changed), 2.5 million had sputum smear-positive pulmonary TB (i.e. 47%), 1.9 million had sputum smear-negative pulmonary TB (35%), 0.2 million did not have a sputum smear done at all (4%) and 0.8 million had extra-pulmonary TB (14%). In other words, nearly 20 years after a global emergency was originally declared, even for those patients who were notified to the WHO as having pulmonary (and not extra-pulmonary) TB, 46% were started on treatment either after not having had a sputum test at all, or after being sputum negative but being judged to have tuberculosis purely on the basis of their symptoms.

The report also estimated that the total of notified cases (a gross 6.1 million in 2012 which included 400,000 who were already notified but who had had their treatment changed) represented 66% of the total global burden, a percentage which suggested in turn a total estimated global burden of 9.2 million incident cases. This missing 3.1 million estimated annual incident cases is well recognised as being a major anomaly and one that needs dealing with urgently if the pandemic is intended to be seriously reduced. The report explains the continued existence of this hidden part of the pandemic as being the result of a mixture of three distinct phenomena:

- "under-reporting of diagnosed TB cases (for instance failure to notify cases diagnosed in the private sector, and
- "underdiagnosis due to poor access to health care and/or
- "failure to ensure that all cases are detected."

Each of these possibilities present their own individual concerns.

The first (especially if it is the largest) suggests that the private sector is still contributing an enormous amount to the epidemic by failing to act in any sort of regulated or co-ordinated way which complies with approved WHO policies. The report, in fact, candidly develops this concern:

> "One of the main reasons for low detection rates in many parts of the world is the existence of a significant private sector, in which care providers frequently diagnose people with TB but fail to notify these cases to national authorities. ***The quality of diagnostic services in the private sector is highly variable.***"

(The last sentence has been deliberately shown in bold type because, as we will be seeing in a later section, it presents particular challenges to parts of the new strategies that are being developed.)

The second and third possibilities listed above suggest that a large proportion of the pandemic remains comprehensively unaddressed and that an enormous number of people with TB are still going untreated. All three factors together, 20 years into an officially announced global emergency, demand that a massive amount more needs to be done to properly get to grips with the pandemic.

We are now racing a little too far ahead, however. We need to turn our attention back to the business of diagnosis by culture.

In co-infected patients more often than not there are fewer organisms present in the lungs than in those with normal disease, even when the disease is pulmonary. Up until recently, the WHO's response to this has included a standard recommendation that culture testing should be performed on samples from any sputum smear-negative HIV-infected patients with any clinical suspicion at all of TB – but it is still impossible for this to be done at any sort of scale in most of the developing world, not just in Africa. In fact it is still impossible anywhere where the disease is rife. The WHO's recommendation that countries with a high burden of TB should rapidly develop such laboratories is entirely logical in that it would certainly improve the diagnosis of TB in HIV-infected patients, but it is generally and practically still an unattainable goal.

The current diagnosis by culture technique involves growing the culture on a broth or on a solid media followed by further microscopy. There are different types of culture material that are approved and available, which include the use of either the Löwenstein-Jensen, Kirchner, or Middlebrook media. This traditional culture method normally takes 2–6 weeks for growth, and any drug-susceptibility testing (DST) can take another 1–2 weeks following on from this, all of which cumulatively creates delays in proper diagnosis as well as similar delays in starting effective treatment if drug-resistant disease is present.

What makes this of most concern is that this WHO recommendation is by far the most critical in any areas where drug-resistant TB is circulating, since culture and drug-susceptibility testing (DST) go hand in hand. The use of these tests' composite results (including DST) allow the avoidance of what is otherwise unavoidable – the indiscriminate misapplication of drugs and a consequential certainty of further spread and amplification of resistant strains. But even if such an impressive development of laboratories were possible in the high burden countries, all of these countries would still have to simultaneously address the shortage of requisite well-trained staff trained in the appropriately extensive technical expertise which accord to the highest international standards required for the quality of such testing to be assured.[72]

The reality is that in resource-poor countries many of the more basic smear microscopy laboratories are already under-staffed. At best they may comprise single-room facilities with poorly maintained microscopes. Furthermore, many of these existing laboratories lack consistent sources of both electricity and clean water. Because of all of this, a desperate need for new, sensitive, easy, and rapid point-of-care diagnostics has for some time been very well-recognised, as has been the need for huge investments in laboratory infrastructure, quality assurance programs, and in those well-trained staff needed to manage it all.

A lot of effort has been expended of late on developing and rolling out a faster and more reliable way of diagnosing both TB and drug-resistance – in fact it's widely accepted that it will be impossible to contain the pandemic of drug-resistant disease without one. New automated faster culture systems have been being developed, though none are yet approved. These include the MB/BacT, BACTEC 9000, VersaTREK, and the Mycobacterial Growth Indicator Tube (MGIT). One other, the Microscopic Observation Drug-Susceptibility assay culture, may also prove to be both faster and more accurate. The method which is now both approved and being rolled out, at least as a preliminary solution to the problem, however, is the LPA GeneXpert device.

Line Probe Assays and the GeneXpert device

Line Probe Assays (LPAs) indirectly detect the presence of *M. tuberculosis* by amplifying the DNA that is present in sputum. This is done by a process known as 'polymerase chain reaction' (PCR). This amplified material is then visualized on to a strip and can then be discriminated as being either positive or negative by the presence or absence of specific bands, very much as is done in a pregnancy test. These bands can then be further differentiated in order to distinguish between the different members of the MTBC (i.e. *M. tuberculosis*, *M. bovis* etc).

---

[72] This entire section is largely sourced from Linda M Parsons et al. – "Laboratory Diagnosis of Tuberculosis in Resource-Poor Countries: Challenges and Opportunities", Clinical Microbioly Reviews, 24, 2 (2011) 314-50.

LPAs can potentially do even more than this, though. They can also potentially simultaneously identify drug-resistance by detecting the most common 'single nucleotide polymorphorism' (SNP) that is most associated with any particular strain of resistance. In other words, these assays look for evidence of mutations at one or more specific places in the DNA.

Such LPA assays have been shown to be highly accurate for the detection of first line drug-resistance, especially so in smear-positive sputum specimens. They are unfortunately demonstrably less sensitive when they are used with smear-negative samples. When it comes to identifying resistant strains of disease, they have also been found to be a little more sensitive in the detection of Rifampicin resistance than with resistance to Isoniazid. With all of this collated knowledge, LPAs were officially first endorsed by the WHO in 2008 for the molecular detection of drug-resistance from samples taken from ***smear-positive*** patients who were also recognised to be at risk of MDR-TB.

Their major advantage is that they can be performed directly on smear-positive sputum samples giving limited results in around five hours without the need for culturing which takes six weeks or more. This is recognised as being something which could make a huge potential difference to treatment outcome – in fact not just to treatment outcome but also to disease prevalence as well. LPAs have two major disadvantages, however: one is that is that they are generally labour intensive and require highly trained personnel and dedicated laboratory space; the other is that they need a continuous electricity supply. Both factors make their widespread implementation in those countries where the disease is rife extremely challenging, at least for the present.

Two commercial LPAs are currently available: the INNO-LiPA Rif.TB test (by Innogenetics of Belgium) and the GenoType MTBDR*plus* test (by Hain Lifescience GmbH of Germany). Both have been officially approved by the WHO.

In 2009 Hain Lifesciences also released a more developed test, the GenoType MTBDR*sl*, intending that it could test for resistance to second line anti-TB drugs as well (i.e. the fluoroquinolones, Ethambutol, and the aminoglycosides and cyclic peptides). It was especially hoped that this test could be used in combination with their MTBDR*plus* test to identify XDR-TB, and so make a huge difference to diagnosis of more extensively resistant strains if rolled out in any quantity where the problems are suspected of being worse. The WHO looked very carefully at this secondary assay but concluded that, with the evidence available, they were unable to suggest this particular line probe assay could be reliably used for detecting resistance to second line anti-TB drugs. In other words, they reported that LPAs cannot and should not be used as a replacement test for conventional phenotypic drug susceptibility testing beyond MDR-TB. The high specificity of the test, however, still allows them to be used as a triage test to guide initial treatment – albeit that they would still be limited to smear-positive sputum specimens and to TB isolates from culture.

In summary then, as far as the WHO is concerned, conventional drug-susceptibility testing remains the only reference standard at least as far as detecting extensively drug-resistant TB (XDR-TB) is concerned until more data becomes available.

The most promising assay of all to have yet been developed and approved, however, is the GeneXpert machine. This device is manufactured by Cepheid, of Sunnyvale, California, USA. The machine is fully automated and runs within a totally enclosed system, performing both sample preparation and real-time PCR together, and produces its results in less than two hours. The Xpert® MTB/RIF test, which is the assay which is designed and manufactured to be used in the machine itself, is capable of determining a specific strain of MTBC while also simultaneously detecting Rifampicin resistance (by targeting the most common location of mutation for this specific resistance – one which is found in the *rpoB* gene).

The assay itself is designed for use with otherwise unprocessed sputum. A sample reagent is simply poured into a tube, incubated for 15 minutes, pipetted into an Xpert cartridge and then inserted into the GeneXpert machine for two-hour processing.

The critical advantage is that highly trained staff aren't needed to run the machine nor to interpret the results meaning that it can be managed in circumstances of much less technical resource than with any method beyond the sputum test. It is also quick and has the potential to be used in only moderately equipped laboratories.

There ***are*** drawbacks, however. The first is that it can only identify resistance to Rifampicin at one particular gene. Rifampicin resistance at any other gene (as is occasionally the case) will be completely missed. It is becoming clearer that the frequency of this occurring may vary dependent upon the strain of disease being examined.

This could be significant. Dr Sarman Singh, professor and head of the clinical microbiology and molecular medicine division at the All India Institute of Medical Sciences (AIIMS) has suggested that, while the GeneXpert may have been initially looking like it might be a revolutionary new diagnostic method, in India it might miss as many as one-third of Rifampicin-resistant cases.

> "The Indian strains have a peculiar gene sequence which is not recognized by the probes GeneXpert has. Hence, if such systems are used routinely, this would give a false impression that India has very low rifampicin resistance thus making the programme managers complacent."[73]

Indian samples were first tested for Rifampicin mono-resistance with a Line Probe Assay and were then cross-checked with the GeneXpert using the newest version of cartridges exactly in accordance with the manufacturer's instruction. Comparative analysis showed that only 64.4% of the LPA determined RR-TB cases were correctly diagnosed by the GeneXpert. The remaining 35.6% were falsely determined to be Rifampicin-susceptible.

The more general drawback – one that applies wherever the device may be used – is that even if Rifampicin resistance is reliably detected, resistance to any other TB drugs will be missed. Nevertheless, given that Rifampicin is the most important TB drug and is also a very reliable marker for possible MDR-TB, this MTB/RIF test has to be recognised as an enormous step forwards.

The assay also cannot be specific beyond diagnosing 'highly probable' TB and only from sputum samples. It is therefore still not accepted as being able to identify extra-pulmonary disease.

Furthermore it cannot identify XDR-TB at all beyond its possibility based on resistance to one single drug (when XDR is confirmed by resistance to at least three others). It also may only be used when a clear likelihood of disease exists because of its cost. Whilst it is relatively cheap, it is simply still not cheap enough. The cost of each test in India has been quoted as being 1,700 rupees (US$28) where it has been suggested that it needs to be as little as 100 rupees (less thanUS$2) for it to be a truly useful tool for getting to grips with the country's epidemic.

---

[73] http://m.timesofindia.com/india/Much-hyped-new-tuberculosis-test-gives-inaccurate-results/articleshow/34217472.cms

Other factors will have undoubted further consequence on its ultimate usefulness – these include the limited shelf-life of the diagnostic cartridges, operational restrictions on its environmental temperatures and humidity levels, requirements for a reliable electricity supply, and the need for annual servicing and calibration of each machine.

But there remains one fundamental disadvantage: it is basically unlikely that it will be able to be used as a point-of-care (POC) diagnostic test in more peripheral settings simply due to poor infrastructures and limited local resources on top of the limited regional or national ones. This, of course, is where much (possibly even most) of the disease occurs and where any form of reliable diagnosis is so desperately needed – in poorly resourced rural health centres.

In 2010, with the WHO's approval the Foundation for Innovative New Diagnostics (FIND) released the Xpert®MTB/RIF TB point-of-care test for a roll-out programme. The FIND-negotiated price for a four testing module GeneXpert machine was then approximately US$17,000 and the costs of the individual Xpert®MTB/RIF tests came in at just under US$17 per cartridge.

By the end of June 2012, Xpert®MTB/RIF had been rolled out in 67 of the 145 countries eligible to purchase instruments and cartridges at concessional prices (so not just in the 22 high burden countries but also in other countries where a need was also being identified). The global average saw 33% of all of these countries having at least one Xpert machines incorporated somewhere in their health service, with 64% of the 22 high burden countries (HBC's) and 50% of the 27 high burden MDR-TB countries having at least one machine respectively. Rather perplexingly, however, only 32% of countries in Africa had yet seen a device at all (in other words, a lower percentage than the global average despite a fairly obvious need).

In August 2012, a public-private partnership was announced between the United States President's Emergency Plan for AIDS Relief (PEPFAR), the United States Agency for International Development (USAID), UNITAID, and the Bill & Melinda Gates Foundation which facilitated a substantial drop in price of the Xpert®MTB/RIF test cartridge from US$16.86 a throw to US$9.98 for use in the public sector of 145 high-burden and developing countries as well as for use by NGOs and other non-profit agencies in these same countries.[74]

By the end of June 2013, 1,402 GeneXpert machines and 3.2 million Xpert®MTB/RIF cartridges had been procured for use in 88 of the 145 countries eligible for this concessional pricing, suggesting that the programme was being developed dynamically. It should be noted how the word "procured" is used in these reports, however. The word falls short of confirming actual delivery and implementation, especially because there has been a backlog in orders because of demand. Nevertheless, 49% of reporting low- and middle-income countries were indicating that WHO guidelines in the GeneXpert test had been incorporated into their respective national guidelines. Most significantly of all, at least at face value, it was reported that South Africa had adopted the machine as its primary diagnostic method for diagnosing TB, with the intention of replacing smear microscopy completely. This country alone now accounts for 43% of all the modules that have been so far procured (amounting to 603 machines) and for 60% of all cartridges. Far behind South Africa in the procurement stakes follow India, Pakistan, Zimbabwe and Nigeria, with the other 83 trailing behind them, with 800 odd machines shared between all of them. This offers more sobering food for thought: apart from South Africa, the global average is still less than ten modules per country that has procured any, three years into a well-publicised roll-out programme.[75]

The GeneXpert machine itself was originally developed as a potential diagnostic for anthrax. It was then approved for rapid molecular diagnosis of TB in Europe and then officially endorsed by the WHO as a potential replacement for sputum smear microscopy for diagnosis of pulmonary TB in both low- and middle-income countries. Widespread excitement has been being expressed concerning this device, particularly because it allows for a diagnosis that can be done in hours, not in days or weeks – all that is needed is the machine itself and individual cartridges for each assay, some sputum and two hours of electricity.

It has to be acknowledged, however, that even a continent-wide distribution of the device may still not be enough to make the difference that is being so desperately hoped for regarding proper identification of

---

[74] WHO - "Tuberculosis Diagnostics – Xpert MTB/RIF Test" (2012).

[75] All data extracted from the WHO's "Global Tuberculosis Report 2013", published 23rd October 2013.

MDR-TB, simply because the GeneXpert only diagnoses resistance to Rifampicin.

Effectively all MDR-TB and XDR-TB strains are resistant to this drug. It is only found to be 'mono-resistant' on its own in around 10% of cases, which makes Rifampicin resistance a very strong indication of poly drug-resistance. Being as this single resistance to Rifampicin is such a reliable proxy for diagnosis of MDR-TB the device is being seen to represent vital diagnostic progress – but it offers no window at all on to the more resistant strains nor, because of this, on to which drugs might be best used in the absence of Rifampicin and Isoniazid in these assumed cases of MDR-TB. So a patient can now almost immediately be recognised as being most probably MDR, but, apart from knowing that Rifampicin will be ineffective if used, that Isoniazid will most probably also not be effective, and that second line drugs will be needed over a much longer treatment period, the diagnosing physician is not, unfortunately, that much wiser.

In one sense, the level of uncertainty of diagnosis has been returned to where it was in the 1990s, when MDR-TB was still in its infancy and XDR-TB was practically unknown. At that time, prescribing first line drugs for patients with limited drug-resistance served to amplify those levels of resistance and helped stoke MDR-TB as a discrete epidemic. Unfortunately, since the GeneXpert cannot identify resistance to any of the other drugs, there are possible similar consequences from its more widespread roll-out which remain of high concern. The diagnosis has in a sense now moved forward, but the disease is outpacing this progress. So similar risks of amplification exist, but now they apply to more extensive and extreme degrees of resistance, though these are still being assumed to be relatively low in incidence. This may not be the case for long, however, and they may even already be being underestimated simply because they are not being looked for. Recent history should be teaching all concerned to be very cautious. Higher levels of drug-resistance than those that are currently estimated within the drug-resistant epidemic almost certainly already exist within the pool of latent disease and this alone is a factor which should not be being trifled with. At least until a better Point-of-Care (POC) device is developed, the necessity for expensive culturing remains sacrosanct as the only proper diagnosis for appropriate treatment of poly drug-resistant TB if it is to be conducted effectively and the growth of more extensively resistant strains is to be contained.

The mobilisation and rolling out of the device has been serially hailed within WHO reports as being "impressive". Given the scale of the challenge, and the average roll-out of 10 modules a country as identified above, it's not certain that such a claim is entirely warranted. South Africa, the leading adopter, will be where the immediate the effects from the device should be being most carefully monitored. Given that South Africa is already recognised as having the highest global rates of XDR-TB should be cause for some concern in itself, the complications of which must be something that the global authorities are already alert to. It might even prove to be the very ***worst*** place on earth for the device to be put it to its first real test.

The WHO's guidelines for using the device have officially been published and:

- **strongly recommend** that the Xpert®MTB/RIF rapid test should be used as the initial diagnostic test in individuals suspected of MDR-TB or HIV/TB, and

- **conditionally recommend** that it may be used as a follow-on test to microscopy in settings where MDR-TB and or HIV is of lesser concern, especially in smear-negative specimens (recognising the major resource implications that may impact upon this recommendation).

Ideally, in a high incidence country this means the following – at least if both extensively drug-resistant and multi drug-resistant strains are to be identified and properly treated rather than dealt with as proxy-polydrug-resistant strains identified only by being resistant to Rifampicin:

> All patients with a positive smear should get a rapid rifampicin test and all smear-negative TB suspects with HIV should have both chest x-rays and culture.
>
> If any such culture proves positive then a rapid Rifampicin test like GeneXpert should also be performed.
>
> All positive Rifampicin tests should also have DST to Isoniazid and Rifampicin, as well as to Kanamycin, Capreomycin and for the fluoroquinolones, the most important second line drugs as well.

Unfortunately the idea that this can be comprehensively conducted at any remotely adequate scale where needed remains a fantasy.

There are other anticipated impacts as a result of this implementation – not all of which, paradoxically, will make the battle any easier although it may at least make the picture clearer.

The first is a probable significant increase in the diagnosis of patients with drug-resistant TB. This expectation has yet to be properly addressed, however, in any published global strategy review.

The second is an expected doubling in the number of TB/HIV cases diagnosed in areas with high rates of TB and HIV (with previous to microscopy diagnosis).

The third is an almost inevitable increase, not only in general incidence rates, but also in estimated rates of confirmed disease prevalence as a result of the extrapolations from the new data that will be being obtained from the device as it is rolled out further, simply because of its increased reliability in comparison to the standard sputum test. In fact if such increases are not revealed, it will certainly vindicate the accuracy of the work of those epidemiologists who have been struggling to develop estimated figures for incidence and prevalence from such a dearth of reliable data.

Results reported by MSF at the 43rd annual Union World Conference on Lung Health in Kuala Lumpur in 2012 generally confirmed these anticipated impacts, and revealed an ever more urgent need to address the growing global crisis of drug-resistant TB. The data presented was collected from 25 MSF projects in 14 countries over almost 18 months. It showed an overall 50% increase in laboratory-based diagnosis of TB using Xpert®MTB/RIF compared to the sputum smear microscopy test. We will look much more deeply at the implications of this report in a later section.

This 50% increase comprised a high variability across their projects (the increases in lab confirmation ranged, in fact, between 10 and 115 percent), something which was not completely explainable. It may have amounted to nothing more than confirmation of the known variability of the AFB sputum testing (dependent as it has been on the care of the technician and the quality of the test) rather than being because of any sensitivity variability of the GeneXpert device itself or of the cohorts that were being tested.

As encouraging as the GeneXpert device is generally being hailed to be, it is definitely still not the whole answer – the ideal TB diagnostic has yet to be developed. Such a device needs to be simple, low-tech, rapid, and able to be used at point-of-care with accurate results that could simultaneously both identify and quantify drug-resistance. In 2009, an expert group led by Médecins Sans Frontières developed a set of minimum technical specifications for such a new POC TB test. The members of the group found that no existing test that met all of its specifications. They could, however, report that the Xpert®MTB/RIF test did meet the majority.

Increased availability of funding and a growing commercial interest in new TB diagnostics have encouraged the development of several other new POC tests for TB, however, so more positive announcements could soon be on the horizon. There are now said to be 50 companies working in this field. This is hardly surprising because there is potentially a lot of money to be made from the right device. Cepheid's (the manufacturer of the GeneXpert) value rose nearly 40% through most of 2013. Such new tests include improved serologic assays, hand-held molecular devices, breath-based assays for the detection of volatile organic compounds, microchip technologies and proteomics-based and metabolomics-based tests. We should certainly hope for more good news soon because it is very desperately needed.

Rats

An unusual test that has been shown in preliminary testing to be more reliable than standard sputum testing is also potentially both economical and appropriate being as it is also extremely low tech. It also comprises an unlikely mechanism – the nose of a species of giant African rat. These rodents, commonly called Gambian pouched rats (*Cricetomys gambianus*) are native to much of Africa and their noses have been put to good use before – being put to the task of sniffing out land mines. They are chunky animals with puffy cheeks, and mature to a disconcertingly large 90 centimetres in length (including their tails).

Since 2008 an apparently crack team of 77 of these giant rats has been being trained to sniff out tuberculosis by the Belgian social enterprise organisation Apopo. In the event they turned out to be much faster and more accurate than the locally trained technicians equipped with their microscopes for standard AFB smear microscopy. Sputum samples from TB patients being treated at 25 nearby clinics were taken weekly to Apopo's lab at Sokoine University of Agriculture in Morogoro, Mozambique. They were then loaded in batches under small holes in the rats' rectangular glass and steel cages. Results were impressive – already accepted to have resulted in greatly improved outcomes for patients whose sputum was tested in this way. The rats were reported to have found more than 3,500 cases missed by the local clinics, improving the detection rates by more than 30%. A subsequent study in 2012 which utilised subsequent culture testing to corroborate the results showed that, when a team of four different rats collaboratively screened in any given batch of samples, the rodents consistently detected the presence of TB in 79.9% of all cases.

It seems therefore that the rats can detect bacteria by smell in significantly lower concentrations than can be visually detected by microscopy, and that their sensitivity and reliability approaches that of the GeneXpert device. The significant advantage associated with this procedure is that it is so low tech.

The rats that are used for this test do have to be captive-bred to be usable. If captured from the wild they remain too feral to be of any use at all, but if they are bred in captivity their development into TB-sleuths appears to be simple and their ongoing practical employment seems to be even more so. They are first taught to recognise the odour of *M. tuberculosis* in sputum samples, and then they learn to seek it out in return for a reward.

Training a TB rat takes around nine months, beginning as soon as the baby rat first opens its eyes at around four weeks. Amanda Mahoney, the head of behavioural research at Apopo has described how:

> "The trainer will put the young rat in a basket in the front of their bicycle, or let them walk around in the dirt and the grass, or take them on a car journey to get them used to different stimuli and experiences."

After this initial socialisation the rodents are trained using a standard technique in animal training to associate a clicking sound with a reward. To start with they are taught to associate the sound with a small reward of banana – ultimately, however, the rat simply associates the sound of the click with the idea of a reward without the use of food at all. In this way, their speed of operation becomes many times more efficient.

They continue to be taught with known samples so that, if they correctly pause for five seconds to smell a TB sample, they are rewarded, whilst lingering over non-TB samples will get them no reward at all. In more advanced training, they learn that they will simply get a click if they stop for an instant over a sample contaminated with the TB bacteria, but get no click if they pause over others. The process of training them has been costed to be around US$7,800 a rat, but they live for up to eight years and are cheap to keep in the meantime.

Once fully qualified, the rats can screen samples devastatingly quickly. Negussie Beyene, Apopo's TB programme manager says that a single technician with a microscope might be expected to complete 25 samples a day; with samples correctly positioned the giant rat can cover 10 samples in just a single minute.

The clear advantage above and beyond the fact that they can effectively diagnose cases which would otherwise be missed is that they can be used to diagnose many times more cases than is currently possible with the existing more technical resource. This is something which could have serious potential value in the fight against this disease where resources are poor. The innovative rat test will need far more rigorous investigation and may well encounter resistance from an organisation as instinctively conservative and wedded to commercial interests as the WHO in the process, but it nevertheless offers a potential and practical opportunity to scale up the necessary response to particular parts of the pandemic.

Drug-susceptibility testing of second line drugs

The importance of being able to accurately diagnose MDR-TB and also the even greater importance of discriminating the level of resistance in XDR-TB cannot be underestimated. Both, unfortunately, are as yet well beyond the abilities of even the most talented rat detective.

TB culture and DST takes six weeks or more due to the slow growth of all of the MTBC organisms. Reliable DST, including second line drug testing, is recognised as being a basic requirement of the Direct Observed Therapy Short Course Plus (DOTS-Plus) second line drug treatment. As we will shortly see, this is the cornerstone of the current strategic response to the MDR-TB epidemic.[76]

It is unfortunately also recognised that the intrinsic accuracy of drug-susceptibility testing (even when performed under the best of circumstances) is not 100%, and varies according to the drug being tested. It is (thankfully) most accurate for Rifampicin and Isoniazid but is proportionately less accurate and inconsistent for Streptomycin and for Ethambutanol, two other 'essential' TB drugs. DST of Pyrazinamide, the

[76] The inclusion of the acronym 'DOTS' in the 'DOTS-plus' title is actually something of a misnomer since it implies that the treatment is still 'short course' which, of course, it is not.

other first line drug, is difficult to perform, as well. Testing for second line drugs can also be difficult.

Any such second line DST is totally unnecessary, of course, if a culture is shown to be susceptible to at least three of the first line drugs. It is furthermore accepted that only laboratories with experience and a well-documented historical competency in performing first line drug testing should perform second line DST at all. This is not just because of its challenges and difficulties, it is also because of the risks from the processes which are known to be high.

As we will shortly see, TB drugs are not only simply classified as being either first or second line; they are also classed into groups based on their similarities. Thankfully, therefore, only one test needs to be performed in any single group of drugs because of almost certain cross-resistance between members of that particular class.

Diagnostics – a summary

The lack of sufficient laboratory facilities in many parts of the world makes the laboratory diagnosis not just of TB but of all infectious diseases in such environments very difficult. In order to address these deficiencies, clinical algorithms have been developed for the syndromic management of some of the more common diseases, and they have been evaluated accordingly. These algorithms amount to being the next best thing to proper laboratory infrastructures. This short-term solution, however, has significant shortcomings for TB, especially because these algorithms have not been properly confirmed with HIV-infected persons nor have they been properly considered in respect of more extensive strains of drug-resistant disease.

The WHO's basic response plan to scale up laboratory capacity to combat XDR-TB can be seen to be ambitious. Whether it is remotely possible, particularly in some of the countries in which it may be most needed, has to remain a matter of conjecture, and there has certainly been little evidence of progress to date. The recommendation has sensibly been for a 'stepwise' approach for middle- and low-income countries, indicating that any decisions at all to develop and implement a liquid culture and DST system should be based on need and should be consistent with other national plans for TB laboratory capacity strengthening and expansion. This makes sense, but the recommendation contains within it something of a chicken and egg dilemma – whether it is possible to identify and then act upon such a need if there is no existing local capacity (and possibly little real inclination) to identify drug-resistance in the first place.

In most circumstances, the first priority is to implement the system inside a national TB reference laboratory. The subsequent expansion of culture and DST capacity would then logically include regional TB culture and DST laboratories, the extent of scale-up being determined by the identified and established need and by the availability of funding and appropriate human resource.

What could be a final stumbling block to such plans is the fact that all of this would be no more than a highly expensive interim solution if a full POC genotypic and/or automated culture and DST is developed as is so desperately hoped for and intended. There may well be a very understandable strategic reluctance to commit any major proportion of funding to these areas as things stand. This could be the case even if funds are available and a need identified, particularly so if such funds are being called upon elsewhere to fight this disease. Conventional culture and DST could turn out to be no more than an expensive and instantaneously out-of-date white elephant if researchers were to suddenly turn up turn up the diagnostic trump card as is hoped will happen.

For now at least, the most recent figures (and for once these are definite figures rather than just estimates) suggest a situation that is vastly out of step with the epidemic. As far as sputum smear microscopy is concerned, the WHO has set a target of at least one centre being available for it to be carried out for every 100,000 population in any country. Globally this target has been met, but it is crazily imbalanced in its regional numbers. Only a dismal 14 of the 22 countries which the WHO itself identifies as having the highest burden of disease met this target in 2012, for instance. In other words, according to the most recent figures, the most basic diagnostic of all is still not yet adequately available in the countries with the most disease.

In 2009 the WHO also recommended the use of the more sensitive fluorescent light-emitting diode (LED) microscopy as a replacement for the traditional Ziehl-Neelsen technique because it's known to give better results. Three years later and only 2% of centres globally have yet made the switch, but what is even more baffling is where this 2% has actually happened. A creditable 97% of microscopy centres in South Africa are now reported to have installed them, and yet, not only is South Africa less than half-way towards matching the global target of one microscopy-centre-per-100,000 population (coming in at just 0.4 per 100,000), but it has also made an official policy decision to replace microscopy with the GeneXpert device. This effectively adds up to an intention to make the LED technology redundant almost as soon as it has been incorporated.

When it comes to provision of DST the WHO is quite candid and we should be equally if not even more worried. The general DST laboratory capacity "continues to be low and is not growing quickly enough".[77] Between 2009 and 2012 the percentage of previously treated TB patients who received DST after their second presentation rose from what was an appallingly low 6% to a slightly better 8.7%. These are the patients who are most at risk of having MDR-TB and are therefore the ones who should be being most targeted. Current estimates suggest that at least 20% of them will be carrying at least an MDR strain. And this doesn't even begin to address the growing number of cases who are recognised to be carrying MDR-TB at first infection. This overall gap between need and provision is still huge and is even probably widening as the provision attempts to catch up with the groing rates of resistant disease. The implications of this are of serious concern. What it suggests is that, even in approved programmes, and even with the notified patients at highest risk of being drug-resistant, far more MDR-TB is being missed than is ever being identified.

The WHO's target for laboratory capacity for culture and DST for at least Rifampicin and Isoniazid is currently one laboratory per five million population. Globally the current global number falls short of this by just 0.1 laboratory per five million (i.e. it runs at 0.9), but in the 27 countries estimated to have the highest burden of MDR-TB it is actually still 0.4 of a laboratory per 100,000 people short. So again this amounts to being less than half the global target where the need is known to be highest.

When it comes to the numbers of DST testing for second line drug-resistance (i.e. spotting XDR-TB or worse) there is no real data available at all despite the epidemic being alive and known to be out there in more than 90 countries. Without such information there can be no proper picture with which we can even begin to judge how the most dangerous part of the epidemic of all is actually being monitored and addressed.

---

[77] WHO – "Global Tuberculosis Report 2013".

Extra-Pulmonary TB

"FROM MY NUMEROUS OBSERVATIONS, I CONCLUDE THAT THESE TUBERCLE BACILLI OCCUR IN ALL TUBERCULOUS DISORDERS, AND THAT THEY ARE DISTINGUISHABLE FROM ALL OTHER MICRO-ORGANISMS."

Robert Koch (1882)[78]

While the majority of TB infections affects the lungs, TB can in fact infect almost anywhere in the body. If the infection is not primarily located in the lungs, it is then most commonly collectively referred to as extra-pulmonary TB – or simply 'EP'.

Extra-pulmonary tuberculosis, apart from laryngeal infection, is generally not communicable, although urine is sometimes infectious in cases of renal tuberculosis. That's pretty much the sum of the good news on the subject, unfortunately.

The bad news is that it's often so difficult to diagnose that treatment starts too late.

EP is estimated to occur in between 10% and 25% of global cases of tuberculosis. This estimate is so varied because certain factors, ones which are often specific to particular regions, make extra-pulmonary infections much more likely in some part of the world.

EP is especially common in people who live with HIV. It is also common in children. As a result, it is more common in countries with a high HIV prevalence (such as in Africa) and also in countries where a lot of children are infected with TB. These are, of course, the countries where the death rates from the disease are also the highest which is almost certainly not coincidental. In a later section we will pay much more detailed attention to the particular phenomenon of TB in children.

It is hypothesised that the reason for the higher rates of extra-pulmonary TB in people living with HIV (PWLH) is because their immune systems are unable to respond sufficiently strongly to a TB infection. As a result they are unable to contain the TB bacilli in the lungs and the bacteria can literally

---

[78] From Robert Koch – "The Etiology of Tuberculosis", Berlin (1882).

leak straight out into the blood stream. The primary location of the TB infection is almost always still in the lungs, but, without containment there, the TB bacilli can spread throughout the body, finding another site or sites where they opportunistically build and multiply. It is widely recognised that those people living with HIV who are also infected with TB are often found to have TB bacilli in their blood, so this hypothesis seems a very reasonable one. TB in the blood is not normal: usually the TB bacilli, unlike the HIV virus, remain contained in the site where they first infect the body and they never gain access to the blood stream at all.

Definitive and rapid diagnosis of all types of such extra-pulmonary tuberculosis is challenging since the conventional techniques that we have already reviewed often have severe limitations in this condition. It is mainly because of this, unfortunately, that extra-pulmonary cases so often remain untreated until it is too late.

People with extra-pulmonary TB initially do, however, commonly have the same systemic symptoms as those with pulmonary TB: fever (90% of the time), night sweats (76%) and weight loss (78%). In addition to these, they may also then develop complaints that are specific to the body site that has been infected with TB, so the diagnosis of disseminated extra-pulmonary TB generally concentrates on those organs most indicated as being likely to be involved. In the presence of HIV, however, these systemic symptoms may not be nearly as evident.

A sputum smear is likely to test positive in around one-third of patients with EP, and even culture testing will only be positive in about 60%. Perhaps even more remarkably still, a Tuberculin Skin Test (TST) is positive in only an average of 45% of patients with disseminated disease. Such percentages offer a clear idea as to just how difficult it is to diagnose these types of TB – and again these percentages are likely to be even lower in cases of co-infection.

It transpires that TB can actually occur just about anywhere in the body, and so EP generally gets differentiated according to the site where the main infection has occurred.

If disseminated TB is suspected, a chest X-ray (or possibly a chest CT scan), a sputum sample for AFB smear and a culture for mycobacteria, as well as first-morning-void urine for AFB should all be obtained; a lumbar puncture and a biopsy of superficial lymph nodes might also done if applicable or if possible. As delays in treatment are so clearly associated with increased risks of mortality, the most rapid diagnostic test possible (i.e. something that is faster than culture results) is always needed.

If sputum smears are negative but the chest X-ray is abnormal, a bronchoscopy with tran-bronchial biopsies is indicated. If these results are non-diagnostic or inconclusive, a bone marrow or liver biopsy could also be done. Both have similar sensitivities, but a bone marrow biopsy may be preferred because of its lower procedural risk.

Because EP is relatively much less common than pulmonary TB, doctors often first think of many other possible causes for the presenting symptoms before first considering TB, particularly in regions where there is generally lower prevalence rates of the disease. This can lose valuable treatment time (for example, a pain in the right ankle will be considered many times more likely to be a sprained ankle than the more remote possibility that it might be TB of the joint itself). Extra-pulmonary TB also often settles in body sites that are difficult to access and which cannot be easily examined or palpated which further adds to the challenges. With extra-pulmonary TB generally only a small amount of TB bacilli can often cause great damage. This is entirely unlike TB in the lungs where the bacilli can multiply for some time before causing any major tissue damage.

Many forms of extra-pulmonary TB are pauci-bacillary which is another reason why the diagnosis of EPTB is so challenging. Acid-fast bacilli (AFB) smears of biological specimens, therefore, often show negative when viewed under a microscope. Tuberculin skin testing (TST) and interferon-gamma release assays (IGRA) are at best adjunctive diagnostic tools in this case; they are never conclusive. Even those constitutional symptoms which are so closely associated with TB, (such as fever, weakness, and weight loss) may also be infrequent, more non-specific than usual or even absent. EP is broadly speaking much less common than pulmonary tuberculosis and is therefore much less familiar to clinicians in many countries and is correspondingly more frequently missed in its earlier stages.

An appropriate level of suspicion is the key to evaluating a patient presenting with any known risk factors, but a firm and definitive diagnosis of TB still requires the culturing of *M. tuberculosis* if it is at all possible. It's also important for drug-susceptibility testing to be carried out if seen as being at all necessary, since resistance may be present and could confound treatment.

Even where resources are good, for 10% to 15% of patients the final diagnosis of TB is based only on clinical grounds. Predictable consequential delays in diagnosis and initiation of therapy are therefore unavoidable and contribute significantly to the recognised increased risks from these types of TB.

Tests for different types of EPTB

As the lungs may still be involved in patients with EP, sputum AFB smear testing and culture are both indicated for all suspected patients. Culture-positive sputum is especially useful when the specimens from the targeted extra-pulmonary sites are culture-negative, and can also add further information concerning the infectiousness of the patient. A chest X-ray should also be a part of any such basic initial work-up which could well show evidence of active or old TB. A tuberculin skin test (TST) should also be done on all patients with suspected EPTB, although its sensitivity may be highly variable depending on the site of disease. As such, a positive TST is certainly helpful for diagnosis, but a negative TST, unfortunately, certainly does not rule anything out. Also a full blood count (FBC) should always be sent for analysis since this might well also show tell-tale abnormalities.

If the suspicion of TB is high, or if the patient is very ill, consideration is normally given to starting TB treatment as soon as diagnostic specimens are taken without waiting for results since any delay could be fatal.

With all of this complicated information under our belts, we can now consider the more common extra-pulmonary sites of infection.

TB lymphadenitis or lymph node TB

This is the most common form of extra-pulmonary TB, especially with HIV co-infection. TB bacilli infect the lymph nodes in the neck and also those above the collar bones, which then swell up with the skin around them becoming inflamed. This is the condition that used to be known as scrofula. The nodes sometimes even end up discharging through the skin forming chronic sinus formations. In fact any lymph node anywhere in the body can become infected, and often these enlarged, swollen lymph nodes can cause other problems as well because of their size.

To diagnose lymph node TB, a sample of the infected node needs to be taken by pricking the lymph node with a syringe and taking out a few cells for examination under a microscope looking for acid fast bacilli.

If the diagnosis remains in question, then a surgical lymph node excision might be undertaken. If the patient has inaccessible lymphadenitis (e.g., mediastinal), an excisional biopsy is obtained with a mediastinoscopy or a thoracoscopy.

Pleural TB

The pleura is a thin skin that envelops the lungs and separates them from the interior wall of the chest cavity. It is double-layered (one layer adhering to the lungs, one layer to the chest wall), and there is a small space in between these layers in which the TB bacilli can sometimes settle and multiply. As a result, the area becomes inflamed and the person infected will have fever and experience pain when breathing. This inflammation leads the pleura itself to secrete liquid, and this liquid then gathers in between the two layers of the pleura, a phenomenon which is called a pleural effusion.

Pleural TB usually presents with symptoms of pleurisy, pleuritic chest pain, cough, and fever. A chest X-ray will normally show a unilateral effusion, which is usually small to moderate in size. Bilateral TB effusions are rare and are strong indications of more disseminated and dangerous disease.

To diagnose pleural TB, a sample of this fluid effusion needs to be drawn off by inserting a needle through the chest wall into the space between the pleural layers and taking out some of the fluid for examination.

Surprisingly, a chest X-ray may show no obvious disease in as many as 50% of patients with pleural TB; furthermore sputum cultures are positive in only 20% to 30% of cases. False-negative TSTs are also quite common in this condition.

Skeletal TB, or TB of the bone and the joint

TB bacilli can migrate either into the bone or a joint, and will then cause pain and swelling of the affected area. More often than not, it won't immediately be thought that this pain is caused by TB – considered more logically and more likely to have been caused by accident or injury.

Such localised pain is the most common complaint with skeletal TB, and those other more general constitutional or systemic symptoms are usually absent. The onset of pain is often gradual (over weeks or months) and, as a result, diagnosis occurs long after re-activation. Local swelling and limitation of movement may also be present, as well as cold non-tender abscesses with leaking sinus tracts.

If the disease is in the spine, it normally attacks and destroys a single infected intravertebral space along with the adjacent vertebrae above and below. This leads to pain, deformity and angular kyphosis, a condition which, when caused by TB, is also known as Pott's Disease. The associated compression of the spinal cord can ultimately lead to paralysis. Lumbar spine involvement also often leads to a tracking of pus down the sheath of the psoas muscle and then to leakage from sinuses in the inguinal region.

If skeletal TB is suspected, the first diagnostic steps are normally by X-ray, but such patients often also need CT scans or an MRI. Diagnosis is then finally based on tissue biopsy. As with the other forms of extra-pulmonary TB, the TB bacilli must be extracted from the site of infection for diagnosis, this time from either the bone or joint by accessing with a needle and withdrawing out a small sample for analysis. A synovial biopsy can also be carried out to diagnose TB arthritis.

AFB smears are unlikely to be positive by microscopy due to probable low bacillary loads, though they are may well prove to be positive if cultured. Between 70% and 90% of such patients may have a positive TST and around a half of such cases will also have abnormalities on chest X-rays that are consistent with TB.

Central nervous system TB

The central nervous system comprises the brain and the spinal cord. TB bacilli can infect both, and most often this causes TB or tuberculous meningitis – an infection of the thin layer that covers the brain. This condition happens, unfortunately, most commonly in children.

The symptoms depend on where exactly in the brain the TB bacilli settle – usually people with TB meningitis become very sleepy, don't react normally, cannot move their hands or feet or walk at all, or may be unable to speak or focus their eyes. Other tell-tale signs and symptoms of meningeal TB include headache, neck stiffness, altered mental status, and cranial nerve abnormalities. Only 38% of children with TB meningitis have fever, with around 9% reporting photophobia. Fewer than half of such patients also have chest X-ray abnormalities consistent with pulmonary TB. Seizures are particularly common in both children and the elderly with this infection.

TB meningitis is both dangerous to the child and difficult to treat. First and foremost it requires a rapid diagnosis. Most commonly, this is established by lumbar puncture – inserting a needle into the back to access the central spinal fluid (CSF) around the spinal cord (which is connected to the brain), and then examining it to see if there are any TB bacilli in the fluid. This procedure may still be inconclusive, however, in which case an increased volume of the sample, or repeated sampling may be required with as many as three lumbar punctures on different days.

In the presence of any meningeal signs at all, the patient should immediately undergo such a lumbar puncture and the CSF should be submitted for differential cell count, glucose, protein, AFB smear and culture. On top of the results from the smear and culture tests, the usual results of such an analysis include a lymphocyte predominance, with accompanying signs of elevated protein, and also of reduced glucose.

Culture, as with all TB, remains the definitive standard for diagnosis but treatment often simply cannot wait until such culture results are available. It may well have to be initiated presumptively based on clinical suspicion, risk factors, and minimal CSF results.

Head CT or MRI scans may also show signs of disease, and could possibly be the quickest available indicative diagnosis. Signs suggesting TB could include oedema, hydrocephalus, basilar meningeal thickening, or tuberculomas. Because of such a generally poor prognosis, treatment based on such inconclusive findings is frequently started in the hope of saving the patient by prompt intervention.

Abdominal TB

The abdominal cavity contains all of the important digestive organs including the liver, spleen and intestines.

If TB occurs within this cavity at all it is generally known as abdominal TB. Abdominal TB includes TB peritonitis and TB of the gastro-intestinal (GI) tract and such patients may have already had the disease for months before a diagnosis is made. Peritoneal disease is the more common abdominal presentation. Chronic abdominal pain is the most common symptom but other symptoms include abdominal swelling, changes in bowel habits and blood-positive stool. TB disease of the bowel often also causes diarrhoea and colicky pain.

A TST may be positive in 70% of abdominal cases and a chest X-ray might also show evidence of old TB.

A CT scan of the abdomen, an ascitic fluid analysis, and a peritoneal biopsy should be initially carried out. Definitive diagnosis is then based on culture growth of *M. tuberculosis* from such ascitic fluid or from a biopsy of the lesion. Such samples are rarely AFB smear-positive from microscopic examination, however. Although the sensitivity of culture from peritoneal fluid is high, results take as long as eight weeks and, given the frequent delay in patient presentation, any delay in initiating treatment is again associated with higher rates of mortality.

Genito-urinary TB

This relates to any tuberculosis in the region of the kidneys, bladder and urinary tract.

The more common symptoms are dysuria, haematuria, and urinary frequency, but symptoms may be absent in as many as 20% to 30% of patients. Genital TB in men may present as a scrotal mass and in women it may be completely asymptomatic or be a cause of non-specific pelvic pain. The more general systemic constitutional symptoms associated with TB are also less common in this condition. Nevertheless, it is a very serious disease, particularly since extensive renal destruction may have already occurred by the time genito-urinary TB is finally diagnosed.

Chest X-rays are abnormal in between 40% and 75% of such patients. TST, however, is found to be positive in up to 90% of them. Urinalysis should be conducted first of all, and the results commonly show pyuria, haematuria, or proteinuria, although urine results may in fact all be normal. Diagnosis normally relies on culturing TB from morning urine samples (three are recommended), although urine culture for TB may be positive in only 80% of such patients.

A definitive diagnosis of genital TB is finally based on tissue biopsy or by biopsy of the lesion itself.

Pericardial TB

Chest X-rays will show cardiomegaly in 70% to 95% of cases, and a pleural effusion in about 50%.

An ECG will be low voltage in about 25% of cases, and should show a T-wave inversion in about 90%. Echocardiography, or CT or MRI scans should show pericardial effusion and thickening across the pericardial space. A proper diagnosis of pericardial TB requires the aspiration of pericardial fluid or, more usually, a pericardial biopsy. Such pericardial fluid will be exudative with increased leukocytes, and an accompanying predominance of lymphocytes. Signs of a haemorrhagic effusion can often also be seen. An AFB smear of such fluid is commonly negative and cultures are only positive in 50% to 60% of cases. A pericardial biopsy offers the highest chance of a diagnosis.

Overall it will be recognised that the diagnostic processes required for the timely diagnosis of each and every type of EP are variable, costly and require a sophisticated medical resource. Even then, they are challenging and often are arrived at too late.

Treating TB

"THE WEARINESS, THE FEVER AND THE FRET
HERE WHERE MEN SIT AND HEAR EACH OTHER GROAN"

John Keats (1819)[79]

A typical procedure following a confirmation of TB in a high-income country might be much as follows:

A written notification of tuberculosis would be submitted to the relevant health authority by the diagnosing doctor. On receipt of such a notification, a public health nurse would be allocated to the patient to provide support, to assist with treatment compliance and to assess the requirements and extent of contact tracing. Patients with pulmonary TB might possibly at this stage be isolated either at home or in hospital until they have been on adequate anti-TB therapy for at least 14 days and their sputum smears are shown to be negative.

The patient would also have provided two samples for smear testing for their initial diagnosis, and a further sample would have been sent for culture.

And, of course, an appropriate directly observed anti-TB chemotherapy for an equally appropriate period of time would already have been implemented. This should result in almost 100% cure rates – at least if there is no drug-resistance.

Appropriate education and counselling, particularly about minimising the risk of transmission of infection, would also be provided to the patients, particularly with a case of pulmonary TB which is recognized to have a high bacillary load. There is normally no restriction on the movement of patients with extra-pulmonary disease because of minimal risks of them infecting anyone else, but there could be enforced isolation in highly infectious cases if it was seen to be warranted. Close contacts would most probably be followed up with skin tests and X-rays, and prophylactic treatment of any confirmed cases of latent infection or early disease in such contacts would be begun if they were identified.

[79] From "Ode to a Nightingale" which was written by Keats while he was caring for his brother Tom as he was dying from TB.

Finally, once the results of the culture tests have been returned, the drug therapy may be altered to suit the results of the test.

These are the collective reasons why so few deaths from TB occur today in high-income countries.

In middle- and low-income countries, things tend to fall a little short of this ideal. The same short treatment regimens are used, but too often they are not completed properly. Sticking to the treatment, as we will see, is not easy, even with first line drug treatment. Shortages of health workers mean that directly observed treatment can be at best haphazard. Drug supply can be interrupted, and even the quality of the drugs themselves may be suspect or deficient. Furthermore, in the vast majority of cases no sample culturing is available to ensure that the correct drug regime is finally prescribed.

Local rates of latent infection may be so high as to make contact tracing meaningless, and in any case prophylactic treatments may well not be available, and in any case may be ineffectual. And where there is resistance to Isoniazid or Rifampicin or to both (as is occurring proportionately more and more in such low-income countries in comparison to higher-income ones) short course anti-TB chemotherapy is not just ineffective and inappropriate, it is downright dangerous.

The ultimate success of treatment relies very heavily on patient compliance which also requires good management of both patient and treatment. Direct supervision is recognised as being an essential cornerstone of any effective treatment programme because patient compliance is seen as being so important in preventing the consequential development of drug-resistant disease. Non-compliance has frequently been blamed on the patient, but more recently it has been accepted that the quality of the medical infra-structure plays as much or more of a part in whether a patient completes his or her treatment as any other.

There can be a very simple reason for such non-compliance with patients undergoing eight month first line drug treatments. One of the major side effects they report is joint pain (or arthralgia) especially focused, according to many patients, in their knees. Why does it affect their knees so badly? In fact it may not even do so, it is just that the pains in the knees affect their lives in ways which have a larger impact on quality than pains anywhere else, so it tends to be complained of the most. Most patients in low-income countries will be accustomed to squatting in order to defecate, often over latrines. Such squatting when the knees are painful becomes a very challenging part of a daily routine so can have a major negative impact on patients, not just on the experience of their treatment, but also on the quality of their life. After a few weeks of treatment, they may notice that their cough has gone, the night sweats have subsided and that they are putting on weight. They may well even be back at work and everything will seem pretty much fine and back to normal – except for this ongoing problem of pain in their knees when attempting to empty their bowels which they know to be caused by their medication. So, somewhat understandably, they stop taking their drugs despite the fact that they have been told that they must continue to take them.

It's hardly rocket science. Most of us will have probably not completely finished a course of antibiotics at some time, even when they had no adverse effects at all on the quality of our lives and were only prescribed for a fortnight. Given that TB drugs can be so difficult to tolerate, it's not at all surprising that so many patients are known to default. What is more surprising is how many of them successfully complete the course.

Anti-TB drugs are now divided into 11 or 12 categories, although there is still no universally recognised set of classifications. Generally these classes represent drugs which are closely related to each other, classified on the basis of their chemical similarity and on the observed frequency of their cross-resistance. What this means is that, if a strain is confirmed as being resistant to one drug within a particular class, it can be expected to be resistant to all of them.

The drugs are listed below set out in accordance with one of the category classifications. Their more common side effects listed in italics alongside them. The first four are also the so-called first line drugs which are normally taken in varying combinations for between six and eight months; the fifth drug (Streptomycin) is regarded as being 'essential' – and as we will see, is often added by protocol to the four first line drugs if treatment is seen to be failing; the remainder are second line drugs which generally need to be taken in varying combinations of six different individual drugs for up to two years – and sometimes for even longer:

1) Isoniazid - *Liver disease, Psychotic symptoms*
2) Rifamycins (e.g., Rifampicin /rifampin, rifabutin, rifapentine) - *Rash with Pruritis, Liver disease, Fever, Arthralgia, Thrombocytopenia, Flu-like symptoms*
3) Pyrazinamide - *Liver disease, Arthralgia, GIT Disturbance, Pruritis, Hyperuricemia*

4) Ethambutol - *GIT disturbances, Optic Neuritis (particularly Ocular Toxicity has been seen in children), Visual Disturbances;* and sometimes Thioacetazone – *which can cause fatal skin rashes in HIV co-infections.*
5) Streptomycin - *Peripheral Neuropathy, Renal Toxicity, Hearing Loss, Dizziness*
6) Second line aminoglycosides (e.g., kanamycin, amikacin) - *Peripheral Neuropathy, Renal Toxicity, Hearing loss, Electrolyte imbalance*
7) Cyclic polypeptides (e.g., capreomycin, viomycin) – *Renal Toxicity, Hearing loss*
8) Fluoroquinolones (e.g., ciprofloxacin, ofloxacin, levofloxacin, and moxifloxacin) - *Arthralgia, Seizures, Psychotic symptoms Peripheral Neuropathy, Dizziness and Insomnia, Photosensitivity, Rashes, GIT Disturbances*
9) Thioamides (e.g., ethionamide, prothionamide) - *Liver disease, GIT Disturbances, Hypothyroidism, Psychotic symptoms*
10) Serine derivatives (e.g., cycloserine, terizido) - *Seizures, Psychotic symptoms, Peripheral Neuropathy, Restlessness*
11) Para-aminosalicylic acid - *GIT disturbances, Hypothyroidism, Liver disease, Coagulopathy*
12) Macrolides (e.g. erythromycin, clarithromycin*)* - *Gastro-intestinal intolerance, Rash, Hepatitis, prolonged QT syndrome, Ventricular Arrhythmias*

Another alternatively used grouping of these drugs is as follows:

Groups	**Drugs**
Group 1	First line oral anti-TB agents: Isoniazid (H); Rifampicin (R); Ethambutol (E); Pyrazinamide (Z), & Streptomycin (S)
Group 2	Injectable anti-TB agents: kanamycin (Km); amikacin (Am); capreomycin (Cm)
Group 3	Fluoroquinolones: ofloxacin (Ofx); levofloxacin (Lvx); moxifloxacin (Mfx); gatifloxacin (Gfx)
Group 4	Oral second line anti-TB agents: ethionamide (Eto); prothionamide (Pto); cycloserine (Cs); terizidone (Trd); para-aminosalicylic acid (PAS)
Group 5	Agents with unclear efficacy (not recommended by WHO for routine use in MDR-TB patients): clofazimine (Cfz); linezolid (Lzd); amoxicillin/clavulanate (Amx/Clv); thioacetazone (Thz); imipenem/cilastatin (Ipm/Cln); high-dose Isoniazid (high-dose H); clarithromycin (Clr)

This classification is most often used to select drugs in instances of resistance, with drugs being chosen and added in a stepwise selection progression through these five groups.

Of all of these TB drugs Ethambutol, PAS and cycloserine are bacteriostatic (i.e. they prevent the bacilli from replicating). All the others are weakly bactericidal (i.e. they have been demonstrated to kill the bacilli). Capreomycin is usually reserved for last resort treatment of XDR-TB because of the severity of its side effects.

Many DR-TB drugs are also difficult to manage given the constraints of health systems in most high-burden settings. PAS, for instance, requires refrigeration, which is an added logistical burden for programmes, particularly in sub-Saharan Africa. The use of injectable products like Streptomycin, kanamycin and amikacin also imposes burdens on the management of any treatment programme because of qualified staff being required for its administration, as well as necessary stoicism and determination being required of the patient herself who must not only undergo six months of daily painful injections but must also get herself to the clinic in order to receive them.

Such treatment is not even always managed at all as might be expected, despite the treatment being supposedly directly observed as its title suggests. Where resources are poor, a common resort with Streptomycin for the so-called 'Category II' treatment is to send the patient home equipped with a week or a fortnight's supply of the injectable drug with the intention that they manage its administration as best they can themselves, which amounts to their finding someone local to them who can safely inject them each day and probably have to pay them. This, then, is a default 'approved' treatment for when a patient's sputum is seen not to be converting as expected from standard first line treatment. It involves daily injection in the buttocks, something which is very painful and also needs to be done at regular times of day. The idea that this might be done either consistently or successfully in the sort of circumstances that is needed is an optimistic one at best. Given that there are also issues of hygiene and needle disposal to be considered, it is almost insane that it might even be considered in any country with a high incidence of HIV. It ***is*** happening, however, although few will acknowledge it. Nearly half a million patients were put on this treatment in 2012.

Treating latent infection

The treatment of latent tuberculosis infection (LTBI) is an essential component of any serious strategy intending to control and eliminate TB anywhere since, if successful, it obviously reduces the likelihood that existing TB infection will later progress to re-activated infectious disease.

Having established a definite probability of latent infection, treatment can be begun – most commonly with Isoniazid. This is a treatment which is generally referred to as IPT (or 'Isoniazid preventative therapy').

The wider strategic goal behind it is not so much to cure the latent infection as to stop those who are most likely to progress to active disease from doing so; in effect those others who are less likely to develop active disease simply don't warrant the treatment. Unfortunately there is still little in the way of definitive predictors for disease progression so that, for now at least, treatment is seen to be best given to almost all cases of latent disease. TST conversion is thought to reflect a more recent infection, and since the risk of progression to disease in such recent infections is known to be that much higher (5% in the first two years), then, treatment is generally recommended with TST positive data, regardless of either HIV status or background of TB incidence. However, for latent infections with HIV who have started HAART (highly active antiretroviral therapy for HIV) TST positive results are treated far more cautiously, since the TST result may be no more than a sign of an immune reconstitution. This significant factor, however, still does need to be carefully weighed against the known increased likelihood of developing disease, so a decision is not always completely clear cut.

As with almost everything else, embarking even on this, the simplest of treatments for TB is not as straightforward is might be wished: it is accompanied with a level of risk and should always be approached with caution.

The first and most important cause for concern is that active TB is absolutely ruled out before any treatment is begun. To give treatment for latent tuberculosis to someone with already re-activated drug-susceptible tuberculosis simply creates the possibility that the patient will consequentially develop a drug-resistant strain of TB because the active bacilli will not be appropriately destroyed being as a single drug is being used.

What is less frequently considered is the possibility that the bacilli in their latent state might be of a strain that is ***already*** resistant to the drug which is being used to treat the latent infection. Such a treatment might then not just be ineffective, but it might also possibly amplify the strain of drug-resistance. Such a possibility is relatively remote in countries like the US where rates of drug-resistance within the epidemic are still comparatively low anyway – and this is where these treatments have been developed and tested. In countries which are recognised as having high rates of MDR-TB, and in many others where no proper surveillance of resistance has yet been conducted, this risk is larger and cannot be realistically ignored. The list below shows some percentage rates of expectation of effectiveness, but these rates may be far from accurate in high burden countries..

These are the various regimes which have been recognised as being effective:

9H — Isoniazid for nine months is considered to be the best default treatment (considered to be 93% effective and widely used in the USA).

6H — Isoniazid for six months might be adopted by a local TB programme based on cost-effectiveness and good patient compliance. This is the regimen currently recommended in the UK for routine use. The US guidance excludes this regimen from use in children or persons with radiographic evidence of prior tuberculosis (considered to be 69% effective).

6 to $9H_2$ — An intermittent twice-weekly regimen for the above two treatment regimens is an alternative if administered as directly observed.

4R — Rifampicin for four months is an alternative for those who are unable to take Isoniazid or who have had known exposure to Isoniazid-resistant TB.

3HR — Isoniazid and Rifampicin may be given daily for three months.

3HP — three-month (12-dose) regimen of weekly Pyrazinamide and Isoniazid.

Only the last could have any effect at all on a patient latently infected with an MDR-TB strain, and it would in any case be unlikely to be effective. MSF and PIH suggest that all HIV-positive adults with no clinical signs of TB should be offered IPT as a matter of course – but that it should last for at least 36 months. Anti-retroviral treatment (ART) is understood to take priority however, and since there's known to be a high prevalence of asymptomatic TB in ART eligible patients they also figure that IPT should be held back for three months with patients being re-assessed continuously to allow undiagnosed active TB to be unmasked by the ART.

Most studies, unfortunately, indicate poor adherence to IHT since patients don't see its point since they don't have symptoms. Poor adherence predicts resistance to Isozianid. But this is only the first problem. It's also a tricky treatment for alcoholics because of hepatic toxicities, and in many high incidence environments alcohol abuse comes along hand in hand with the disease.

The percentage success rates (where they are identified above) may, in fact, also not be accurate anywhere where the disease is rife simply because they do not allow for the risk of re-infection which can be especially high in any high incidence country. A Cochrane review from 2000 analysed the results from 11 double-blinded, randomized control trials involving a total of 73,375 patients. It depressingly concluded that there was a relative risk of 0.40 for development of active tuberculosis over two years or longer for patients treated with Isoniazid whether it was for six or for 12 months.[80]

Of the 33,000 in the control (placebo) group, 1.7% were seen later to develop disease; of the 40,000 in the IPT group, 0.6% went on to develop disease. As such, the absolute reduction of later developing infectious disease by using IPT turns out to be only just over 1% which hardly sounds that significant. Nevertheless it seems to have reduced the actual risk of re-infection by a third which is far from being insignificant. The development rate of 0.6% in the IPT group may also be very significant since it implies a possible incidence rate of re-activated disease in such cases which may be several times higher than the general incidence rate naturally occurring even within high incidence communities.

There is probably slightly stronger evidence for some consistent protection from TB with the use of IPT in TST-positive subjects with HIV. Unfortunately, there are so far no studies at all which consistently show direct evidence of the efficacy of IPT based on IGRA results, although there is said to be some indirect evidence now emerging and this could change things in the future.

---

[80] Smieja MJ., Marchetti CA., Cook DJ, & Smaill FM – "Isoniazid for preventing tuberculosis in non-HIV infected persons", Cochrane Database of Systematic Reviews (Online), 2;2 (2000).

One recent study in Botswana has shown that long-term IPT in TST-positive persons with HIV/AIDS does have a strong impact on survival. The study has also shown that Isoniazid appears to have little benefit at all in HIV-positive individuals who are TST-negative, however, so simple blanket treatment across a high incidence HIV-positive population would not seem likely to be of any benefit. [81] In fact, if there was also any significant rate of drug-resistance in such a community, it could prove to be devastatingly counter-productive. In a later section we will see what happened in a large study which attempted exactly this in South Africa – the so-called Thibela Study.

Rather worryingly, when it comes to treating latent infection for persons with known exposure to MDR-TB no evidence base exists at all, nor, unfortunately, does any consensus yet exist on optimal treatment.[82] Worst of all is the unfortunate fact that no existing test for LTBI can diagnose drug-resistance within it so with MDR-TB the entire endeavour is founded on uncertainties. A regimen consisting of Ethambutol and PAS has occasionally been used on such suspect cases but no good data has been harvested. If the treatment under consideration is being considered as part of a case-finding exercise from a known index case of MDR-TB, the best approach would seem to be a combination of antibiotics based on the defined sensitivities of the bacillus in the particular index patient. Such a regimen would need to have been defined by their DST, but it would be an uncertain treatment without any existing evidence base. The American Centers for Disease Control and Prevention (CDC) have recommended a combination of Pyrazinamide and Ethambutol, or Pyrazinamide with a fluoroquinolone for more general cases with recognised high risks of having drug-resistant latent TB. According to these recommendations, immuno-competent cases should be treated for six months and immuno-compromised ones for 12 months.[83]

---

[81] Samandari T, Agizew TB, Nyirenda S et al. - "6-month versus 36-month isoniazid preventive treatment for tuberculosis in adults with HIV infection in Botswana: a randomised, double-blind, placebo-controlled trial", The Lancet, 377; 9777 (2003) 1588–98.

[82] Passannante MR, Gallagher CT, Reichman LB - "Preventive therapy for contacts of multidrug-resistant tuberculosis: a Delphi survey", Chest 106; 2 (1994) 431–4.

[83] ATS/CDC Statement Committee on Latent Tuberculosis Infection – "Targeted Tuberculin Testing and Treatment of Latent Tuberculosis Infection", Mortality and Morbidity Weekly Report, 49; RR06 (2000) 1–54.

As we will discuss in more detail later, such complexities present enormous challenges to the necessary concerted efforts which are now needed to confront the ocean of latent infection in South Asia and Africa.

Treating drug-susceptible TB and the 'Category II' regimen

Treatment of what we might now call 'normal' TB (tuberculosis which is susceptible to drugs) today employs a standard regimen of first line drugs (Rifampicin, Isoniazid, Ethambutol, and Pyrazinamide, with the occasional additional use of Streptomycin).

In many parts of the world patients treated with first line drugs are divided into two significantly distinct categories:

Category I TB patients are patients who test sputum-positive for TB for the first time.

The slightly different drug treatment regimens used on such patients are denoted by their acronyms as 2HERZ/6HE or 2HERZ/4HE. The letters and numbers denote both the drugs used and their durations. Both are standard first line treatment regimes used in different countries depending on local expert opinion for newly diagnosed patients who have no previous history of infection.

In each case the treatment is divided into two phases. The initial 'intensive phase' is 2HERZ. The duration of this phase is two months, and the treatment uses Isoniazid (H), Ethambutol (E), Rifampicin (R) and Pyrazinamide (Z). Dosages are varied dependent upon the patient's weight. During this phase, the patient should quickly respond in terms of their symptoms, and within a matter of weeks should show sputum negative (and therefore should no longer be infective).

The subsequent 'continuation phase' is either 6HE or 4HE. The duration of this phase is six or four months. Drug treatment is daily, with Isoniazid (H) and Ethambutol (E).

Given the emerging pandemic of drug-resistant disease, a particular risk of this continuation phase needs some consideration. This continuation phase used in isozianid-resistant patients effectively amounts to ethambutol monotherapy which would promote resistance to ethambutol. It is recognized that as many as 20% of sputum-positive patients in some parts of South Africa are isozianid resistant, so this can no longer be considered a small risk.

In fact, in such areas with known high Isozianid resistance the standard Category I treatment should really not be used at all without drug-susceptibility testing. If this were not available (which is likely at the sort of scale that would be needed) then MSF believe that Ethambutol should be added to the continuation phase in the hope of reducing the chance of drug-resistance increasing, despite the fact that many patients would be receiving Ethambutol unnecessarily.

Category II TB patients are patients who are known to have relapsed, who fail treatment, or who are identified as having defaulted. This default treatment is generally used in low- and middle-income countries where around a million people in over 90 countries may be being treated with it, with around half of these being treated with National Treatment Programmes approved by the WHO. This number constitutes 8.5% of the current estimated total of prevalent cases under treatment.

This Category II drug treatment is denoted as 2SHERZ/HERZ/5HER. In this regime Streptomycin (administered by injection) is added to the regime which is divided into three phases.

The 'initial phase' (2SHERZ) lasts two months. Drug treatment is with Streptomycin by injection (S), Isoniazid (H), Ethambutol (E), Rifampicin (R) and Pyrazinamide (Z).

The next phase is one month duration HERZ. Drug treatment, as with the initial phase of the Category I treatment, uses daily Isoniazid (H), Ethambutol (E), Rifampicin (R) and Pyrazinamide (Z).

The final phase is five months with Isoniazid (H), Ethambutol (E) and Rifampicin (R).

This treatment does not rely on drug-susceptibility testing at all, simply because it is assumed that it will be unavailable, although drug-resistance may quite possibly be present. In fact, of course, this is a very reasonable probability.

Unlike Category I treatment, the Category II regimen has never been evaluated for efficacy either in randomized clinical trials or in cohort studies. In other words there is no gold standard evidence base for its use.

The WHO formulated the recommendation to add Streptomycin to the four first line drugs from expert opinion only which is now highly questionable. It was a recommendation which significantly occurred both before the emergence of more widespread drug-resistant TB and before more prevalent HIV co-infection. More recent WHO guidelines correctly recommend drug-susceptibility testing (DST) prior to retreatment of ***all*** confirmed treatment failures or treatment of suspected multidrug-resistant TB cases. Since access to DST and to second line TB drugs remains so poor in all high-burden and low-income countries, however, the Category II retreatment regimen remains the general mainstay for treating nearly all failing patients in the national programmes in resource-limited settings.

It should also be well noted that this method of re-treatment (which is out of a perception of necessity still endorsed and accepted as a default by the WHO) can be logically predicted to potentially promote the development of both MDR-TB and XDR-TB. This is because the regimen amounts to the addition of just one drug to an already failing regimen, something which is known to potentially amplify the level of drug-resistance.[84] This treatment breaks one of the golden rules of TB chemotherapy: ***never to add a single drug to a failing treatment regimen.*** In fact the WHO's "Guidelines for the Programmatic Management of Drug-Resistant Tuberculosis - Emergency Update" of 2008 was explicit that Streptomycin should actually be avoided as an additional drug "even if DST suggest susceptibility, because of high rates of resistance with DR-TB strains and higher incidence of ototoxicity". The document recommends only starting Category II treatment "while awaiting DST". It begins to look like the treatment has been being very widely misapplied.

It's impossible not to reflect on the immortalised words of Hippocrates in relation to this – "As to diseases, make a habit of two things—to help, or at least to do no harm."[85]

It should also be noted that this treatment requires much closer management than the Category I treatment because of the first part of the treatment which requires daily injection in the buttocks. Although it is rarely discussed, it is doubtful that this treatment is being as well managed

---

[84] Yanis Ben Amor , Bennett Nemser, Angad Singh, Alyssa Sankin, and Neil Schluger - "Underreported Threat of Multidrug-Resistant Tuberculosis in Africa", Journal of Emerging Infectious Diseases, 14; 9 (2008).

[85] Hippocrates - "The Epidemics".

as it should be in many (if not most) instances, something which has to be of particular concern in countries with high levels of HIV co-infection.

The WHO's own surveillance data has suggested that this re-treatment regimen is successful in about 70% of patients, but other retrospective studies have shown much more variable treatment responses with success rates ranging wildly between 26% and 92%. These studies, however, generally have only assessed outcomes at the ***completion*** of the re-treatment regimen so they may be well undervalued anyway. Furthermore few studies have examined the risk of TB recurrence from the treatment, especially in people who are also infected with HIV and so are recognised to be much more likely to experience it. This is the key issue, of course, in Sub-Saharan Africa, a region where Category II treatment is very widely used.

In a study based in Uganda,[86] researchers conducted a prospective cohort study to assess treatment and survival outcomes in patients previously treated for TB who were put on Category II treatment. Given the overwhelming contribution of HIV infection to mortality rates in Uganda, the researchers elected to categorize their survival analyses by their HIV status. The researchers encouragingly found that only 20% of HIV-uninfected patients had unsuccessful outcomes, but a higher rate of 26% of HIV-infected patients had unsuccessful treatment outcomes from this regimen. There were, unsurprisingly, no successful outcomes at all with patients with existing identified MDR-TB, and the risks of amplification of resistance is thus highest in these patients exactly as would be expected. The overall results from this study are a little confusing, however. What the researchers did conclude was that, given that this regimen was devised before the growth of MDR-TB and HIV co-infection, it remains an "inadequate" regime in countries with high incidence of either disease.

Both the 2012 and 2013 WHO reports suggest that it is still being used widely. 400,000 patients were notified as "previously diagnosed TB patients whose treatment regimen was changed" in both of these reports. (In other words they were changed to Category II treatment). A total of 20,000 (or 5% of the 400,000) might possibly have been put on second line drugs but

---

[86] Jones-López EC et al. - "Effectiveness of the Standard WHO Recommended Retreatment Regimen (Category II) for Tuberculosis in Kampala, Uganda: A Prospective Cohort Study", PLoS Med 8;3 (2011).

this is unclear from the information that is available. This serves up an idea of the scale of this "inadequate" treatment that is potentially fuelling rates of drug-resistance.

There is also a Category III treatment which is still occasionally used. It is intended for patients who are diagnosed sputum smear-negative and who are "not seriously ill". In other words, there may be a clinical suspicion of TB but the patient does not show any serious symptoms. In this case the regimen is 2HRZ/4HR – as Category I, in effect, but without Ethambutol in the first intensive phase. There are no current figures on how often this regimen is applied and it seems likely that it is more widely applied in the private unregulated health sector.

Treating drug-resistant TB

Effectively, treating TB of any type today anywhere in the world without additional sophisticated diagnostics amounts to an unenviable game of epidemiological Russian roulette.

The same basic principle of diagnosis for TB has been most commonly for the majority of cases ever since Robert Koch identified the bacillus 120 years ago: a modified process of gram staining is used on sputum samples, after which the bacilli (if they exist in sufficient numbers) can be identified through a microscope. The process is simple and, theoretically, it can be done in minutes.

The problem, as we have already identified, is that this process is not only known to be unreliable but it also fails to identify if the subject's bacilli is resistant to any of the existing first line drugs used in the treatment of TB. Without this knowledge, the clinician is left with no option but to prescribe blindfold with whatever drugs are available, in the full knowledge that, if the strain is resistant, such treatment might not just be ineffective, but that it might also stoke or amplify an existing drug-resistant strain into becoming that one step more resistant (in other words from single-drug-resistant DR-TB to MDR-TB, or MDR-TB to pre-XDR-TB etc.).

Furthermore, patients who are co-infected with HIV have a higher rate of failure to test positively for TB using the sputum test, meaning that, if reviewed dispassionately, the sputum test can today be reasonably regarded as being both unreliable and largely unfit for the purpose of both diagnosis and for formulation of good treatment in almost all of Africa. At least it certainly seems unlikely that it won't be seen that way in the future with the benefit of hindsight.

In the world of higher incomes further testing is done automatically by sending suspect samples for culturing, a process which will identify whether a straightforward six- or eight-month first line drug regimen will work, or whether a tailor-made second line treatment lasting as long as two years will be needed. Full susceptibility testing of a selective range of drugs will identify exactly which drugs should work and which shouldn't be used.

There are three inconvenient catches to this treatment principle which explains why it is too rarely used in many of the countries where MDR-TB is most rife.

One is that the fact that the process of culture testing takes six weeks or longer.

The second is that these diagnostics require well-equipped laboratories which are expensive – so expensive that they have yet to be made available at any scale in any country with a known need.

The third is that the drugs which may be identified as being needed will, unfortunately, often not even be available or may have delayed delivery problems because of the quirkiness of the current system of ordering them to match demand.

The global laboratory capacity for drug-susceptibility testing (DST) is unequivocally identified by the WHO as being "low", although all 29 WHO approved Supranational TB Reference Laboratories now routinely perform DST to detect MDR- and XDR-TB. Only four of these supranational labs are in Africa (only two of which are in the Sub-Sahara) – while 12 are in Europe, so there is plainly a very serious imbalance of resource. These WHO supranational TB laboratories are generally expected to offer both technical and training support to regional TB laboratories in other countries and thus are expected to contribute to a strengthening of the worldwide TB laboratory network. More regional laboratories will further add to the global laboratory resource, but nevertheless they substantially vary in their capacity to perform DST to any level of extensive drug-resistance beyond MDR-TB which is increasingly being required. Currently, the future format of the supranational TB reference laboratory network is under discussion. It is foreseen that the future network will consist not just of these supranational reference laboratories but also of other centres of excellence intended to have more regional scopes of operation. What all of this adds up to is that moves are afoot to improve the situation, but also adds that they are being made much later than might have been expected.

After confirmatory diagnosis of MDR-TB, patients can be treated with either a standard MDR regimen or an individually tailored regimen which is based on their drug sensitivity tests. In most cases it will be by the former. Effective treatment regimens in either case are always intended to contain at least three drugs with certain efficacy (and preferably four).

Any patient who does not respond to the treatment of Category I or III, any Category II patient who remains smear-positive at the end of the fourth month of treatment, and all close contacts of confirmed MDR-TB cases are considered to be "MDR-TB suspect". Every single one of these should, in a better resourced world, be immediately tested by culture sensitivity tests for drug-resistance.

If such a suspect is then confirmed as being a non-MDR-TB case, then Category II or Category I regimens are recommended to be continued, but if MDR-TB is confirmed then a Category IV regimen should be started immediately.[87]

Although any such treatment should be reliant on appropriate identification of resistance through DST, treatments are most often simply started based on probabilities calculated from experience. The Revised National Tuberculosis Control Programme (RNTCP) of India, for instance, uses a standard Category IV regimen for the treatment of MDR-TB.[88] This treatment includes an intensive phase (IP) of six drugs for 6-9 months. This phase has been widely considered to be ideally conducted in an isolation unit since the patient may remain infectious for most of this period although this philosophy is now in a state of flux internationally. This intensive phase in India is comprised of the following drugs:

four bactericidal:
- ofloxacin (or levofloxacin)
- kanamycin
- ethionamide

[87] Naveen Chabra, et al. – "Pharmacotherapy for multidrug resistant tuberculosis", Journal of Pharmacology and Pharmacotherapies, 3; 2 (2012) 98–104.

[88] RNTCP - "DOT Plus Guidelines", http://www.tbcindia.org/pdfs/DOTS_Plus_Guidelines_Jan2010.pdf

Pyrazinamide
- and two bacteriostatic drugs:
  Ethambutol
  cycloserine

It is then followed by four drugs during the 18 months of the continuation phase (CP):

ofloxacin (or levofloxacin)
ethionamide
Ethambutol
cycloserine

PAS is included in the regimen as a default substitute if either any one of the four bactericidal drugs or if any of the two bacteriostatic drugs is not tolerated.

After the first six months of treatment, the patient is then reviewed and the treatment changed to CP only if the fourth month culture result is negative (the fourth month culture results normally being available at the end of the sixth month). If the fourth-month culture result remains positive the IP treatment will be extended for at least a further month. Extension of IP beyond seven months is generally decided by the results of the sputum cultures of the fifth month (available at the end of seventh month) and then of sixth months. The IP can be extended up to a maximum of three months on based on such culture results (i.e. the maximum duration of IP is effectively nine months) after which the patient is normally initiated on the CP irrespective of the culture result.

The standard duration for the CP which follows is then 18 months regardless of the length of duration of the IP.

MSF and PIH have a slightly simpler model for treating MDR-TB than the Indian RTCP. The core design of their MDR-TB treatment include at least four group 2-4 drugs including one that is injectable – plus Pyrazinamide. They believe that the most effective four drug combination that can be developed from this protocol should include a fluoroquinolone, one injectable drug, ethionamide, and cycloserine or PAS with Pyrazinamide added to make it five drugs.[89]

---

[89] PIH & MSF - "Tuberculosis – Practical Guide for clinicians, nurses, laboratory technicians and medical auxillaries" (2014) http://refbooks.msf.org/msf_docs/en/tuberculosis/tuberculosis_en.pdf

South Africa has recently been favouring a different regimen again: six months of kanamycin, moxifloxacin, ethionamide and terizidone, with a further 18 months continuation phase using Pyrazinamide, moxifloxacin, ethionamide and terizidone.

The following extract is a sobering summary of the existing evidence base that is available for some of the currently-used second line drugs. It was prepared as part of a case which was being promoted to try to fast-track approval of bedaquiline, a new TB drug, in South Africa. The section is included in its entirety since it gives as good a picture as any of the deficiencies of the past few decades in the research and development of treatment of DR-TB

> "All the recommendations [for second line treatment of drug-resistant TB] are graded ***very low quality evidence*** which is the WHO's lowest level of evidence. This grading effectively means that 'any estimate of effect is very uncertain'.
>
> "The side effects of the standard drugs used to compose MDR TB regimens are awful. In one South African MDR TB cohort, more than half the patients taking aminoglycosides [kanamycin or amikacin]) became hearing impaired [and such impairment is normally permanent]. In another, 28% on SLDs had severe adverse events recorded. In a Turkish cohort, side effects were severe enough to cause drug changes in more than half the patients.
>
> "The South African MDR-TB treatment guidelines recommend a regimen that includes kanamycin, ethionamide, Pyrazinamide, levofloxacin and terizidone. Other drugs like linezolid are also often used for MDR-TB. The efficacy of Pyrazinamide has been well established [however].... we searched for controlled clinical trials of the remaining drugs to treat TB, i.e. kanamycin, ethionamide, levofloxacin, terizidone and linezolid.
>
> "**Kanamycin** – We can find one clinical trial of kanamycin in people with TB, though it is more accurate to describe it as a prospective case-controlled study. It was published in 1958 and compared kanamycin to Streptomycin in 162 patients. It does not appear to have been randomised and the two groups of patients appear not to have been matched at baseline. The data showing the effectiveness of kanamycin is no better, and perhaps worse, than the data on bedaquiline. The available data shows that the side effect profile of kanamycin is much worse than bedaquiline. Kanamycin causes hearing problems in 3% to 10% of patients and it also causes kidney problems.

"**Ethionamide** – A tiny clinical trial of 27 people compared ethionamide against thiacetazone in 1963. Cycloserine was given to patients in both arms. Nine out of 14 versus three out of nine patients on the ethionamide and thiacetazone arms respectively had what the authors call "bacteriologically quiescent disease" after one year. The authors state that the ethionamide arm performed statistically significantly better than the thiacetazone one. A Japanese controlled clinical trial that compared ethionamide against prothionamide was published in 1968. However, since all patients also received Isoniazid and Streptomycin and nearly all patients sputum-converted in all arms of the trial, it is impossible to calculate the effectiveness, if any, of ethionamide in this trial. There are other clinical trials of drug-resistant TB patients that use ethionamide as part of a treatment regimen, but we can find no other clinical trial evidence in people with TB in which ethionamide is tested against a control. Ethionamide is associated with serious side effects. Liver toxicity in particular is common and may continue even after patients stop taking the drug. It is also associated with peripheral neuropathy.

"**Levofloxacin** – Besides a seven day early bactericidal activity trial, we can find no clinical trials of levofloxacin that have considered the drug for the treatment of MDR TB. It also has several side effects, including phototoxicity, glucose disturbances, QT prolongation and others.

"**Terizidone** – We can find one reference to possible clinical trials of terizidone in a 1972 paper written in Croatian, but we are unable to get the paper. The evidence base for terizidone is poor.

"**Linezolid** – Linezolid has been used in South Africa for drug-resistant TB for some time. Yet the first randomized controlled trial of linezolid in patients with drug-resistant TB was only published in October 2012 and it was a smaller trial (n=41) than the Phase II bedaquiline trial described above. The results are promising and significantly more patients taking linezolid sputum-converted compared to the controls, but the drug was also associated with more serious adverse events than bedaquiline.

It seems that the most reasonable conclusion to be drawn from the above is that, if any of these drugs were being proposed for the first time for the treatment of MDR-TB today, they would almost certainly not be approved without much better evidence.

Another of the thorny problems confronting clinicians faced with treating MDR-TB is that there is also literally no evidence in terms of controlled research studies that support the use of one management protocol over another. The last trials of combination therapy for these drugs date back decades, and then they were only testing them as first line drugs for what was indisputably drug-susceptible tuberculosis. With the advent of new drugs this situation is changing, but for now the best advice that doctors can rely on when using these current drugs are guidelines based on expert opinion and/or clinical experience.

Such experience, as hard won as it may have been, may well be principally dependent upon where it has been gained: with TB environmental and epidemiological variations are known to potentially make significant differences to clinical outcomes. In other words, if a protocol is worked up and seen to create positive results in Eastern Europe, it cannot be assumed that it will have the same effect in Sub-Saharan Africa or India. Such an idea clearly does not suit the DOTS-type 'one-size-fits-all' approach, but it is a probable reality which potentially confounds any similar approach with DOTS-Plus protocol treatments.

When it comes to the treatment of XDR-TB and the more extremely resistant strains of the disease, the rule books have to be thrown out almost as extensively as the diagnosed strain of disease. With no real diagnostic infrastructure to fall back on, nor any real research data, treatment often simply has to become as intuitive as it may be properly informed.

Strictly speaking, in fact, 'straightforward' XDR-TB should not perhaps be quite as challenging to treat as it is generally accepted to be. Prior to the development of Rifampicin and the fluoroquinolones in the 1960s, such basic XDR-TB as we see it today would equate to resistance to just three drugs (Isoniazid, Streptomycin and PAS), and not to four or five. Such resistance would still have been challenging to treat, but there are records of patients with such combinations of resistance being successfully treated with a three drug combination in certain countries in an era in which local rates of both susceptible and resistant TB were not being recorded as rising.

If disease which might have equated to cases of XDR-TB as we see them today really was successfully treated in the 1960s, it suggests that other things almost certainly must have been helping as well. A core issue to consider would what such 'other things' might have been, and, if they are properly identifiable, to decide whether or not they might then be worked into the current strategy, such as exists, to contain the XDR strains. It might simply have been that those cases were being caught a lot earlier so treatment was more likely to succeed. Nevertheless such a historical heterodoxy challenges the current belief that the only way that this morphing pandemic can be defeated will be with new drugs. Something extra that was perhaps implicit in previous treatment regimens may also be needed today with XDR-TB, to the extent that such 'somethings' could be critical to the quality of programme management and treatment outcome. We certainly know that TB is a perniciously multi-factorial disease. It just may be that some of these contributory factors may be being underestimated wherever XDR-TB is on the rise simply because of the knee-jerk fear of the prospect of pharmaceutically untreatable disease. Other tools in addition to new or existing drugs could and should very definitely be considered as a way of helping to contain the pandemic, and so both save lives and reduce rates of disease. Such add-ons most probably still won't be enough to effectively eradicate such extensively resistant strains, but they could well help contain it at more acceptable and manageable levels.

Somewhat similarly to the way in which it was finally realised that sanatoria were not the answer that they had been believed to be, there is currently a movement away from the hospitalisation and isolation of MDR-TB patients in some settings in the developing world. This has not as yet been endorsed by results from clinical trials (and may never do so), being driven more by simple and equally empirical *realpolitik* – an attempt to address the simple but daunting question as to how any financially constrained health system might hope to cope with the growing burden of drug-resistant TB. Based on the success of projects run by Médecins Sans Frontières and Partners in Health, the WHO has now recommended that:

> "…where possible, patients with MDR-TB should be treated using ambulatory or community-based care rather than models of care based principally on hospitalization."[90]

The wisdom of such a statement, however, is dependent entirely on the quality of community care that can be sustained in such programmes, although it is undeniable that MSF and PIH are both experts in administering and engendering them. Whether this success can be easily replicated in wider programmes is still highly debatable.

Until 2011, South African health guidelines were requiring that patients with multi drug-resistant-TB received their treatment as in-patients in one of the country's handful of dedicated TB hospitals. New cases of DR-TB had been significantly outstripping the bed capacity for some time, so the government had no real alternative but to re-think its policy. The director

[90] WHO – "Global Tuberculosis Report 2013".

of TB, DR-TB and HIV in the South African national health department, Dr Norbert Ndjeka told a United Nations news agency in 2013:

> "We will never have enough beds in our lifetime to admit all the MDR-TB cases and we can't keep building more hospitals."

His words reveal the decisive logic behind the WHO's 2013 statement. South Africa is said to have 2,500 beds for DR-TB patients at 63 sites. In 2012 there were 14,161 laboratory diagnosed cases of MDR-TB and 1,646 XDR-TB cases, adding up to nearly ten times the bed capacity that would be needed. Incidence rates of MDR-TB have doubled in the five years between 2007 and 2012, and nearly quadrupled for XDR-TB in the same period.[91]

Both MSF and PIH, who are effectively the flag-bearers for this innovative approach, almost certainly have as much or more experience in the treatment of MDR- and XDR-TB than any other NGO. And both of them see the situation the same way – that the only realistic hope of managing MDR-TB in resource-poor environments is to use ambulatory patient-centred care rather than by hospitalisation. PIH has described a continued reliance on any hospital-centred model as being "self-defeating" since the NGO sees it as being guaranteed to "stymie" any possible scale-up of second line treatments simply because the need and demand for them so consistently outpaces bed capacities in hospitals. PIH accepts that the justification for hospital treatment has most often been primarily to remove infectious MDR-TB and XDR-TB patients from their communities. It also points out, however, that, if bed supply cannot keep up with demand, all of those infectious patients awaiting admission will still be out there in their communities infecting family and neighbours. In the longer run this experienced organisation believes that this growing cohort of patients awaiting treatment will be far more dangerous to the epidemic.

An emerging belief is that delivering MDR-TB care in the community may in fact have many benefits beyond a potential overall reduction of transmission, although it simply ***must*** be appropriately managed if it is to work. For one thing, it is seen as being much less disruptive for patients and their families. It is also considered to be the best way to identify and address those social and economic needs that almost always coincide with the medical ones. These NGOs also see that there are invaluable potential

[91] Dr Robert Ndjeka - "Strategic Review of Multi Drug-Resistant Tuberculosis", Department of Health, Republic of South Africa.

opportunities within this model to better educate communities in the issues of the disease, as well as to reduce some of the stigma associated with it.

PIH, at least, is also convinced that, not just any global MDR-TB treatment scale-up, but also any proper introduction or inclusion of bedaquiline or any other new drug will ultimately be totally dependent upon such modifications of approach.

The Business of Vaccination

"IN VIEW OF THE EPIDEMIOLOGICAL SITUATION IN GERMANY, THE LACK OF EVIDENCE FOR THE EFFECTIVENESS OF THE BCG-VACCINE AND THE NOT UNCOMMON SEVERE, UNDESIRED SIDE EFFECTS OF THE BCG VACCINE, THE STIKO [THE PERMANENT VACCINATION COMMISSION IN GERMANY] CAN NO LONGER SUPPORT THE RECOMMENDATION FOR THIS VACCINATION."

The Robert Koch Institute (1998)[92]

The BCG vaccine, as we have already seen, first began to be developed from a live but attenuated bovine strain of tuberculosis by Albert Calmette and Camille Guérin in 1906. It was first tested on a human being in France on July 18, 1921.

No new or better vaccine has appeared since.

Clinical vaccine trials using *M. bovis* were first conducted in Italy in the late 19th century – but with disastrous results because *M. bovis* in an unattenuated form was found to be just as virulent as *M. tuberculosis*. The key to the safety of the BCG vaccine itself was down to the systematic attenuation of the bovine strain.

BCG, however, has not been one of the most successful vaccines ever developed. It has been shown to have what is rather euphemistically described as "variable protective efficacy". This is not because of any reduced potency as a result of the attenuation, but it is mainly simply because of the limitation of the acquired resistance to tuberculosis after its administration. At its very best, the BCG vaccine has been promoted as being 80% effective in preventing tuberculosis for a duration of 15 years; however this claim is doubtful and its protective effect varies massively according to geography and demography, and is also dependent on the type of TB.

What this really means is that it doesn't really appear to protect adults at all from any strains or types of the disease. It ***is*** agreed that it protects kids – but even for them only against specific forms of the disease. As a result of

[92] The Robert Koch Institute in Germany is the central federal institution responsible for disease control and prevention and is therefore the central federal reference institution for both applied and response-orientated research as well as for the Public Health Sector.

such limitations, the vaccine is not recognised today as being of any real use at all in developed/industrialised countries where the incidence of TB is low, and as a result the practice of BCG vaccination has been widely dropped in these countries. The reason, as much as any, is because both seed and soil (in terms of the epidemics) in these countries has changed so dramatically – certainly it is not because it is regarded as a dangerous vaccine.

Given how relatively ineffective the vaccine has been shown to be, it is ironic that, whenever a story appears in the press in a low incidence country relating to a local outbreak of TB, a popular suggestion almost invariably appears in the media that BCG should be re-introduced either locally or nationally to address the problem. That such a suggestion isn't dismissed immediately simply on the grounds of the fact that it reveals such a limited understanding of both the disease and the vaccine, is itself something of a mystery. It is as if it remains somehow expedient to maintain a myth that this vaccine has and can perform like other more successful ones. Such an outbreak might occur in a school – perhaps in an inner city community with a high incidence of first generation immigrants. The BCG vaccination is completely unrealistic as a way of protecting a wider community in such a case, or indeed the school in question, because both would be at risk from aerosol-born pulmonary disease which the vaccine offers no real protection against at all.

What the vaccine ***is*** recognised as being usefully protective against is maternally-transmitted TB, as well as bovine TB from unpasteurised milk. It may be recalled that the very first successful proven use of the vaccine back in 1921 was on a new-born infant with an infectious mother. Perhaps not that much has ever really changed.

It may well come as something of a surprise that this vaccine is really so unreliable in protecting anyone much older than a new born against pulmonary TB given that this is the type of tuberculosis which accounts for the majority of the infectious disease wordwide. Actually, with the benefit of knowledge and a little hindsight, it really should come as no surprise at all. It might even not be that unfair to suggest that BCG should ***never*** have been regarded as an effective vaccine against tuberculosis – but rather that it just might have been the most ineffective vaccine that has ever been widely implemented. It has been used continuously for over 90 years and it is said that it has had the highest coverage of any human vaccine – and yet the current estimate of latent infection globally is quoted as running at 32% of mankind, or one in three people. This is in spite of several billion doses of it having been administered across the decades, although its administration has varied widely.

India, for instance, started a mass BCG campaign to combat TB in 1951, one which has been continued right up until today. It was the first nationwide campaign against TB and yet latent infection rates in India run today at an estimated 40%. Has it helped? Yes, it must have done. Has it helped anywhere near as much as hoped? No. Did it play a part in helping to bring down or containing rates of TB? Most certainly, yes, but not anywhere near the desired or mistakenly believed amount – nor as much as has been needed.

There is some scientific evidence of exactly how effective (or more accurately ineffective) this vaccine has been. Most earlier studies had been restricted to the new born and young children, generally assessing efficacy of anywhere between 0% and 80%, but there was one large community-based controlled trial of the BCG vaccination which was conducted between 1968 and 1971 in southern India. This trial reported on the effect of BCG vaccination on 360,000 people in 29 villages and in one small town – enrolling the entire resident populations with the exception of a single infant who was less than one month old. Two different vaccine strains were used (as well as a placebo), both strains being considered to be the most potent available at the time. The general conclusion was that no real protective efficacy in either adults or children was demonstrated five years following the mass vaccination. The recipients were then re-evaluated 10 years later, at which time the protective efficacy in persons who had been vaccinated as children was assessed as being 17% whereas no protective effect was seen at all in those participants in the study who had been vaccinated as adolescents or adults.[93]

It might still be reasonably argued that the BCG vaccine may have contributed to bringing down a residual rate of latent infection in India by as much as half what it might more normally run at in an otherwise unprotected population. Surveys of children in England in the early 20th century suggested that latency was then running at around 80% – and this was at a time when there was also far higher incidence of infectious disease in the wider population. If the latency rate is currently running at 40% in

---

[93] Tripathy SP - "Fifteen-year follow-up of the Indian BCG prevention trial", International Union Against Tuberculosis, ed. Proceedings of the XXVIth IUAT World Conference on Tuberculosis and Respiratory Diseases. Singapore: Professional Postgraduate Services International (1987) 69-72.

India after 60 years of vaccination, in a country with a current comparative of infectious TB to that of the England a hundred years ago, it would certainly suggest this argument might be valid, although other factors may have been involved as well.

If we compare the BCG vaccine with the more successful targeted vaccination campaigns against smallpox and polio, a truly sobering picture emerges being as current global rates of TB disease remain so very high. With these other two diseases, concerted vaccination campaigns have seen both diseases driven either into total or near total submission. Nothing similar can yet be said of tuberculosis

More recently the WHO has published annual country-by-country estimates for BCG coverage worldwide. Their records range from 1980 until the present – a period of 30 years. They offer us fairly salty food for thought. Only 13 countries have not vaccinated at all during at least a part of this period – but all of these same countries had minimal incidence rates of tuberculosis over this period so vaccination was unnecessary and would have made no difference for any of them. The vast majority of countries worldwide, however, have continued vaccinating throughout this period – with coverage in some instances claimed to be as high as 99.5%. In fact it was estimated that over 85% of the world's children received the vaccine in 1990 – and yet, we must remind ourselves, the estimated figure for latent infection worldwide still sits at 32%.[94]

The WHO does now recommend vaccinating all at-risk HIV-uninfected infants. (HIV infection simply confers too much risk of active infection from the attenuated vaccine which, although attenuated, is still live.) This policy is viewed as being by far the most effective way of reducing TB meningitis in children of less than five years of age, as well as of reducing death in babies in countries of high TB prevalence. Based on what is known about the vaccine, this has to be a judicious recommendation.

Unfortunately, for reasons which may possibly be associated with existing endemic mycobacterial bacilli in local soils being a little too similar either to

[94] WHO - "Reported estimates of BCG coverage", http://apps.who.int/immunization_monitoring/en/globalsummary/timeseries/tscoveragebcg.htm
The countries who have not vaccinated are Andorra, Australia, Bahamas, Belgium, Canada, Cyprus, Germany, Granada, Iceland, Lebanon, Netherlands, New Zealand and the USA.

the tuberculosis or the bovine bacilli, the existing vaccine simply doesn't work so reliably in some parts of the tropics. As a result, in some of those very parts of the world that is being most devastated by the disease, it is sometimes suggested that this vaccine isn't even that effective for infants either.

This anomaly has been explained by a suggestion that exposure to other environmentally occurring mycobacteria might result in nonspecific immune responses against mycobacteria generally which might in turn somehow reduce the efficacy of the BCG vaccine. In other words, administering BCG to someone who already has a nonspecific immune response against similar mycobacteria would not be expected to augment the response which already exists. Such an effect is known as 'masking'. In some parts of the tropics the effect of BCG might be being masked by prior exposure to exactly these other environmental mycobacteria. Some clinical evidence for this phenomenon has been revealed in a series of studies which were carried out in parallel with adolescent school children in both the UK and Malawi.[95] The UK school children were shown to have a generally low baseline cellular immunity to mycobacteria which was then seen to increase after administering BCG; in contrast, the Malawi school children were seen to have a high existing baseline cellular immunity to mycobacteria and this was not significantly increased by BCG at all. Whether this existing natural immune response might also be protective against *M. tuberculosis*, however, is unfortunately not known, but, based on epidemiological evidence it is unfortunately probably unlikely.

Despite all of this, until recently no real effort at all had been made regarding the development of new vaccines for TB whilst there has been much effort expended on developing vaccines and vaccination programmes for other diseases. There have been several reasons for this.

In 2008 the World Health Organization undertook a prioritisation exercise to better focus new research and development in the field. What appeared at the top of their list was a perceived need for new influenza vaccines. The bitter experiences of the 'flu pandemic just one year later only seemed to support their conclusions, apparently proving how valuable it would have been to have had an existing influenza vaccine that was cross-protective against all strains and which could thus generate long-lasting immunity from the constant on-going threat from ever-mutating highly infectious

[95] Rodrigues LC, Diwan VK, Wheeler JG - "Protective Effect of BCG against Tuberculous Meningitis and Miliary Tuberculosis: A Meta-Analysis", International Journal of Epidemiology 22; 6 (1993) 1154–8.

influenza. It still does remain unclear, however, exactly how feasible such a cross-protective vaccine might be.

In fact, if the prioritisation for development of new vaccines had been finalised purely on the basis of the existing global burdens of disease, and most particularly concerning mortality rates, then HIV, tuberculosis and malaria should all be at the top of any list, not influenza, so the prime candidacy of influenza in the WHO's poll has to be, to some degree, a perplexing choice.

A supposedly innovative finding solution was developed to help promote such general vaccine development. It is known as "Advanced Market Commitment" (AMC). This involves a donor or group of donors agreeing to subsidize the future purchase of a new vaccine if it can be developed effectively and is then being demanded by developing countries. Such an agreement is intended to be legally binding as long as the final product is successfully developed, the idea being to incentivise the private sector to develop a product for the public good. As donors to the development of the product, governments promise to purchase a certain quantity of the future vaccine at a set price, and then after a pre-agreed number of vaccines had been purchased, the originator companies would have to provide the vaccines at a pre-agreed price.

This model must have been seen by many as an exciting way forwards, since it promised to promote research but still put a high risk on the developers who have to design a treatment that meets a prior specification at their own cost whilst the donor only has to pay for results. It has hardly proved to have been an overarching success, however, with some of its principle features sometimes mysteriously disappearing into the mist.

A pilot AMC was launched by the GAVI Alliance in 2009 and paid for by Italy, the UK, Norway, Russia, Canada and the Bill & Melinda Gates Foundation, with the aim to accelerate the roll-out in developing countries of a vaccine for pneumococcal disease. It offered US$1.5 billion as an incentive for the development of a new pneumococcal vaccine under the terms of an AMC. Somehow this AMC shifted from incentivising the development of a new product that had not yet been invented (as intended), to purchasing two vaccines that were already in development, one produced by Wyeth and one by GlaxoSmithKline. Because these two vaccines were already substantially advanced, the AMC didn't have to match the costs of their early stage development meaning that the financial commitment that had been made had been grossly over-estimated. At one point, MSF estimated that the total sum put forward for the AMC would result in about one billion dollars in profits for Wyeth and GSK – of which at least six hundred million dollars constituted excess profits over and above what the companies would have usually generated. MSF's analysis also suggested that this pilot AMC has not paid enough importance to ensuring any proper competition from developing country producers, even though such competition can lower vaccine costs and would have been a desirable outcome.

As a mechanism to incentivise new development to meet a specific need, then, the AMC had patently failed, although, it's possible that the two vaccines would never have made it through to the final stages of development without the AMC being available. Either way, the two companies made handsome profits for their shareholders out of the wheeling a dealing.

To date no AMCs have yet been struck on new TB vaccines. The situation regarding researching new vaccimnes has been changing, however. In 2012, Dr Peter Small from the Bill and Melinda Gates Foundation summed the situation up as follows:

> "Ten years ago, all the TB vaccine researchers in the world would have fit into a minivan."

Meanwhile he reckoned that as many as 500 researchers worldwide had been switching their focus and moving into this field of research. "The awareness has changed," he reported.

As many as ten new candidate vaccines against TB are said to be currently moving through developmental stages, and two immune-therapeutic vaccines are in trial as well.[96] Today, 107 years after the initial development of the BCG vaccine, a new, effective and affordable TB vaccine certainly could present the world with a major new tool with which to control the disease. From the perspective of its manufacturer, a newly patented vaccine should be an extremely profitable product, particularly if the progress gained in reducing the general burden of global disease reverses as is feared by some – or more probably if the perceived threat from drug-resistant disease remains the same or grows, as it almost certainly will. One thing is for sure, though – modern ethical standards make such research many times more challenging than they ever were for Jenner with his cowpox, or indeed for Calmette and Guérin with their BCG.

---

[96] WHO - "Global Tuberculosis Report 2013". (This number has recently been reduced: it was 11 in the previous 2012 report.)

But there are other implicit problems which may make such possible profit extremely hard to come by. One is that, unlike many infectious diseases, acquired immunity to TB does not seem to be lifelong – and in fact may be not much more than transitory. Another is the simple frustrating fact that someone can be infected by TB and can then develop either primary or re-activated TB, and can have such active disease for months or even years without showing any serious symptoms: any slow-burning disease like this has to be massively harder to control or eradicate by vaccination than are the far faster developing diseases like smallpox or measles.

Until recently it was being genuinely hoped that there might be a new vaccine available by 2019. There was particularly high anticipation being promoted in late 2012 for one which was being developed by the so-called the 'Oxford Group', or more formally the 'Oxford-Emergent Consortium'. Both Phase I and preclinical trials of the vaccine had looked very promising, but a Phase II 'proof-of-concept' trial in South Africa which studied the response in nearly 3,000 infants offered no statistical differences between the group who had received the vaccine and the one which had received a placebo. The only good news seemed to be that it was proved to be safe. The results sent the research team back to the drawing board, determined not to see the fruits of their hard work totally dismissed.

Their vaccine was administered (for ethical reasons) to all of the children a few months after receiving the BCG vaccination, and it has been validly argued that this earlier vaccine may have provided an existing plateau of protection which effectively skewed all of the anticipated results. Also rates of TB in the Western Cape of South Africa are recognised to be so exceptionally high that such a high force of infection "may be difficult to address with any vaccine".[97] In view of this, it has been proposed that the trial was not conducted in the best environment, and that these same results might not be seen in another population of children somewhere else, nor possibly in older subjects (and these also present the greater risk of infecting others since children are rarely infectious so might be as valid a target group for a vaccination programme). In response to both of these ideas, the vaccine is being simultaneously re-evaluated in HIV-infected adults in both Senegal and South Africa.

From the perspective of the developing world, however, where latent infection runs so high, it has to be recognised that the benefit of a new vaccine might be largely inconsequential for at least a generation – apart from for infants. Its impact could still be substantial however. A recent

[97] WHO - "Global Tuberculosis Report 2013".

study modelled the potential impact of a new vaccine with just a 60% efficacy rate in children if it was administered in South East Asia and it was suggested that it could "contribute a significant decline by 2050". And if a vaccine could be developed and administered to both adolescents and adults as well, then the impact on the pandemic would be "much larger". A subsequent remodelling of this same study assessed the global impact of a new adult/adolescent vaccine with this same 60% level of efficacy and it resulted in an estimate that potentially 30-50 million new cases could be averted over a 25 year period.

Such a positive possible prospect can hardly sniffed at if a vaccine of this type can be developed, but there is honestly not that high a degree of optimism about this. The most recent WHO report suggests that there is currently too much similarity in the immunological strategies that are being pursued for much progress to be likely to be made and encouraged the alternative investigation of a "different and novel immunological space", whatever that might ultimately prove to be.

If four out of every five people in Africa are already latently infected with TB, no conventional vaccine in the world can hope to protect the majority of the continent's existing population, and any short term impact would almost certainly be low. Vaccines simply don't normally work by protecting people from an infection which they already have; they work by preventing people from an infection in the first place (something which is technically referred known as 'pre-exposure' vaccination). This same problem, of course, applies to the other one-and-a-half billion people worldwide who are currently estimated to be latently infected.

There is only one real answer for these 2.3 billion people who are estimated to be at immediate risk of developing the disease. It would need to be a vaccine that would be able to prevent primary re-activation of TB into infectious disease from latency. This is what is known as a 'post-exposure" vaccine.

These are the types of vaccines which are very effectively used, for example, with rabies or tetanus infections, when they are applied immediately after initial exposure. It's pretty clear when one has been bitten by a dog, or trodden on a rusty nail – the experience is immediate and it is obvious. But after sharing a bus with someone who coughs a little carelessly? Or after being in an elevator with someone who looks a bit pale and who sneezes as she passes by?

TB, as we know, can take years to develop to the stage when symptoms become obvious and for that initial moment of infection to finally reveal itself as active and potentially lethal disease. A post-exposure vaccine would have to be applicable and effective possibly years after the initial infection for it to be effective for tuberculosis. It would almost certainly constitute one of the most remarkable medical discoveries of the century if it can be achieved. Exactly this ***is*** being attempted nevertheless. The best report of progress so far has seen a slight delay in disease development in animals.[98] This slowing down of disease progression was also unfortunately only determined to be transient to the extent that no final differences in long-term survival were seen. In fact, given that the disease seems to harvest advantage from its slow development, such a further slowing down just might even do a further favour to the bacilli as much as it might favour the host as is intended. It might not do so, of course, so even such a limited response should not be rejected out of hand. In the event of a particular virulent or volatile poly drug-resistant or extremely drug-resistant outbreak, for instance, such a post-exposure vaccine could potentially slow down disease progression long enough for drug-susceptibility testing to be appropriately completed and for effective chemotherapy to be initiated in time for better outcomes.

Finally, the somewhat uncomfortable reality, which should not be ignored, is that any new conventional vaccine would paradoxically be of most benefit to those who are least threatened by the disease since they would by definition be living in environments that are less exposed and have lowest rates of existing infection in their communities and, therefore, also much lower prevalence rates of latent infection. As such, a conventional vaccine would still offer remarkable immediate potential for such populations, not least in terms of profitable return to the owners of its patent and to their shareholders since it could thus be marketed for the benefit of those best able to afford it at a good price. This would be particularly the case if fears of resistance or new virulent strains could be appropriately promoted or manipulated. Large batches could then be ordered either to be stock-piled or administered as required. Something very similar almost certainly occurred with the Tamiflu anti-viral drug, whose initial manufacturer (Gilead Health Sciences) had Donald Rumsfeld on its board. Rumsfeld was repeatedly requested to step down from his post on the board because of conflicts of interest as US Secretary of Defence, but he resisted the pressures and chose not to do so.

---

[98] Henao-Tamayo M et al. – "Post-exposure vaccination against Mycobacterium tuberculosis", Tuberculosis (Edinburgh) 89;2 (2009) 142-8.

It should also be recalled that new and untested vaccines were very rapidly implemented at the behest of the WHO during the recent H5N1 scare, with potential liabilities having to be shared by the national health authorities as well as by the drug companies who manufactured them as would normally be the case. The European Medicines Agency (EMEA), for instance, granted marketing authorisation to two swine flu vaccines (Focetria produced by Novartis, and Pandemrix produced by GlaxoSmithKline). This authorisation was given in spite of the fact the vaccines, according to some authorities, had not been properly tested. The EMEA itself was said at that time to be two-thirds funded by pharmaceutical companies so there were incontrovertible conflicts in its actions. And Pandemrix, at least, has been identified to have created adverse effects in the years since this rushed introduction.

Multi Drug-Resistant and Extensively Drug-Resistant TB

"THE ONLY THING [THAT MDR-TB] HAS IN COMMON WITH THE OLD TB IS THE LETTERS 'T' AND 'B' – THE DRUGS ARE NEW, THE WAYS OF MONITORING PATIENTS ARE NEW, AND THE PATIENTS ARE MORE DIFFICULT TO TREAT."

Dr Ernesto Jaramillo[99]

Multi drug-resistant tuberculosis (MDR-TB) is defined as tuberculosis disease which has confirmed simultaneous resistance to both Isoniazid and Rifampicin, the two strongest TB drugs. Essentially this means firstly that it is resistant to more than 50% of the therapeutic package delivered by the four first line drugs, and secondly it means that that the older and harder-to-tolerate second line drugs need to be resorted to along with much longer treatment regimes.

Extensively drug-resistant tuberculosis (XDR-TB) is defined as MDR-TB with additional resistance – firstly to any fluoroquinolone and secondly to at least one of three of the injectable drugs used for TB treatment – capreomycin, kanamycin, or amikacin.

These are currently the only two 'official' classifications of drug-resistance, although there are further unofficially recognised terms describing degrees of resistance which we will look at shortly.

The insidious development of bacterial drug-resistance is sometimes rather chillingly described as if it is almost a skill which can be passed between bacilli, as if they were super intelligent mini-organisms. Whilst there ***is*** evidence that bacteria can communicate with each other to the extent that resistance to a drug can sometimes be acquired by one species of bacteria by its having previously been acquired by another, there is little or no evidence that this occurs with TB. In the case of *M. tuberculosis* the resistance is believed to occur when individual mutant bacilli, which occur naturally in any bacterial population, turn out by chance to confer natural resistance to a drug which might be being used against them, and so are then further naturally selected by either inadequate or interrupted drug

[99] WHO Medical Officer in charge of MDR-TB policy.

treatment which allows them to flourish whilst other non-mutant bacilli are otherwise destroyed.

Such mutation can occur in various ways. It often initially happens, for instance, as a result of a chance collision between a part of a strand of DNA and a stray particle zipping in from outer space, or indeed from radioactive particles from closer to home. At other times such changes occur as a result of chance errors occurring whilst DNA is replicating. Quite infrequently they may also occur in the course of transfer of DNA among bacteria. Whatever the source or the cause, the effect is the same – a tiny change takes place in the inherited DNA which most often is of no consequence at all so no self-selective advantage is acquired by the mutated organism from the event. More often than not, in fact, such a mutation actually leaves it with a handicap, or an environmental disadvantage, so that the mutated gene will simply not survive at all in subsequent generations. Sometimes, however, a mutation creates a genetic change which can make a real difference from that generation onwards. If it gives it some specific competitive advantage over its fellow life forms the chances are that the mutation will be passed on naturally again and again.

Exactly something of this nature happens from time to time to TB bacilli: they can be randomly changed by a tiny chance mutation in a way which leaves them incrementally less vulnerable to the drug which has been developed, tried and tested to destroy them – and as a result they proportionately flourish instead of succumbing to the targeted chemical assault that is made against them, in contrast to their non-mutant fellow bacteria which succumb to the drug as intended. Clinically significant resistance is defined as allowing *in vitro* growth of bacilli in the laboratory in the presence of a critical concentration of a particular drug – growth which is equal to or greater than 1% of the growth in the absence of the drug which hardly sounds an awful lot. It seems that mutant TB bacteria need little in the way of opportunity to develop into a serious problem.

The use of antimicrobial TB drugs offers any targeted bacteria what amounts to an unnatural man-made selective device which can favour mutant organisms if they are rendered resistant as a result of the mutation, and, as a result, the resistant bacteria may come to dominate and the standard treatments begin to be seen to fail. In complete contrast to the initial mutation (which involved a random genetic event) this subsequent development of the resistant strain is entirely pre-determinable, and generally reflects the extent of the use of the drug, the way it is used or misused, and the effectiveness of any accompanying infection control.

Once established they may then develop into an infectious basecamp for a new strain of potentially untreatable disease to infect others

Such mutations may be spontaneous but the probability of them occurring has been calculated so as to be mathematically predictable. What this means is that mutations which cause resistance to a single drug occur in about 1 in 10^8 replications of bacteria. Such mutations are totally unlinked in terms of their resistance to different drugs, so such a development of resistance is usually totally irrelevant for another unrelated drug, or at least for another drug group as they are usually classified. The probability of spontaneous mutation causing resistance to two drugs together at the same time (i.e. both Isoniazid and Rifampicin to confer the strain the status of being MDR-TB for instance) would thus be $10^8 \times 10^8 = 10^{16}$. The fundamental fact that such mutations are not pharmaceutically linked underpins the cardinal principle underlying the current multi-drug chemotherapy of TB because the survival of a strain that is resistant to a single drug is logically many times more likely to occur if only a single drug is used, and is mathematically far less likely to occur when two or more drugs are used. It is even less likely to happen if a combination therapy of four drugs is applied, especially if they are applied rigorously, since strains which by chance become resistant to one of the drugs being applied are almost guaranteed to be destroyed by the other three active drugs before being able to really develop into any form of infectious colony of mono-resistant bugs or to mutate further to become poly drug-resistant. Such mutations are therefore highly unlikely to ever successfully or substantially propagate. If these drugs are not applied rigorously, however, the chance of such propagation happening becomes much higher, and the likelihood of multi drug-resistant strains emerging increases incrementally.

One logical assumption that can be made from this all of this is that any mutation is more likely to occur in a patient with a higher bacillary load simply because there will be more bacteria replicating and therefore a higher likelihood of mutation occurring. This does not always seem to be the case, however, since HIV-positive TB cases with low bacillary loads are widely recognised to have an especially high risk of developing drug-resistant disease.

We already know that *M. tuberculosis* replicates slowly in comparison to other bacteria, so all of this takes time to happen. The risk is cumulative, however, and it soon evolves into a process that, unlike the first mutation, is far from spontaneous – it is completely predictable: the more treatment courses patients are given which are not comprehensively completed, the stronger and more widespread the resistance is likely to become. In Eastern

Europe and in Asia widespread pharmaceutical malpractice made emergent multi drug-resistant strains totally predictable and also that much more common. At first this was far less likely to occur in a region such as Africa where, despite the pandemic already being more appalling, the newer drugs were being introduced much later and were being much less used.

Resistance has been seen to develop at identifiable points on the bacteria's DNA. Since this knowledge helps diagnosticians know where to look for it most efficiently with their newer diagnostic tools it remains a challenging task. Attempting to properly understand this very quickly becomes both more technical and more complicated.

Getting straight down to the technicalities, Codon 531 of the *rpoB* gene (rpoB531) has been found to be the most frequent mutation associated with Rifampicin resistance (an estimated 97% of the time in fact).[100] Codon 315 of the *katG* gene (katG315), however, is found to be the most frequent mutation associated with Isoniazid resistance (90% of the time). Other genes in which mutation for Isoniazid can occur, however, are *ahpC* and *KasA*. Both Isoniazid and ethionamide (one of the second line drugs) also share a common resistant target gene which is the *inhA* gene, and so, as a result, resistance to Isoniazid due to *inhA* mutation is also associated with possible resistance to ethionamide. All in all there are in fact six codons (rpoB531, rpoB526, rrs513, rpsL43, embB306, and katG315) which are recognised to be the main locations responsible for MDR-TB.

Meanwhile mutations in other *rpsi* and *rrs* genes are responsible for Streptomycin resistance and a mutation in one of the *embB* genes can be responsible for Ethambutol resistance while changes in the *pncA* gene can make for resistance to Pyrazinamide. But, frustratingly, as many as 120 different Pyrazinamide-resistant mutations have so far been identified.

What this adds up to is that, if you want to look for resistance to Rifampicin (the most effective drug) you may only have to look in one place. But if you want to really look for MDR-TB and XDR-TB with any degree of certainty you have to look in a few other places as well. This has huge implications for the other new PCR diagnostic methods. It explains as well, not just the reliability of the GeneXpert device in confirming

[100] The recent finding that a third of Rifampicin resistant cases are potentially being missed in Indian strains of TB is probably because of the resistance occurring at a different location in the gene. If this is so this particular estimate will require revision.

Rifampicin resistance, but also why it is unable to confirm resistance to any other drug.

It may also be that resistance may be seen at low concentration of a drug, but that using higher concentrations of the same drug is still useful. Such an approach is often used with Isoniazid, one of the most effective first line drugs, particularly since it has been found to be the best of the essential anti-TB drugs in preventing resistance in companion drugs due to its high bactericidal activity and its large therapeutic margins.

> "What's so frustrating about this progression is that it is a totally man-made disease"

So says Dr Lucica Ditiu, the current Executive Secretary of the WHO's Stop TB Partnership whilst expressing her frustration at the resistant bacteria's growing proliferation in the presence of the man-made drugs that are intended to kill it.

> "The doctors, the health care workers, the nurses, entire health care systems have produced MDR-TB. It's not a bug that has come from nature. It's not a spontaneous mutation. It came about because patients were treated badly – either with poor quality drugs, or not enough drugs, or with insufficient observation so the patient didn't finish the treatment course."

Even this may be an over-simplification, however, because multi drug-resistance is now recognised as being able to develop even when adherence to treatment and patient care is excellent. It just may be that the non-compliant patient has been the easy scapegoat to avoid confronting far more complex phenomena than had been previously considered.[101]

Several such factors have been suggested to potentially explain this, including 'active efflux', 'pharmacokinetic mismatches' between individuals, or even instances of localised immunopathology in a patient's lung (resulting in sub-optimal drug penetration into granulomas and cavities). All of these might drive site-specific drug concentrations below the minimum concentrations which are vital to inhibit the development of resistance.

'Active efflux' is an intracellular mechanism which removes toxic substances (which can include antibiotics) out of the cells, pumping them

---

[101] Calver AD, Falmer AA, Murray M et al. - "Emergence of increased resistance and extensively drug-resistant tuberculosis despite treatment adherence, South Africa", Emerging Infectious Diseases 16 (2010) 264-71.

out through specific 'efflux pumps'. Most antibiotics are easily recognized by such pumps which, if activated, then reduce their effect. Some efflux systems are drug-specific, while others can accommodate multiple drugs simultaneously – so these could contribute to multi drug-resistance with just a single pump.

Such low level efflux pumps effectively protect the bacilli during several rounds of their replication, allowing the eventual generation of mutations associated with high-level acquired drug-resistance to occur. It is a process which has been called the 'antibiotic resistance arrow of time', with (at least in the laboratory) sub-therapeutic drug concentrations initiating a one-directional sequence of events. The first step induces the action of these efflux pumps, the final step sees the development of genetic mutations which might be drug-resistant.

This 'arrow of time' model assumes that efflux pumps will be induced within hours of the occurrence of a low concentration of one or more drugs. Within days this can have amplified to a low-level resistance created by several efflux pumps being at work together allowing bacteria to replicate in the face of what amounts to a monotherapy. Within weeks this can escalate to high level resistance due to mutations developing at specific locations on the gene amounting to a viable mutant sub-population of as little as 1% of the total bacterial population.

The phenomenon of 'pharmokinetic mismatches' presents a further complication. These can, at least theoretically, occur in any combination drug treatment and,in such scenarios, several factors interplay. One relates to a shorter half-life of one of the drugs in the combination treatment. This creates a fluctuating chemotherapeutic potency, leaving one companion drug (the one with a longer half-life) temporarily holding the fort as a mono-therapy.[102] Another factor relates to the natural variability in rates of drug metabolism between patients, creating possible sub-therapeutic concentrations of each drug as well as variability in absorption rates.

Together, these variables appear to lead to low drug concentrations of one or more drugs in the available regimen in some patients (again effectively becoming equivalent to a monotherapy). The bacteria can then adapt to these concentrations, initially through the induction of several of those efflux pumps. Such situations are now accepted as being able to cause

[102] Mitchison DA - "How drug resistance emerges as a result of poor compliance during short course chemotherapy for tuberculosis", the International Journal of Tuberculosis and Lung Disease, 2 (1998) 10-15.

sequential acquisition of drug-resistant mutations, with multidrug-resistant and even extensively drug-resistant tuberculosis developing due to an accumulation of mutations acquired one at a time. Such theoretical ideas have arisen from data from laboratory experiments, from clinical trial simulations, and from prospective clinical studies. When viewed together they provide support for a growing suspicion that such biological variabilities may be as much the main culprit for the emergence of multidrug-resistant tuberculosis as treatment mismanagement, although such an idea is far from universally accepted. If this idea is true, however, then innovative new methods are going to be needed to optimally dose patients.

It will require further studies to establish just how significant these technical factors may have been in the emergence of drug-resistance so far. It may prove to be not much more than a technical smoke-screen intended to take some of the pressure off the patient who has been so consistently blamed by many experts for the development of disease. To some degree this has already been done by increasingly recognising that it has been as much or more the fault of the system of treatment implementation as it may have been the fault of the recalcitrant patient. There still remains institutional resistance, however, to such revisionist ideas especially from those who have most political investment in the systems already in use.

It should be well remembered that, for some years in the 1990s and after, it was being entirely illogically argued by many experts that DOTS alone could control the growth of MDR-TB. Experts can be expected to get things wrong from time to time.

Whilst acquired drug-resistance has been known for several years now to occur even under strict supervision, many public health researchers and doctors still choose to believe that poor adherence accounts for most cases of acquired drug-resistance. Recent studies, however, have challenged this - directly examining the role of lack of adherence in emergence of drug-resistance during standard short-course chemotherapy. Their findings were surprising and they continue to challenge the fundamental ideas which underpin most orthodox understandings of the drug-resistant pandemic. Therapeutic failure was seen to occur only when more than 60% of doses were missed, but no multi drug-resistant isolates were reported in patients with lack of adherence except for some transient mono-resistance which was seen to disappear with time.[103] Findings from a follow-up study that used animals also showed no emergence of multi drug-resistant tuberculosis from subjects with high rates of non-adherence.[104] Such findings, together with those reports of acquired drug-resistance even under strict supervision seriously suggest that pharmacokinetic variability could possibly be the main cause for acquired drug-resistance.

Further complexities arise in consideration of the strains of disease themselves. Findings from a 2013 study showed that 'lineage 2' (to which the so-called Beijing strain belongs) had much higher mutation rates than did 'lineage 4' (which has been more common in Western Europe and the USA).[105] In view of this finding, the emergence of MDR-TB has been calculated to be a worrying 22 times more likely for lineage 2 than for lineage 4, to the extent that multi drug-resistance can even be predicted to pre-exist in some patients originally infected with a drug-susceptible strain even before therapy has been initiated.[106]

Ruth McNerney, an expert on tuberculosis at the London School of Hygiene and Tropical Medicine, added a warning of her own regarding DR-TB in 2012.[107]

> "We can't afford this genie to get out of the bag. Because once it has, I don't know how we'll control TB."

---

[103] Srivastava S, Pasipanodya JG, Meek C, Leff R, Gumbo T - "Multidrug-resistant tuberculosis not due to noncompliance but to between-patient pharmacokinetic variability", Journal of Infectious Diseases, 204 (2011) 1951-9.

[104] de Steenwinkel JE, ten Kate MT, de Knegt GJ, et al. - "Consequences of noncompliance for therapy efficacy and emergence of resistance in murine tuberculosis caused by the Beijing genotype of Mycobacterium tuberculosis", Antimicrobial Agents and Chemotherapy, 56 (2012) 4937-44.

[105] The issue of the 'lineages'of MTBC will be discussed further in a later section.

[106] Ford CB, Shah RR, Maeda MK, et al. - "Mycobacterium tuberculosis mutation rate estimates from different lineages predict substantial differences in the emergence of drug-resistant tuberculosis", Nature Genetics, 14 (2013) 784-90.

[107] http://www.reuters.com/article/2012/03/19/us-tuberculosis-idUSBRE82I0D820120319

The likelihood is, unfortunately, that the genie almost certainly had already escaped a significant time before she made this statement and a long time before these more sophisticated understandings of the development of drug-resistance were developed. This is even more likely in relation to the invisible epidemic of latent disease because a further problem exists in respect of this part of the pandemic: no current test can identify drug-resistance in a latent case. As a result the amount of drug-resistance which exists within the huge pool of existing latent disease remains immeasurable and generally unestimated. We will see in a later section what possibilities may exist because of this.

Furthermore, since drug-resistance develops gradually as bacilli populations fluctuate, both resistant and susceptible bacilli can be readily expected to be present together in a patient during the early stages of the development of resistance. This can make it very difficult to identify resistance in the early stages of its development in any active case.

What is becoming very clear is that the fundamental dynamics of the development of resistance are still far from universally understood or accepted. Without far better understandings, along with relevant public health policies to address them, it is difficult to see how any genie could have ever been be kept in any bag. The epidemiological situation, much like the fluctuating populations of susceptible and resistant bacilli in a patient, is itself in a state of flux – and it is one that is far from easy to judge at any moment given that so many variables may be at play, not least of which is the matter of there being different levels of resistance.

Definitions of resistance

"It's like dealing with a new disease."

Dr Ernesto Jaramillo[108]

Before we take a more in-depth look at the potential issues which begin to reveal themselves as this drug-resistant phenomenon emerges from its murky genetic depths, we must deepen our general understanding of DR-TB a little further. We need to be able to discriminate a little in order to

[108] WHO Medical Officer in charge of MDR-TB policy.

appropriately distinguish and properly appreciate the varying forms in which this resistant phenomenon of disease can manifest – variations that have huge impact on how we should be interpreting the signs within the current epidemic, as well as on how such resistant disease might possibly best be treated where resources are endemically deficient.

A drug-resistant patient must first and foremost be fundamentally classified as to how his or her resistance arose. Such an infection is classified essentially either as being 'primary' or 'acquired'. 'Primary' resistance occurs in a patient who has never received any anti-TB treatment previously. 'Acquired' resistance is that which occurs as a result of, or at least subsequent to specific previous drug treatment for TB.

The WHO and the IUATLD have recently reclassified both of these terms – replacing the term primary resistance with the more self-evident '**drug-resistance among new cases**', and replacing acquired resistance with the term '**drug-resistance among previously treated cases**'. These definitions may seem clumsy but the implicit differences between these two types of resistance are not just made clearer with these terms, they highlight the immensity of their epidemiological differences as well. The first term indicates the existence of a strain of drug-resistance that is loose in a community because it has almost certainly been caught off someone else and then gone through the usual process of disease development before showing itself; the second is a strain which may not yet be in the community because the resistance may have developed within the patient during previous treatment (although it could technically still be a re-infection from an individual in the community).

We next need to look at the further various degrees of drug-resistance, each of which could themselves be either acquired or primary. Various terms have been proposed and used but a usable set of definitions is, rather surprisingly, still not agreed upon. Some of the commonly used terms, in fact, remain, at least for now, controversial. They are listed below, along with a short commentary against each.

We can start by simply defining disease which is NOT known to be resistant to any existing drugs. This is straightforward, **drug-susceptible TB** or **drug-sensitive TB (DS-TB)** which can be expected to be effectively treated by the four first line drugs. This category also could include discrete mycobacterial strains of tuberculosis, as defined by culture testing, some of which are much more common (and more dangerous) than others. *M. africanum* would be an example.

The first definition of resistance itself is also the most general and simple. It is just **drug-resistant TB (DR-TB)** which offers us a broad and non-specific description of any strain with known drug-resistance.

The next descriptor defines tuberculosis which is specifically resistant to just one single drug – usefully termed **single drug-resistant TB** or **mono drug-resistant**. This could technically be Rifampicin resistant TB as identified by the GeneXpert device. The GeneXpert has in fact spawned the separate acronym RR-TB (for **Rifampicin-resistant tuberculosis**). If the diagnosis is made with the GeneXpert the possibility that the case is MDR–TB must not be excluded and is even indicated as a likelihood. The GeneXpert can only identify resistance to this one drug, however, but it has been found to be only rarely mono drug-resistant. Should this strain indeed be resistant to ***only*** Rifampicin it may well succumb to the other first line drugs, three of which will remain effective, although it will most probably require longer treatment periods for full cure. Resistance to Rifampicin in particular also offers a poorer prognosis for the patient compared with the other possibilities contained within this definition of mono drug-resistance since Rifampicin is the strongest of the existing TB drugs.

Such single drug-resistance as picked up by the GeneXpert, however, also means that the strain is probably resistant to another one of the most commonly used first line drugs including Isoniazid (with this second resistance remaining completely invisible to the GeneXpert).

To complicate things a little further, one particular type of mono drug-resistant TB could actually just be 'normal' bovine TB (*M. bovis*) which is known to be unresponsive (and therefore effectively already resistant) to Pyrazinamide.

The next loose term is **poly drug-resistance (PDR-TB)** which can usefully describe any strain of disease which is resistant to more than a single drug.

Multi drug-resistance (**MDR-TB**) comes next in a growing list of escalating complexity. MDR-TB represents the most common problematic type that presents real challenges to treatment. It is also an official classification, and is defined as any strain that has confirmed simultaneous resistance to both Isoniazid and Rifampicin, the two strongest and most effective TB drugs. Essentially this means that this strain is resistant to more than 50% of the therapeutic package delivered by those four first line drugs.

Extensively drug-resistant tuberculosis (XDR-TB) is the next – defined as MDR-TB with two additional specific resistances, and this is the only other official classification of drug-resistance. Firstly it is resistant to any fluoroquinolone and secondly to at least one of three injectable second line drugs used for TB treatment – capreomycin, kanamycin, or amikacin. This strain is less common, but is also much, much harder to treat with far higher rates of mortality.

Dr Mario Raviglione, the Director of the WHO Stop TB Department, has chillingly suggested that:

> "XDR-TB is probably the worst thing we could ever have imagined."

Current success rates in its treatment are unfortunately very low.

It will be observed that there is a further category that falls between these last two types – these patients who are MDR-TB but who are also resistant either to another first line drug or to one single second line drug. A study in 2012 showed that, of 1,278 patients with MDR-TB, some 43.7% had resistance to at least one second line drug as well, but they did not have resistance to the requisite two of the second line drug necessary for them to be categorised as XDR-TB. The percentage of actual XDR-TB identified in this study was at a far lower level at 6.7% so this 'in-between' level of resistance may well involve a huge number of cases.[109]

It has been very reasonably suggested because of this study that the extent of MDR-TB with additional resistance to a single second line drug may well be being dangerously ignored, as well as remaining un-represented in almost all surveys. Apart from creating possible additional challenges to clinical management, this 'in-between' level of drug-resistance also adds understandable confusions as *ad hoc* terms are adopted in response. Most importantly of all, however this 43.7% (if it a typical proportion) provides a potentially lethal pool for one further mutation into more deadly XDR-TB. It is certainly a category that is insufficiently discussed or sought out. The rather vague term proposed for this a category is "**MDR-plus TB**" – and another possibly more useful term which is occasionally used is "**pre-XDR-TB**". Neither of these terms is officially accepted or adopted however.

---

[109] Dalton T - "Prevalence of and risk factors for resistance to second line drugs in people with multidrug-resistant tuberculosis in eight countries: a prospective cohort study", The Lancet, 30 August 2012. www.thelancet.com/journals/lancet/article/ [last accesses 30/4/2013].

There is a logical reason why this pre-XDR phenomenon appears to be so neglected, and it is to do with clinical treatment and predicted patient response to approved treatments rather than simply because of semantic oversight. With MDR-TB, a total of six drugs are used for the intensive phase of treatment, with four of them still in the mix for the longer continuation phase. The intention is that the intensive phase of all treatment regimens should, similarly for the treatment of drug-susceptible TB, always contain at least four drugs with certain effectiveness, but, if this is not possible, then at least three of them should definitely still be effective. Such is the case with mono-resistant strains when only three of the four drugs will be effective, but it is essentially the same thing with pre-XDR-TB. This same three-drug scenario can be assumed to be the case using a standard MDR-TB treatment; with full-blown XDR-TB, however, this is definitely is not the case, so additional modifications to treatment protocols are needed.

Patients might even be resistant to three or even all four of the first line drugs, of course. In such cases the same principles would apply – the four active second line drugs introduced as a package for treating MDR-TB (which this would still be defined as) would be assumed to be adequately effective as a combination to treat such a condition.

What remains concerning, however, about the epidemiological neglect of this level of pre-XDR resistance is that, as a result, a very important question associated with this particular resistance commonly gets ignored: exactly how did such patients who have developed resistance to any single second line drug acquire it in the first place – or rather, exactly how did the MDR-TB bacillus experience sufficient exposure to a second line drug to develop such resistance? The question may not be relevant to the treatment of the individual patient, but it is highly relevant to the local epidemic, and is particularly pertinent in any environments in which such second line drugs are not in common use for TB, because it implies several possibilities. One is that the drugs may be being dangerously mismanaged in the treatment of TB or even other infectious conditions, either by clinicians or by pharmacists. Another is that this resistance may have been primarily acquired from an infectious source – potentially, for example, from migrant workers who may have been in a country where second line drugs are more regularly used or misused – and who are therefore technically on the loose in an essentially vulnerable community without available second line drugs, capable of infecting others with a potentially untreatable strain of TB which carries a mutational advantage over local strains of disease.

From here, we move on to further levels of resistance. Dr Raviglione's suggestion that XDR-TB might be the worst thing imaginable seems to be rendered a little optimistic given that there are worse levels still, though all of these currently remain only unofficially defined.

The next level of resistance attempts to identify strains of disease which are more resistant still than XDR-TB. This is an unofficial term known as **extremely drug-resistant TB** (**XXDR-TB**) – disease which is resistant to more than four of the drugs as defined by XDR-TB – in other words, which is even more resistant still. This is a more recent classification reflecting the way the DR-TB has been developing but it has been around for years nevertheless. It remains a loose one. There are a total of nearly 20 compounds which are recognised as being in some way effective for treating the disease, though most, as we have seen, tend to be co-resistant so are classified into groups. There is therefore plenty of theoretical scope for potential combinations of 'extreme' resistance, any of which should generally be predicated by the quantities of any individual anti-TB drug which is in use in a community.

The final classification has been used most recently both by the media as well as in some medical papers. It is used to describe the potentially apocalyptic strain of disease which is called **totally drug-resistant** (**TDR-TB**). Sometimes such a strain is also referred to as being **pan-resistant**. Effectively it is a strain which is pharmaceutically untreatable. Such strains can be best defined as being resistant to all current drugs that are known to be effective in the treatment of TB. Patients infected with what has thus been called TDR-TB have been positively identified in India in 2012, and also possibly previously to this in both Iran and Italy. Further cases have since also been identified in South Africa.

In March 2012 the WHO convened 40 experts to discuss the implications of this strain. They particularly wanted to decide whether current evidence made it necessary or even possible to officially define patterns of drug-resistance beyond extensively drug-resistance TB (XDR-TB) and, if so, whether better guidance on appropriate treatment options for these patients was possible as well. While the group acknowledged that patients such as those described in Mumbai pose a formidable challenge to clinicians and public health authorities, no reliable definition beyond XDR-TB could be agreed upon or proposed. There were no references at all to such cases in the 2013 report, a silence which suggests that, at least for now, these categories are being officially ignored.

This may seem baffling, since it would appear to offer the bacillus an opportunity to lumber off ahead of the clinicians in desperate pursuit of it. To some extent there exists an understandable reluctance for the medical community to publicly accept that such a strain might exist since it indicates the realisation of an extreme pharmacological nightmare that has been genuinely dreaded by the WHO – one that is genuinely worse than what was being anticipated by Dr Raviglione.

Certainly, until its appearance, its possible development was viewed by most as a mathematical improbability. A few years before the confirmation of the existence of such strains, however, the mere possibility that they might occur had already been recognised and had prompted Dr Margaret Chan, the Director General of the WHO, to call such a phenomenon the "return to the pre-antibiotic era".

In fact, whilst the concept of resistance to all standard anti-TB drugs might appear in retrospect to be both logical and easily understood, the mathematical possibilities for such mutations occurring really remain extreme. The fact that they have occurred at all must cast a terrible shadow over TB management. Furthermore actually defining total drug-resistance is challenging because so few laboratories can test all of the current drug groups, and there is also no consensus list of all anti-TB drugs anyway, with some as yet unapproved drugs believed to have some level of effect against the TB bacillus. Furthermore, the drug-susceptibility testing of some of the second line drugs is known to be not that reliable even in good laboratory conditions, since retesting the same isolate has been seen to give different results in many cases.

Given the possible development of a pipeline of new drugs, this TDR-TB definition constitutes something that can be anticipated to be a moving target as any new drug comes on stream. What might be defined as being totally drug-resistant on one day, in other words, might not be by the end of the month.

One other rather ugly factor stands embarrassingly tall in any sensible definition of total drug-resistance as well – a factor which relates to the actual availability of the drugs themselves. Depending on the day-to-day availability of drugs in any specific country, it does not actually matter a jot for many patients (or to their physicians) whether resistance to 11 categories of drugs is detected or just to two. If a strain is resistant to all of the drugs that are available, then it is *de facto* functionally equivalent to total drug-resistance already from the perspective of both patient and health care provider if other drugs are unavailable. Given the availability of the drugs and the cost of their supply, this is patently far more often the case than for the handful of confirmed 'totally' resistant cases in Mumbai.

This situation presents the flip-side to the argument that the term TDR-TB should not be used because new drugs will make such a term automatically redundant. In essence, wherever strains of resistance occur to degrees beyond the capacity of any locally available treatment to effectively cure, it can arguably already be defined as being totally drug-resistant.

Total drug-resistance, in these terms, in fact already constitutes the majority corporate reality of the drug-resistant pandemic in the 21st century, however much we might be tempted to play around with the terminology and believe otherwise.

Treating 'really' drug-resistant TB

With the global emergence of XDR-TB the rule book to some extent has already had to be thrown away. Some clinicians have resorted to administering so-called third-line drugs, for instance, some of which are also classified by WHO as Group 5 drugs, because of their *in vitro* effect against *M. tuberculosis* or because of their known activity against other species of mycobacteria. These third-line drugs include amoxicillin/clavulanic acid, clofazimine, linezolid, metronidazole (and other imidazoles), thioridazine (and other phenothiazines), macrolides, and monobactams (imipenem, meropenem). Clinical trials of some of these drugs have been undertaken to attempt to measure their effectiveness against both drug-susceptible and drug-resistant disease, but only one study to date has taken this further to develop the ever-important possible new drug combinations that are needed.

We have listed the second line drugs in an earlier section. They were included in a list of the 11 (or 12) classes of drugs that are recognized as having some sort of effect on the bacillus. It's worth always reminding ourselves, however, that, whenever a clinician has to resort to second line drugs he/she is generally employing older drugs with weaker effects and also ones with more pernicious side effects – effects which, if they occur, will have to be suffered by the patient for a treatment period that will probably be four times longer than a course of first line treatment, and one with a far less certain outcome.

The current WHO guidelines recommend a protocol for treatment of MDR-TB which, as far as possible, comprises a standardised treatment regimen for empirical treatment in patients who have previously received only first line TB drugs. This standardised regimen includes (ideally dependant upon known resistance determined by drug-susceptibility testing) a mixture of what are termed 'essential' drugs (Rifampicin , Streptomycin, Pyrazinamide, Ethambutol and Isoniazid) and 'second line' drugs as they are deemed needed to complete a safe and effective combination. Such drugs would properly be selected based on culture testing of samples taken from the patient at diagnosis of drug-resistance. In reality, they are more often selected based on what is believed to be the most probable strain circulating in the locality.

Such a treatment typically uses six drugs over a period of two years – something which has been variously calculated by MSF to comprise a total of anywhere between 8,700 and 11,000 toxic pills (MSF have quoted both, and they are probably the best authority in the world on the subject) and daily intra-muscular injections for as long as six months. Often this adds up to as many as 20 pills a day. The side effects are often debilitating, and (again particularly highlighted by MSF) survival is low – in South Africa their success rate from this regime for MDR-TB is as low as 52% and the global success rate is 48%.

When it comes to XDR-TB things are even bleaker still. The WHO's Global Tuberculosis Report of 2013 stated that of 623 XDR-TB who completed treatment in South Africa in 2102, only 18% had a positive outcome from the treatment. This figure does not, of course, include XDR-TB patients who never got to treatment.

In stark contrast, the Partnership's target for 2015 has been that 75% for ***all*** estimated cases of drug-resistant TB should be being successfully treated. The current gap between target and reality is almost impossibly large.

DR-TB can, at least theoretically, be cured, but patients often endure intolerable side effects which include nausea, severe vomiting, depression, aggressive behaviour, hallucinations, vertigo, hearing loss, diarrhoea and lethargy. Success may well also depend upon how quickly the disease is picked up, which was exactly what was found to be the case in the pre-drug-resistant era of TB in the 1950s when combinations were first being developed.

The story of Dr Uvistra Naidoo, a South African doctor, offers us a graphic idea of the challenge of such treatment. He initially contracted his disease whilst working with TB patients in a paediatric clinic in Cape Town. His illness began with 'flu-like symptoms and chest pains but, despite losing 30 pounds in weight, he did not seriously consider it a possibility that he might have contracted TB. When he went finally in for an X-ray, it was found that his entire right lung had filled with fluid. Within a matter of weeks, he became gravely ill and it was clear that he wasn't responding at all to first line medication.

Dr Naidoo survived because an individual treatment regimen was found to work for him, but he was in and out of hospital for three years in the course of his treatment, and, in his particular case, the drugs' side effects were truly extreme. He developed something called Stevens-Johnson Syndrome, a complication that causes layers of skin to separate from each other and which itself can be deadly. He also regularly bled from his eyes. He gave an account of his experiences in the South African media:

> "The TB doesn't feel like it's killing you, but the drugs do. I am a doctor and was informed that the drugs you take make you feel worse. My case was three years long. I don't think the average patient has that kind of patience."[110]

Patience or resilience – take your pick – but most important of all must be intensive care. The antiquated drug regimen available for DR-TB treatment poses what has been described as a "cruel conundrum" for both patient and doctor: take the treatment and risk symptoms such as psychosis or permanent deafness with perhaps a 50-50 chance of survival at best; or refuse the treatment and most probably die.

Dr Jenny Hughes, a DR-TB expert with MSF, offers her own expert insight:

> "I can talk about side effects until the cows come home…These drugs were first produced decades ago for normal TB. They have developed better drugs since then, which they now use for normal TB, but because DR-TB is resistant to those drugs, we have nothing else and so we have to use these old drugs against DR-TB and they're horrendous.

---

[110] "Doctors Struggling to Fight 'Totally Drug-Resistant' Tuberculosis in South Africa", http://www.usnews.com/news/articles/2013/02/11/doctors-struggling-totally-drug-resistant-tuberculosis-south-africa

> "To tell a patient that you have to stop working, you have to walk to your clinic every day, take an average of 20 pills and an injection which makes you go deaf – every single day for two years, it's impossible. So you need to find ways to enable patients to do that."

Dr Hughes' observations, along with those of other expert doctors in the field, has been informing the way that MDR-TB is being treated by MSF, not just in South Africa but in many other countries where the NGO is at work as well – in the process becoming a vanguard in the development of patient-centred models for treating the disease more effectively and efficiently. It's still generally accepted by them, however, that as many as a third of their patients may default on treatment at some point in the two years so what they've developed is still far from being a solution. "It's complex, there are lots of different reasons [for defaulting]" says Hughes. "It's never just one, but I do think that side effects is quite high up there."

Hughes sums up what is accepted by nearly everyone:

> "You can try to think of all sorts of different strategies to help people take their treatment, but in the end, you need a better drug regimen."

By "better" she means drugs that work much faster (requiring treatment regimes of two or maybe four months at a push), ones that are more effective, and ones which are free from some of the dreadful and dreaded side effects.

By comparison, treating what Dr Hughes calls 'normal' TB may seem relatively simple, sometimes with only two or three tablets a day, but because people feel so much better after three or four months, even with these shorter regimes and their more limited side effects, it is too often still a huge challenge to ensure that even this gets completed.

No-one anywhere is fooling themselves with the idea that treating drug-resistant tuberculosis is easy, but actually, it may be revealing itself to be even more complicated still.

Multiple strains

Although most specimens collected from patients with tuberculosis show the presence of only a single strain, some patients can be predicted to be potentially infected with more than one strain of *M. tuberculosis* during any given episode of drug-resistant TB. This may seem unlikely, but as long ago as 2006 a really worrying average of 17% of the new tuberculosis cases in a high incidence setting were being shown to contain multiple infections.[111]

The basic principle of diagnosing resistance by culture becomes significantly more complicated by this possibility of there being more than a single strain of TB in any specimen sample since they may be difficult to spot and differentiate. Such possible complications unfortunately arise largely because of the slow speed in which the disease progresses.

Such multi-strain phenomena cannot just seriously confuse any subsequent interpretations of drug-susceptibility testing results, they can also muddy interpretations of epidemiological contacts between patients.[112] There is still totally insufficient data on this subject for any definite clarification to be yet attempted – the one agreed idea being that a high incidence setting is probably the most likely predetermining factor for such events to occur.

If such multiple infections occur exogenously, and particularly if they are seen to be occurring more frequently, they must present some degree of challenge to the current strategy for treating tuberculosis. It certainly must put paid to any surviving assumption that infection with TB confers immunity against exogenous re-infection in a high incidence setting, for instance, and this alone must have implications for the development of any new vaccine that would be expected to protect reliably in such environments.

There is another aspect to this, however, and that is the likelihood that multiple infections might develop endogenously in the course of treatment, and, if so, proportionately fluctuating bacterial populations might be predicted to occur.

Such possibilities offer huge hypothetical challenges to current clinical treatments, and they are ones that appear to remain as yet almost completely unexplored. If we accept that two strains can exist together, we must also accept the probability that they could each also have differences in their susceptibilities to individual drugs. If the two strains are both susceptible to first line medication then no problem really presents itself. If

---

[111] Linda M Parsons et al. - "Laboratory Diagnosis of Tuberculosis in Resource-Poor Countries: Challenges and Opportunities", Clinical Microbiology Reviews, 24; 2 (2011) 314–50.

[112] Braden CR et al. - "Simultaneous infection with multiple strains of Mycobacterium tuberculosis", Clinical Infectious Diseases, 33 (2001) 42–47.

not, however, then several possible mechanisms present themselves which could result in fluctuating patterns of resistance emerging during the course of a therapy which in turn could demand changing patterns of treatment.

Let us assume that a patient with two strains presents initially as a drug-susceptible patient. In such a case, the susceptible strain could be assumed either to be the first infection (and therefore the more established of the two) or simply a fitter strain. Alternatively, the patient might be a retreatment case. In either case, these susceptible bacilli will show up more readily during testing since they will be proportionately larger in number. Initially such a patient may well test sputum-positive, and first line treatment will be started. At four weeks the probability exists that they will test sputum negative, and everything will be assumed to be going well. Since the dominant or fitter strain of bacillus is the more populous of the two, even drug-susceptibility testing (if it were carried out) would almost certainly have confirmed that the proportion of bacilli killed in the presence of first line drugs would have been sufficient for the cultured bacilli *in toto* to have been recognised as being drug-susceptible.

During this initial phase of treatment the first line antibiotics will predictably reduce the population size of the drug-susceptible strain, but this will also allow the minority drug-resistant strain population to slowly grow since they would remain unaffected by the treatment, thereby effectively finally converting the patient from an apparently drug-susceptible tuberculosis case into an MDR one. Sooner or later the patient will again show sputum-positive with the second strain now showing under the microscope. If DST were to be repeated at this point, he or she would now be diagnosed drug-resistant.

If this first line antibiotic pressure were now to be removed, however, either by poor treatment adherence or by default, then the underlying drug-susceptible strain could then slowly re-emerge as the dominant population. The patient would then again essentially be diagnosed drug-susceptible. This has actually been observed in the laboratory when drug-susceptible and drug-resistant populations were cultured *in vitro* and in macrophage cell lines. Such a re-emergence of a drug-susceptible population would suggest that the initial period of therapy in these patients may simply have been insufficient to enable complete sterilization of the site of disease. As such, this phenomenon fully accords with the accepted necessity for complete adherence to a full course of therapy including its continuation phase – in fact it serves to prove how vital it is, even if there is a second strain of DR-TB lurking in the background.

But let us assume that the patient is adhering to their short course treatment regime as required, but is subsequently identified as becoming drug-resistant, either after showing new symptoms of disease or after retesting sputum-positive. This could possibly be the result of a second exogenous infection with a drug-resistant strain of disease. In a high incidence environment this is far from being a remote possibility. But it could also be the second strain slowly showing its face as the susceptible strain succumbs.

At this stage the treatment would be switched to second line drugs and, unless the full course of first line drugs had been properly completed, the underlying drug-susceptible strain population could now possibly re-emerge as the fitter strain as the antibiotic pressure was changed by the introduction of this slower second line therapy. Second line antibiotics are known to have lower bactericidal activities when compared with first line antibiotics and therefore we can suggest a mechanism of selection due to what would effectively be a reduced antibiotic pressure on the fitter strain. The patient might then be subsequently re-confirmed as being drug-susceptible.

This second scenario is probably less likely, but the first one – that an apparently susceptible patient may emerge as a resistant one – is a reasonable probability in any environment with a high incidence of MDR-TB, a possibility which must make any sort of effective chemotherapy potentially more complicated and a lot harder to manage. It might even explain some of the lower success rates in treatment regimens which use some of the older drugs in comparison to what they would appear to have been when they were first developed.

There is further evidence of such possible phenomena available for us to consider in a paper entitled "How many sputum culture results do we need to monitor multidrug-resistant-tuberculosis (MDR-TB) patients during treatment?" Its authors speculated that discharging am MDR hospital patient after a single negative sputum culture might save money, but it might also be a disastrous strategy. The study reported that, after initial AFB sputum conversion to negative status in 336 South Africans patients, 11.6% and 5.4% reconverted to a positive diagnosis either one or two months after leaving hospital, respectively.[113] Such results might be readily explainable if we consider the possible presence of multiple strains.

[113] Janssen S et al - "Mycobacteriology and aerobic actinomycetes: how many sputum culture results do we need to monitor multidrug-resistant-tuberculosis

There is one further hypothetical aspect to this complexity which deserves consideration because the above examples assume that the multiple strains exist only in re-activated disease. What are the implications if they exist when the disease is still in latency? The certainly would seem to be possible. The trigger that promotes the critical moment of re-activation is still far from understood. It seems quite possible that some strains might respond rapidly to this trigger whilst others respond more slowly, leaving a reserve of mycobacteria still in their latent state. Logically, it should be hoped that they would still be finished off during DOTS chemothapy, but what if they were resistant?

There may even be more than a single trigger at work, with one trigger being more specific to one strain and a second trigger more specific to another – in other words, while two strains may co-exist in latency they will show as a single infection. Only one strain might re-activate initially, leaving the other with the potential to re-activate later.

Perhaps the only useful conclusion we can draw without much more detailed evidence is that the successful treatment of MDR-TB in high incidence environments may require substantial review, and might well require a fuller range of antibiotics than that which is currently approved – ones which target both drug-susceptible and drug-resistant sub-populations together and do so quickly. Furthermore, regular re-testing of cultures and also ongoing modifications to treatment based on the results are probable necessities in order to optimize and improve treatment success rates.

(MDR-TB) patients during treatment?" Journal of Clinical Microbiology, 51; 2 (2013) 644-646.

A Resurgence, an Emergence - or had it ever gone away?

"THE NEGLECT OF TUBERCULOSIS AS A MAJOR PUBLIC HEALTH PRIORITY OVER THE LAST TWO DECADES IS SIMPLY EXTRAORDINARY. PERHAPS THE MOST IMPORTANT CONTRIBUTOR TO THIS STATE OF IGNORANCE WAS THE GREATLY REDUCED CLINICAL AND EPIDEMIOLOGICAL IMPORTANCE OF TUBERCULOSIS IN THE WEALTHY NATIONS."

C.J.L. Murray[114]

It is, perhaps, worth us briefly reviewing the story so far.

As much as death rates may have dropped so dramatically in the more developed nations, TB was still recognised as being the greatest infectious killer in the world right into the 1990s, with the current global emergency being officially announced by the WHO in 1993. These factors alone may make what developed before 1993 and what has developed since as puzzling as anything for future medical historians, since, surely, more could and should have been being done about it. For at least a decade 97% of the world's cases had been occurring in non-industrialised countries[115] and there was (and still is) significance in this. The disease was remaining endemic in those populations most cursed with poverty and amongst those who endured the poorest living conditions. Even today, 95% of all deaths from TB are estimated to still occur in the developing world.

But it is a complex disease, which means that there can be no simple medical solutions:

> "Tuberculosis is a social disease, and presents problems that transcend the conventional medical approach. On the one hand, its understanding demands that the impact of social and economic factors on the individual be considered as much as the mechanisms by which tubercle bacilli cause damage to the human body. On the other hand, the disease modifies in a peculiar manner the emotional and intellectual climate of the societies that it attacks."

---

[114] Professor of Global Health, University of Washington.

[115] Bloom BR, Murray CJL - "Tuberculosis: commentary on a re-emergent killer" Science, 257 (1992) 1055-64.

René Dubos wrote these words with his wife Jean back in 1952. Dubos was one of the giants of 20th century medicine – his wife subsequently tragically baceme a victim of the very disease they were writing about.

The Dubos' words resonate across more than half a century, and they are perhaps even more pertinent today than they were when they were written 60 years ago. Overcrowding, poverty, social alienation, refugee crises, increased incarceration rates in prisons, homelessness, and HIV/AIDS (the 'deadly alliance') are combining to overwhelm what were already essentially unco-ordinated and under-resourced public health responses. An important consideration in respect of some of these contributing factors concerns the fact that some of them also contribute not just to the highest risks of transmission, but also to the highest risks of acquiring drug-resistant strains, and the highest risks of not completing treatment.

It is tempting to suggest that today's resurgence of TB as a global health problem has been mainly caused simply by the new hard-to-treat strains of drug-resistance or by the complications created by HIV/AIDS, but this has to be too simplistic a view. For one thing, from the perspective of the developing world the disease actually hasn't resurged at all but has remained exactly the "captain of the men of death" or the "dread disease" that it always was. Furthermore, the global pandemic of the 20th century initially checked from its downward trends and began to rise as early as in the mid-seventies, a full decade before either HIV or drug-resistance ever poked their heads above the parapet, and only a decade after the discovery of Rifampicin .

We should be very wary of being too judgemental in hindsight, but we should also be on high alert to the mistakes that may have been made in recent decades in case we end up repeating them. It seems almost a certainty that, if the concerted and co-ordinated case-finding, surveillance and treatment programmes that clearly ***did*** work in the developed world had been properly implemented globally, the problem would not be as it is today – in fact TB might possibly not really be a problem at all. But combatting TB is never, it seems, as simple as might be wished, largely because the causes of TB are so multiple. Exposure to the bacillus is one thing; the environment in which the exposure occurs is another; and the constitutional state of the person exposed to it is possibly the most important of all. Those ideas of Hermann Brehner, the German doctor who first developed the sanatorium movement, may well seem naïve to us today, but although his theories may never have been properly tested, they were nevertheless effective to some degree. Simple isolation may have significantly contributed to the containment of the disease. Good food, another essential part of the sanatorium movement, must also have made a difference. A healthy diet is rarely something that is enjoyed by those exposed to and enduring constant poverty, and it is beyond doubt that this is one reason why poverty itself is one of the principal risk factors for tuberculosis. It simply offers an ideal opportunity for the bacillus by creating a far higher disposition for its development into infectious disease.

Particular factors contributed to this wave of risk as the 20th century spun out towards its end. One was the worldwide economic crisis in the 1970s, particularly because, in this same period, outbreaks of civil war, violence and instability resulted in many national health budgets being negatively affected.

The Alma-Ata Declaration of 1978 attempted to address this problem, championing a new idea of integrated primary health care instead of focusing energies and resources on single disease programmes like those previously rolled out for TB. It was an idea that was optimistically developed further by the 1979 "Health for All by the Year 2000" initiative. The eradication of smallpox had been announced the previous year, and this alone seemed to be as good a reason as any to be hopeful: the future of international public health was genuinely looking promising.

Then, in 1982, however, things took a turn. The Mexican government defaulted on some of its loan payments, which in turn triggered debt crises in other countries with similarly weak or even weaker economies. As a result, international donors and policymakers began to get nervous and started questioning what was being seen as the over-ambitious agenda set at Alma-Ata. Instead influential policymakers began to gravitate towards an alternative idea – one of more selective primary health care, specifically including programmes which involved discrete, targeted, measurable and most of all ***inexpensive*** (or at least cost-effective) interventions.

And in almost exactly this same period poorer countries were becoming increasingly reliant on loans. The World Bank was one of the main provider of such loans, and it was also soon seen to be similarly basing its own health agenda on the core principles of 'cost-effectiveness', modifying Alma Ata's general call for 'health for all' to one which was for '***affordable*** health for all'.

Such selective primary health care programmes promised better potential return on health investment, something which held particular appeal to donors who were beginning to worry about the risk of investing in countries which might be on the brink of default. Several leading causes of disease, disability and death thus simply came to be seen as being just too costly and complex to be addressed in resource-poor settings at all, and so found themselves largely excluded from this emerging, more focused agenda for effective health investments.

Almost unbelievably, TB was considered to be one of these conditions. In 1979, two of the architects of selective primary health care wrote that:

> "Leprosy and tuberculosis require years of drug therapy and even longer follow-up periods to ensure cure. Instead of attempting immediate, large-scale treatment programs for these infections, the most efficient approach may be to invest in research and development of less costly and more efficacious means of prevention and therapy."[116]

It may have seemed an intelligent approach at the time but surveillance, diagnosis and treatment of TB all suffered as a consequence and there can be little doubt that it was a disastrous idea. Mario Raviglione, the WHO Stop TB Tuberculosis Officer, summed it up as follows:

> "During this period [1977-88] WHO, many international agencies, most ministries of health, and academic institutions were perceived to have lost interest in tuberculosis control."

This period in fact has been rather more emotively identified as including:

> "..a woeful inadequacy of funding for tuberculosis control activities by the World Health Organisation."[117]

The focus of lung specialists had also comprehensively switched from tuberculosis to lung cancer during this same period, as the proportional rates of each flipped in a period of 20 years in the industrialised world. At this time only foreign-born ethnic minorities constituting any sort of meaningful reservoir for infectious tuberculosis in these richer countries, and, where they were occurring they could be effectively managed. The result of this was not only a common national neglect of the disease, but also a new complexity – a potentially misleading association of the disease with issues of immigration and economic migration. Wherever outbreaks

---

[116] Walsh JA, Warren KS - "Selective primary health care: an interim strategy for disease control in developing countries", New England Journal of Medicine, 301 (1979) 967-74.

[117] Philip Hopewell - "Mycobacterium Tuberculosis - an emerging pathogen?" Western Journal of Medicine, 164; 1 (1996) 33–35.

were occurring in the developed world the resultant debates were centring on whether the disease was simply a consistent factor in what was effectively a residual social underclass or whether it was a direct result of the proportion of a local population originating from countries with known high incidence rates of TB. The longer term broader implications of high incidence rates of a generally suppressed disease surviving anywhere in an age of increasing globalisation appears to have been being missed by everyone – something that can perhaps best be explained by the fact that wherever TB was occurring it was occurring well away from, and out of sight of, the mainstream of society.

The global problems of public health, meanwhile, were being aggravated by refugee crises in the 1980s and 1990s, with camps full and overflowing in both Africa and Asia. These crises were characterised by unpredictable influxes of peoples escaping conflict or political dangers, as well as being a consequence of natural disasters and famines. Vaccinating young children in such circumstances could go some way to protect the young against disease, but it could do nothing to prevent wider sickness and transmission of disease in adult age groups.

Then HIV/AIDS entered the equation, and it first entered global consciousness to a very large degree in the USA. There were explicit signs, even then in the richest country of all, of deadly these two diseases could be when they worked in concert: in 1990 half of those hospitalised in New York for TB were identified as also being HIV-positive.

That year a WHO report prepared by its Geneva-based Tuberculosis Unit (which had by then reportedly been reduced down to being just a two-man operation) attempted to make a belated and fresh assessment. Their report suggested that there were 7.5 million new cases of disease in that year and 2.5 million deaths "making this disease the largest cause of death from a single pathogen in the world." Africa, even then, was recorded as having the highest estimated infection rates at 272 per 100,000.

The following year a WHO meeting in Geneva concluded that, on the basis of recorded results from skin testing, as much as a third of the global population could be anticipated to be latently infected with the disease. A full 20 years later, and this same fraction is still being quoted by both the World Health Organisation and by a host of other expert authors who publish papers on the disease. What this implies is that, if the fraction is still correct, the ***actual numbers*** of those who are latently infected will have increased proportionately to the increase in the world's population, and will now be about 2.3 billion.

It was also being estimated that 30 million might die in the next ten years running up to the millennium if nothing was done, and it was being further suggested that at least 10% of these would be on account of HIV.

In every sense, therefore, however much it was being believed that that the disease had gone way, it was now clear that it never had at all – in fact it had just been getting worse, and that (in certain countries at least) it had now found a new and deadly friend.

As far as Africa was concerned it should have been simple to have swiftly linked TB with HIV, this new disease which was by then being seen to be really ravaging the continent – but in countries with more developed economies where latent infections had become residually prominent only in more elderly patients, and where HIV was primarily affecting young males, the two diseases remained epidemiologically distinct from each other. As a result, the true significance of this link was generally ignored, particularly because TB infection rates were still remaining relatively stable and low in the developed world. There seemed little cause for concern.

This lethal link between HIV and TB, and the serious consequential epidemiological risk from co-infection, was certainly not being missed by everyone, however. In August 1991 the Lancet had published a provocatively entitled article simply called "Is Africa lost?". It was written by three eminent bacteriologists, J.L.Stanford, J.M.Grange and A.Pozniak. The article starkly concluded by suggesting that the world might just be facing one of the greatest public health disasters since the bubonic plague. More than 20 years later, this remains a suggestion that has yet to be proved to have been incorrect.

The first identifiable signs of yet another dangerous extra layer to the problem, however, also emerged in 1991. That year the acronym MDR-TB began to be used for the first time as strains of disease that were resistant to the two strongest drugs began to be seen more commonly in actual circulation. That year as well, Professor John Murray of San Francisco General Hospital, announced that there had been a global resurgence of TB with a particular explosion of disease being seen in South Africa in the previous five years. Generally, however, both his warnings and the existence of the phenomenon of MDR-TB itself were being ignored by those with the power to do anything meaningful about them.

Because of the limited responsiveness of drug-resistant TB to available antibiotics, mortality rates among patients with DR-TB were, unsurprisingly, suggested to be similar to those of TB patients in the pre-antibiotic era (50-70%) – but with HIV co-infection they were now being seen to be higher still. As TB historian Helen Bynum has chillingly observed:

> "Drug-resistant tuberculosis in an HIV-infected patient is about as bad as it gets."

The general picture in more developed countries across the world reflected the same patterns: older cases were native born and were more often than not re-activations of latent infections contracted as long as 50 years earlier; younger cases, in the meantime, were most often foreign-born – either that or they had HIV, used drugs and alcohol, or were destitute. In other words they were the easiest of all to dismiss with a wave of stigmatisation.

How accurate all the figures from this time really were is impossible to say, because it was also being identified at the time that many national control programmes were in the process of unravelling or in fact had already done so. As such, accurate information on any part of the disease at the time has to be assumed to have been totally inadequate.

In 1991 the WHO issued a new resolution: it decreed that by 2000 all national TB programmes (NTPs) should be detecting 70% of all cases in all countries and have 85% of all sputum-positive cases in treatment.

In 1993 the World Bank began to employ the phrase "disability-adjusted life-years" as a way of determining which health interventions were worth supporting and which ones weren't. The term adds up to being accountant-speak to calculate the relative cost-effectiveness of a given health intervention by taking morbidity, mortality, and age into account.[118] Using this methodology, short-course chemotherapy[119] for tuberculosis was unexpectedly deemed to be a highly cost-effective intervention and, as such, support for better programmes of treatment rapidly gained momentum.

---

[118] Murray CJL - "Quantifying the burden of disease: the technical basis for disability-adjusted life years", Bulletin of the World Health Organisation, 72 (1994) 429-45.

[119] 'Short course' is a relative term. Treatment was still 6-8 months, but this was comparatively significantly shorter than earlier drug regimens.

Seizing the opportunity, the WHO ramped things up – the organisation now officially called this 'new' threat of tuberculosis a "global emergency" and called the governments of the world to arms to fight it. It also offered its own systematic solution which was organisationally branded in 1995 as DOTS. DOTS (or 'directly observed therapy, short course') was what the WHO was now advocating that all countries should use as their prime tool to fight the disease. DOTS was officially endorsed by the World Bank the same year, which described it as being "one of the most cost effective of all interventions". Things were starting to roll.

According to the WHO strategy, the diagnosis of active disease was to be made with the use of smear microscopy only – in spite of its insensitivity and the inability of this technique to detect drug-resistance. Furthermore, the treatment approach was to be based on the empirical use of first line essential anti-tuberculosis agents without second line drugs.[120] It was at heart a highly pragmatic solution. It is also a policy which has been clung to ever since. It seems in retrospect that the idea that it might be a one-size-fits-all solution to what was emerging as a multi-faceted problem has been both its greatest strength and also its most vulnerable underbelly.

As Helen Bynum identifies, DOTS was from the outset far more than just 'directly observed treatment'. There was a five-point strategy that came with it:

- diagnosis of self-referring patients through sputum-smear microscopy
- standardised short-course directly observed therapy
- government commitment to sustainable TB control
- functioning systems of drug supply
- recording and reporting systems allowing proper assessment of results.

Any sort of facility-based infection control was, however, never part of the general DOTS strategy, nor was active case finding.

Despite this reliance on first line drugs and on the unreliable sputum test, DOTS was a massively important development. Because of it, there can be no doubt that many lives have been saved and many new cases averted. However, for children with tuberculosis, for people with both tuberculosis

[120] Kochi A - "Tuberculosis control – is DOTS the health breakthrough of the 1990s?", World Health Forum, 18 (1997) 225-32.

and HIV, for patients with disease which could not be detected by sputum testing, for patients who (for many reasons) might fail to self-refer, and for the slowly increasing proportion of patients infected with strains of tuberculosis that were now drug-resistant, the DOTS strategy never promised that much in terms of either diagnosis or cure.

DOTS was quickly being seen to help bring the recent rise in rates of drug-susceptible TB in New York under control, however. By 1995 there were 1,282 enrolled on DOTS treatment in the city as opposed to just 137 two years before. This came at a great price, however – at a cost of US$400 million which was somewhat at odds with the assessments that had been made by the World Bank. To be so truly effective, was it really quite so economical as the World Bank had considered it to be?

Meanwhile, DOTS was not getting so well rolled out elsewhere, particularly where resources were deficient. By 1996 it was estimated that only about 11% of TB patients worldwide were being treated this way, and that it wasn't even being widely used in the 22 high burden countries which had been identified as being where 80% of the world's cases were supposed to be.

As a result, in 1998 the WHO TB programme was restructured and renamed the 'Stop TB' initiative. It had the same goals (the detection of 70% of infectious cases and the successful treatment of 85% of them), but the targets' completion date was now revised from 2000 to 2005.

By the year 2000 the number of new cases was estimated at 8.2 million, a little higher than nearly a decade earlier, and the tide still seemed to be rising. In Amsterdam on March 24th that year the 'Global DOTS Expansion Plan' was launched, supported by low interest loans from the World Bank. The loans arose from their calculations that, in developing countries like India, TB accounted for a quarter of all avoidable deaths. The Global Drug Facility (GDF) was also founded that year to address the recognised problems in supply chains of drugs.

Throughout this period, however, one major component part of the global emergency was still to be addressed at all – that of drug-resistance. Unfortunately, this component of the pandemic simply didn't fit neatly enough into the brand that had been created. In fact it was looking like a little too much had been expected of the brand itself anyway so there was still too much work to do developing DOTS further, let alone allow other distractions to interfere.

There was already adequate official awareness of the threat, however. Back in 1994 the Global Project on Anti-Tuberculosis Drug-Resistance Surveillance had been set up, and its first report had revealed a growing and widespread trend in resistance, not just to single drugs but also to a common occurrence of resistance to two drugs or more.

The Project was established mainly by the WHO and the International Union Against Tuberculosis and Lung Disease (known simply as "The Union"). It had been awarded well designated spheres of activities:

- Technical assistance to countries in design and implementation of anti-tuberculosis drug-resistance surveys or the strengthening of existing DR-TB surveillance systems
- Training of specialists at country and regional level to ensure running of high quality surveys/surveillance and proper analysis and interpretation of the results
- Periodic collection and analysis of global DR-TB data and publication of results
- Provision of regular updates on anti-TB drug-resistance surveillance methods

The Global Project was essentially established to respond to the lack of standardisation of data on drug-resistance, as well as to estimate the global prevalence of resistance. Nearly 20 years later on these factors alone, let alone on the designated activities listed above, it is hard not to be harsh in judging its actual achievements.

Since 1994, the Global Project has been collecting and analysing data on drug-resistance from surveys of sampled patients and from national surveillance systems from an increasing number of settings around the world. Unfortunately it has revealed the same two-speed weaknesses that have characterised almost all of the more recent TB initiatives: whilst it uses sophisticated computer engineering back at base to check and cross-check data from across the world, it has been impossible to collect the appropriate quality of data that these systems demanded. Practically speaking, the Project has remained impossibly dependent upon the relatively primitive and inadequate collection of unreliable data from sputum samples and occasionally from their growth on culture plates which have also almost invariably been impossibly uncertain – even in those official high burden countries.

In the late 1980s and early 1990s, limited outbreaks of MDR-tuberculosis were being reported in the United States. One outbreak occurred in a New York City hospital. During that outbreak, 32 patients caught MDR over the course of a few months and 29 died. The outbreak was contained, but it was reported to have finally cost the city an estimated US$1billion. As such, there was good early evidence of just how challenging containing DR-TB might be even if a well-resourced city.

Subsequent genetic analysis of these drug-resistant strains had also proved that airborne transmission of undetected and untreated strains had played a role in these outbreaks, although opposing ideas (that resistance stemmed solely from "sporadic pill taking") were persisting. These specific successful experiences in New York were also suggesting alternate methods of response that were entirely different to the simpler DOTS strategy. These consisted of specific diagnosis using mycobacterial culture with drug-susceptibility testing, and an appropriate longer-term directly observed treatment using second line drugs, along with a programme of proper infection control rolled out behind it thoroughly following up on all possible contacts.

In complete contrast to this newer strategy emerging for treating patients in the US, the WHO (understandably perhaps) was continuing to advocate the use of both sputum smear microscopy and first line anti-tuberculosis treatments as the only way to combat all epidemics in resource-poor settings, even if they were known to include drug-resistant cases. Some policymakers simply considered that treating MDR-TB in any other way was simply impossibly expensive and complex and, perhaps as importantly, that it could also put at risk the newly branded DOTS strategy.[121]

Fresh evidence in the United States and more particularly in several countries from the former Soviet Union was now suggesting, however, that short-course chemotherapy was not just basically ineffective against strains which were shown to be resistant to half of the drugs on which such therapy was based, but that it also ran a substantial risk of amplifying the resistance both in both quantity and degree.[122]

---

[121] WHO report on the tuberculosis epidemic (1997).

[122] Frieden TR, Fujiwara PI, Washko RM, Hamburg MA - "Tuberculosis in New York City – turning the tide", New England Journal of Medicine, 333 (1995) 229-33.

A serious and significant outbreak of MDR-TB was then identified in a shantytown in northern Lima, Peru in 1995. Many patients were being identified as being infected with strains of TB with broad-spectrum resistance to first line drugs – so standard DOTS based treatment could be predicted to be ineffective for them, and was being seen to be so. An earlier campaign to promote the basic DOTS strategy in Peru, however, had been highly successful in making TB treatment more available across the country and as a result the country's leaders were politically attached to DOTS as being the best way to fight their tuberculosis problem. The WHO, meanwhile, was still arguing that DOTS alone could rein in the mutant bacteria. In consequence, the advice was given to the Peruvian government to adopt the low-cost, standardized DOTS regimen for the treatment of their MDR cases of tuberculosis rather than adopting protocols based on the results of any sort of drug-susceptibility testing. In the absence of the necessary tailored therapy, many hundreds of deaths occurred, occurring among some of Lima's poorest people – and, as was being predicted by some experts, an associated amplification of drug-resistance was occurring as well.[123]

Non-governmental organizations stepped in to help out. They used Partners in Health (PIH) as their flagship, and began working with the Peruvian Health Ministry to try and apply the sorts of standards of care that had been successfully used in New York. PIH had been working in former Soviet countries and had had as much experience as any in confronting the problem of drug-resistance. The strategy that had been used in New York was also tellingly modified to include the provision of community-based care and not hospitalisation, however, and it began to show good results.

It's very difficult not to conclude that the risks of drug-resistance have been repeatedly sacrificed to the perceived needs of the DOTS programme. With the benefit of hindsight, the whole story appears to have developed into an ever growing tragedy of missed opportunities given the fact that DOTS should ***never*** have been considered as in any sense being able to address MDR-TB. Different reasons were being proposed to try to explain the problem as much as anything was actually being seriously done to address it. It's arguable that, to some degree, this is a situation that still exists: blame the victim (who had obviously defaulted); blame the poor implementation of the national DOTS programme; or blame the structural design of the

[123] Vasquez-Campos L, Asencios-Solis L, Leo-Hurtado E, et al. - "Drug-resistance trends among previously treated tuberculosis patients in a national registry in Peru, 1994-2001", International Journal of Tuberculosis and Lung Diseases, 8 (2004) 465-72.

DOTS programme which ignored the possibility that there could be much primary transmission of drug-resistant TB. Paul Farmer and his colleagues in Partners in Health were already accurately identifying the paradoxical "amplifier effect of short course chemotherapy" in the presence of existing drug-resistance nearly 20 years ago, and steps should have been taken there and then to address this well before things were able to get further out of hand.

The first alternative effort to properly address this emerging divergent drug-resistant disease was developed in 1998, and it was directly as a result of the Peru experience. The strategy was called 'DOTS-Plus' – first initiated by Paul Farmer and Partners in Health. This innovative approach included implementing both the vital drug-susceptibility testing and the additional use of second line drugs. PIH however, was also providing something else which may yet prove in the long run to be just as important: community care along with extra food programmes and other support.

The tensions which quickly developed between proponents of DOTS and the more complex interventions were well summed up by Farmer and Keshavjee, both of PIH, in 2012:

> "Such protocols [as DOTS] helped standardize tuberculosis treatment around the world – a process that was sorely needed – but they hamstrung practitioners wishing to address diagnostic and therapeutic complexities that could not be addressed by the use of sputum-smear microscopy and short-course chemotherapy or other one-size-fits-all approaches. These complexities, which now range from pan-resistant tuberculosis to undiagnosed paediatric disease, account for more than a trivial fraction of the nine million new cases of tuberculosis and the almost two million deaths from this disease that occur around the globe each year....
>
> "The history of divergent policies for combating drug-resistant tuberculosis shows that decades of clinical research and effective programs in high-income settings did not lead to the deployment of similar approaches in settings of poverty. Achieving that goal demands a commitment to equity and to health care delivery. The U.S. response to the outbreaks of MDR tuberculosis in New York City and elsewhere was bold and comprehensive; it was designed to halt the epidemic. A similar response has not yet been attempted in low- and middle-income countries. Instead, selective primary

> health care and 'cost-effectiveness' have shaped an anaemic response to the on-going global pandemic."[124]

By the end of the 1990s, facing mounting evidence that MDR-TB could not be controlled or countered simply by the use of DOTS in resource-poor settings, a multi-institutional mechanism, the 'Green Light Committee', was created to both encourage and learn from specifically approved pilot projects for treating MDR-TB. This initiative coincided with a grant from the Bill and Melinda Gates Foundation to scale up treatment of MDR-TB in Peru and elsewhere as well as to review global policy towards the disease.

The true reality, in fact, was that the TB pandemic had already begun to diverge into separate sub-pandemics, with each one requiring their own response if they were to be appropriately confronted – if, in Farmer's and Keshavjee's words, there was to be anything more than an "anaemic" response to the DR epidemic. Essentially today there are now several different discrete diseases each flying the flag of tuberculosis, with each one now requiring different approaches to both diagnosis and treatment.

These are:

- TB (drug-susceptible)
- Poly drug-resistant TB (which comes in several forms itself)
- TB with HIV
- Drug-resistant TB with HIV
- Bovine TB
- Bovine TB with HIV
- Multiple strain TB

Drug-resistant TB can thus be defined to have been an emergent new disease, and drug-susceptible TB as a resurging one. It may seem both tragically ironic and perplexingly paradoxical that one of the oldest of diseases should today also be determined to be an emerging one, but it is a mistaken view. What is perplexing, however, is that such a constant killer which, even at the time that its so-called 'resurgence' was still being

---

[124] Salmaan Keshavjee and Paul Farmer, - "Tuberculosis, drug-resistance, and the history of modern medicine", New England Journal of Medicine, 367 (2012) 931-936.

identified as the single most dangerous global infectious killer, was simultaneously being so singularly and self-evidently neglected.

In 2007, based on surveys conducted in over 110 settings over a decade, the WHO was estimating that nearly half a million active TB cases were MDR, resulting in 130,000 deaths up to that time. In fact it was almost certainly more because, according to their figures, only 27 countries were apparently accounting for 85% of all such cases. The countries that were ranking first to fifth in total numbers of MDR-TB cases in 2007 were India, China, the Russian Federation, South Africa, and, rather curiously, Bangladesh.

In addition, estimates for the even more worrisome XDR-TB were by then already about 50,000 (or 1% of active MDR-TB cases), and the majority of these were fatal. By November 2009, over 50 countries and territories had reported at least one case of extensively drug-resistant TB (XDR-TB). By 2012 this was 92 countries, and the percentage of MDR-TB that was XDR had risen to 9.6%. Between 2007 and 2012 (a period of five years) percentage rates of MDR-TB that were XDR were being estimated to have risen by nearly 1000%.

The true prevalence of poly drug-resistant TB might be best highlighted by a study in the Lancet published in 2012.[125] Researchers tested cultures from 1278 confirmed MDR patients from eight countries. They then tested these for resistance to 11 different first line and second line anti-TB drugs. What they found offers us very bitter food for thought.

Whilst 92% of the patients had previously received treatment with first line drugs, only 195 had ever received treatment with any second line drugs. We might therefore reasonably expect (and hope) that only 195 (or 15%) might be carrying strains which might be resistant to any individual second line drugs, since they would have been the only patients enrolled on the study who would have been exposed to them. In fact 44% (or 562) of the whole cohort demonstrated resistance to one of the second line drugs (i.e. they were MDR-plus or pre-XDR-TB depending on your preferred unofficial terminology). This is nearly three times as many as might be expected to have been the case. This finding suggests the likelihood that strains that are more dangerous than MDR must be actively circulating at least in these eight countries but also probably elsewhere as well. Furthermore, 20%

---

[125] Tracy Dalton et al. - "Prevalence of and risk factors for resistance to second-line drugs in people with multidrug-resistant tuberculosis in eight countries: a prospective cohort study", The Lancet, 380, 9851 (2012) 1406-17.

(256) overall were resistant to one of the three injectable drugs – again more than might be expected, also suggesting similar infectious transmission. The most startling statistic, however, related to findings in the Eastern Cape of South Africa where a terrifying 49% of MDR-TB cases were found to be resistant to ***all three*** second line injectables (which are rarely, if ever, administered together), suggesting that this region is already inflicted with a terrible burden of extensive drug-resistance.

The other surprising finding was also (for once) good news – that, of the 1278 patients overall, XDR-tuberculosis (i.e. resistance to Isoniazid, Rifampicin, and at least one drug within the fluoroquinolones and one anti-tuberculosis injectable drug) was found in only 86 (6.7%) of the cohort. This added up to being a little less than the estimated global average

Since 2007 the WHO has been collecting surveillance data of its own on cases of MDR-TB with additional resistance to the fluoroquinolones. In most cases, quite logically, only the compound most commonly used in the country is tested for such susceptibility, usually ofloxacin, moxifloxacin or levofloxacin. In total, 62 countries and three territories have reported representative data on the proportion of MDR-TB cases that had additional resistance to these fluoroquinolones. Combining their data, the proportion of MDR-TB cases with additional resistance to fluoroquinolones was established to be 14.5%, a percentage which included cases of XDR-TB. This result suggests that the previous study may have overestimated the problem given that it tested cases from fewer countries, but it also tested more second line drugs. It certainly begs the question as to whether countries which do not use the second line fluoroqinolone drugs, but which have migrant workforces which routinely travel to neighbouring countries which do, would have been included in such surveys. Such countries would particularly include those which border South Africa which has uniquely high rates of reported XDR-TB.

The Green Light Committee

"WHEN A VIRUS (HIV) AND A BACTERIA (TB) CAN WORK SO WELL TOGETHER, WHY CAN'T WE?"

Michel Sidibé[126]

Following the conceptualisation and subsequent development of DOTS-Plus as a feasible response to MDR-TB, the WHO set up its "Green Light Committee" in 2000 to see how subsidised and quality-assured second line drugs could be best supplied in a targeted way to patients with drug-resistance. It was formally established under the Stop TB working group on MDR-TB. The Committee itself was and still is comprised of an independent group of experts who serve the WHO in a technical advisory capacity.

It certainly must have felt like a very good start towards belatedly getting to grips with the growing problem of drug-resistance. Only four years before, in 1996, in a publication entitled "Groups at Risk" the WHO had been officially speculating that "MDR-TB is [simply] too expensive to treat in poor countries; it detracts attention and resources from treating drug-susceptible disease".

The GLC was promising a change of heart, and it arrived on the scene with its own bold and uncompromising mission statement – "to achieve a world free of drug-resistant TB". Its goal was "to accelerate scale up to achieve universal access to prevention, early diagnosis and effective patient-centred treatment for drug-resistant tuberculosis by 2015". These were unambiguous statements.

In order to reach this goal, the new global framework which included the GLC was intending to provide:

---

[126] Executive Director of UNAIDS, the Joint United Nations Programme on HIV/AIDS, and Under-Secretary-General of the United Nations since 1 January 2009.

- Increased levels and diverse models of technical support from partners to assist countries to plan, implement, manage and monitor the required scale-up of MDR-TB services.
- Increased access to high-quality, affordable second line drugs (SLDs) for the treatment of MDR-TB.
- Strengthened advocacy for the accelerated scale up of the response to MDR-TB.
- Regular and supportive monitoring and evaluation of country performance in accelerating access to MDR-TB treatment and care, to inform assessment of global progress, to propose improvements to the global, regional and national approaches, and to pursue advocacy activities tailored to country needs.
- Regular updating of international policy and guidelines relating to programmatic management of drug-resistant TB.
- Provision of advice to funding agencies, on their request, ensuring that the effective treatment of patients with MDR-TB is done in accordance with international standards.

The current members of the Green Light Committee are:

- Partners In Health (PIH)
- The American Thoracic Society (ATS)
- Hospital General de "Francisco J. Muniz", Argentina
- The International Union Against Tuberculosis and Lung Disease (IUATLD)
- The KNCV Tuberculosis Foundation
- Médecins sans Frontières (MSF)
- The State Agency for TB & Lung Disease, Latvia
- The Indus Hospital, Pakistan
- The World Health Organization (WHO) – as a standing member

It's not unfair to suggest unfortunately that, 13 years after its founding, things can hardly be said to be going according to plan.

Superficially at least, it looked as if the GLC was being set up with the specific responsibility of addressing the pandemic of drug-resistance. In fact it would appear that this was not quite the case at all. The overall responsibility appears rather to have been spread unhelpfully between agencies, and as a result the opportunity to get on top of the disease before it really took off may have been missed and the world may be left with the problem of somehow playing catch-up as a result. The fact of the matter is that those with most interest in the outcome of the disease still have far too little power over it, but worse, those with the most power may still be too reluctant to adopt appropriate responsibility for a proper resolution. Certainly, we can at least conclude that those parties who have most influence currently do not seem to be seeing completely eye to eye on what should be done, nor on how it can be done best.

In 2012, Dr Salmaan Keshavjee of PIH offered a stinging critique of the situation. He identified that, in fact, the GLC had, in fact, not been created as a mechanism for scale-up *per se* at all. Rather it had been formed only:

- To receive and approve applications for DOTS-Plus pilot projects
- To make drugs available at low cost to DOTS-Plus pilot projects
- To help these projects successfully treat MDR-TB
- To provide data to the WHO to help inform and/or change policy.

In other words, the GLC was only enabled to work with individual approved 'projects', and not to roll out treatments in any sort of scale at all. And he identified some major problems even with this – ones which had revealed themselves since the GLC's founding.

The first related to getting second line drugs procured at low costs. At a Global Fund Board Meeting in 2002 it had been agreed that: "To help contain resistance…all procurement of medications to treat MDR-TB must be conducted through the Green Light Committee." Keshavjee saw this as having been a huge strategic mistake, not least because it granted the GLC an effective monopoly which created what he defined as a moral hazard. But there were other reasons as well.

He identified that, whilst the GLC handled the applications, it was the GLC secretariat that handled the administration and it was the Global Drug Facility (GDF) that handled drug procurement. As a result, he suggested that there had been a lack of the necessary direct relationship between the targeted countries themselves (where the pilot projects were taking place) and the drug manufacturers, and as a result the system had become unnecessarily long-winded and time consuming.

Almost unbelievably, the system that had been created had also failed to incorporate any sort of pooled procurement – entirely unlike what was happening at the same time with HIV drugs, as well as with TB first line drugs. To some degree this might have been an understandable decision – the GLC, after all, was set up to attend to pilot studies, not to large scale roll-out programmes. But this second line drug procurement was set up through the Global Drug Facility which did have proven experience of bulk buying, so it is baffling that this anomaly was not being properly addressed as much as a decade ago. Effectively, these vital SLD drugs for drug-resistant disease were, on every single occasion, being purchased piecemeal per project – not even per country. Worse still, there were simply not enough companies involving themselves in their manufacture to ever develop a reliable and competitive supply, and no-one was doing anything to attend to this either. There were drug shortages with no strategies for preventing them; there were no price negotiations and no plans being developed to bring down prices. As a result, the drugs themselves remained essentially unattractive to their producers whilst they remained excessively expensive to the purchasers – in fact, because of the piecemeal system of ordering, their manufacture was being seen as more of a nuisance than any sort of commercial opportunity (which it surely should have been), and their pricing effectively reflected this.

What soon happened was that some of the SLDs, rather than reducing in price as had been specifically intended, in fact began to rise. During the period 2001-2009 – a period in which in-patent HIV drugs were seen to drop in price by around 50% because of strategic procurement – the price of these out-of-patent SLDs actually ***increased*** by an overall average of approximately 25% (some individual ones dramatically so). In 2011 MSF published their own figures in relation to this, listing the prices that were available for some of them on their own GLC-approved programmes in 2011 compared with prices paid in 2001. It makes for disconcerting reading.

Products	**July 2001 (lowest price US$)**	**March 2011**	**% Difference**
Amikacin 500mg	0.11	1.20	+991%
Kanamycin 1g	0.36	2.58	+617%
Cycloserine 250mg	0.14	0.59	+321%
Capreomycin 1gr	1.02	4.00	+292%

MSF offered the same general explanation for the price hikes as Keshavjee – a total lack of co-ordinated negotiation.

Keshavjee also chose to publish excerpts from specific pieces of correspondence on the subject – ones which seem to reveal a dreadfully dysfunctional gap of understanding developing between agencies and individuals who should have been working closely and co-operatively with each other. On 17th October 2007, for instance, the Working Group of the Stop TB Partnership wrote to Mario Raviglione (of the WHO) and to

Marcos Espinal (then Executive Secretary of the Stop TB Partnership). The letter said that:

> "The crisis [in drug management of SLDs] directly affects approved GLC projects and hampers the anticipated scale-up of MDR-TB treatment programs…The evidence of the procurement crisis is seen in the severe shortage of second line anti-TB drugs and impossibly long times for delivery of drugs to countries… These shortages and delays pose a significant threat to patients; they are undermining TB projects throughout the world and will certainly contribute to the creation of more XDR-TB cases."

Broadly speaking, this letter reflected Keshavjee's analyis. The language was measured but plain-speaking: it is clear that, seven years into the life of the GLC, things were definitely going seriously wrong.

Yet the GLC's own Executive Committee Summary Report of March 2007 had been surprisingly exhortative in tone:

> "In 2006 the GLC initiative has reshaped, streamlined and strengthened its processes to respond to increasing demand…and provide for the targets outlined in the Global Plan to Stop TB and the Stop TB Strategy."

It added that the Green Light Committee with "its expertise and unique procurement mechanism for quality assured second line drugs…calls for countries to scale up access to treatment of drug-resistant TB".

Two separate realities seem to have been emerging.

The GLC's Executive Committee's report of 2007, in fact, only really contained one cautionary sentence, suggesting that: "despite [these] encouraging trends…the current status covers less than 5% of patients with drug-resistant TB worldwide".

Even that may have been optimistic. Paul Farmer and Salmaan Keshavjee have separately estimated that this figure may be adrift by a factor of ten. They quoted a WHO report of 2010[127] which suggested that MDR-TB had killed an estimated 1.5 million people between 2000 and 2009 (an annual rate, incidentally that was 10 times that of the H1N1 influenza virus), and that, during this same period, of the estimated five million who had become

[127] WHO - "Multidrug and extensively drug-resistant TB (M/XDR-TB): 2010 global report on surveillance and response".

ill with MDR-TB, barely 0.5% had received treatment with quality-assured second line drugs. One-in-20, or one-in-200? Did anyone really know?

Something that we do know is the following: the Global Drug Facility – the international pooled procurement mechanism for TB medicines and diagnostics – procured DR-TB treatments for less than 20,000 people in 2011. This number amounts to only 6% of the WHO estimated 310,000 MDR-TB cases in their 2012 Global TB Report. In fact it's hard even to be sure of this statement, however, since MSF's report from a year earlier had reckoned that just 6,000 of the 440,000 (or 1%) new MDR cases in 2010 were treated on GLC-approved programmes. Had the numbers infected by the disease dropped so dramatically, and/or the treatment so dramatically increased? Or were there simple semantic niceties being employed in these choices of words – the WHO listing the number of patients who had had drugs "procured" for them, and MSF identifying the number of patients that were actually "treated"? And in any case, those 310,000 were only "among those notified patients with pulmonary TB", and there was over 300,000 more out there somewhere even by the WHO's own estimations, meaning that only just 3% were possibly getting approved treatment. Included within this number as well, there also has to be (at the very least) 60,000 XDR-TB cases (if 9% of the MDR-TB burden is XDR as the WHO itself currently suggests). Given this "alarming outlook" and all of the other confusions, MSF were considering it imperative that DR-TB be immediately officially declared a public health emergency.

By 2009 the GDF had been reporting to the GLC's secretariat delays of an astonishing ***average of 54 weeks*** between GLC approval and actual arrival of medicines at a country/project. Three years later and this had only slightly improved, as confirmed by MSF in their 2012 report on TB drugs:[128]

> "Orders for DR-TB drugs placed with GDF are often small and need to be pooled by manufacturers before they produce a new batch, leading to four to six months standard lead times, from order placement to receipt in country."

At the same time PIH was also reporting that prices were rising because there were not enough suppliers and because there was no pooled procurement. On May 15th 2009, Partners in Health, as a member of the

[128] MSF - "DR-TB Drugs Under the Microscope" http://www.doctorswithoutborders.org/publications/reports/2011/DR_TB_Drugs_Under_the_Microscope.Full%20Report.pdf

GLC, wrote to the MDR-TB Working Group of the Stop TB Partnership. Their letter included the following:

> "The Green Light Committee …have expressed repeated concerns ...about the stock-outs, repeated delays and outright shortages of second line MDR-TB drugs ...members [of the GLC] now fear that the poorly functioning …procurement system …threatens the entire functioning of the GLC initiative."

A fortnight later Stop TB's perplexing response of 29th May 2009 to PIH suggested that Dr Espinal knew "no WHO member country that had made any complaint" regarding the performance of the GDF and even went further, suggesting that "no issues had been raised at previous meetings with GLC and the GDF".

Something clearly wasn't working.

The consequence of an inadequate TB drug supply is chillingly predictable. Either the patients receive no treatment and probably die – or they do their utmost to obtain what they can when they can wherever they can. An article in the Journal of Infectious Disease from 2012 summed this up:

> "Individuals with suspected MDR-tuberculosis who cannot access second line treatment in the public sector may turn to private providers who may supply drugs, but of variable quality and without appropriate medical supervision, and the risk of amplified resistance and the risk of XDR-TB are high."[129]

In the mess that was evolving, players appear to have been beginning to wriggle uncomfortably and try to shift blame. Again Keshavjee helps illustrate these issues by describing how he himself saw the different roles of some of the key protagonists at the time:

- The WHO was carrying the overall responsibility for helping countries and for setting global standards but it had a direct conflict of interest regarding reforming the system from which it was receiving money itself on account of its existing strategies. Its funds were providing political leverage over countries and were therefore a source of power as well as a means of facilitation.

[129] Alimuddin Zumla et al. - "Drug-resistant tuberculosis—current dilemmas, unanswered questions, challenges, and priority needs", Journal of Infectious Diseases 205 Supplement 2 (2012) 228.

- Furthermore, the WHO appeared to be content with taking credit for the progress that had been made in the global fight against TB but was remaining tellingly reserved on the subject of MDR-TB and had added little or nothing to its targets connected to drug-resistance. The organisation certainly went so far as to acknowledge that the problem was or might well be growing, but it was resisting developing strategic targets for dealing with it.

- The Global Fund did not appear to want to take any responsibility at all for XDR-TB (hence they had casually passed the monopoly to the GLC); nor did it have in-house technical expertise on MDR-TB so was content to stay away from it; and worse still it feared any conflict with or within the WHO because of the potential negative effect this might have on donors.

- The Stop TB partnership's co-ordinating board was being undesirably unresponsive to the MDR-TB SLD price- and supply-problems even though these problems could usefully benefit from the size and scale that GDF operations could give it.

- UNITAID, created to scale up access to treatment for HIV, Malaria and TB, appeared to have been unable to do anything with second line drugs at all.

- Neither PEPFAR nor UNICEF included universal access to MDR-TB treatment as part of their global strategies.

- Donors did not appear to want to be seen as exerting influence on the WHO or other multilateral bodies; it seemed probable that the politicians concerned knew that doing so might incur huge political risk if they were seen to in any way shifting away from an existing policy (DOTS) that had already cost millions and was being hailed as having been a success.

- Patients were essentially being collectively unrepresented in this system. Individually they were still essentially being stigmatised within it, having little in the way of rights, and they knew that they might lose what little they got if they complained.

- The countries most affected by MDR-TB had existing national TB programmes which were already linked to WHO and they were essentially unwilling to jeopardise either this relationship or the funding that came with it. In a nutshell, they figured that they could lose vital donor money if they were seen to be rocking the boat.

This last may seem unlikely, but something similar may have happened in Uganda in 2012. In March that year the supply of first line drugs mysteriously dried up completely, and stayed that way for an unbelievable three months before the flow was in any way properly restored. No final official explanation has ever been offered. The Minister of Health had sacked three senior members of staff at the start of March for substantial financial improprieties which definitely included purchase of TB drugs, but there were subsequent public assurances that the drug supply had not been affected by this action. It may have been down to several factors combined with this, one of which was almost certainly connected to a cancellation of Round 11 of the Global Fund the previous autumn, whilst another may have been administrative inadequacy as well this evidence of corruption which has been since kept quiet. Either way, nobody rocked the boat, whilst for at least a full three months TB bacilli were merrily mutating in untreated Ugandan patients.[130]

The WHO defines a "defaulted" patient as being one whose treatment is interrupted for two consecutive months or more. By this definition, the ***entire national cohort*** of TB patients in Uganda at the time (one of the 22 high burden countries) defaulted through no fault of their own. What is

[130] There is food for thought here if we contrast this under-reported episode of potentially genocidal negligence with the more recent international political and media response to the same country's repressive anti-homosexual legislation. During the 2012 drug-supply disaster, neither the WHO, the UN, international politicians nor donor nations either reacted or took action; in contrast, the repressive Ugandan anti-homosexual legislation has attracted the regular attention, not just of the world's media, but more recently also of the President of the United States. The US has been threatening to freeze its aid to the country or at least to bypass the usual government pipelines (such as the Health Ministry) to NGOs. In 2013 this financial aid included US$411 million which went directly into health programmes including ones for TB. The Ugandan legislation is undeniably repressive and is also a contravention of international human rights; it has resulted in at least one death and 17 arrests, as well as persecution of individuals which has been stoked by a hostile tabloid press. But the Ugandan legislation is actually not as repressive as that which exists in Saudi Arabia which neither the White House nor the world's media seems interested in taking public issue with. It is sometimes very difficult to fathom out the collective agenda of the world's political and media elite.

interesting is that this event was neither measured nor reported in the 2013 global report. Will it show in the 2014 report? We will have to wait and see.

A further question arises from this: was this particular situation unique. Could it, or something like it, happen even more easily in another low-income country that isn't one of the 22 HBCs? It seems entirely possible.

MSF protocols insist that all patients with a break of two months in their treatment should receive drug-susceptibility testing when their treatment is resumed. They should also be given new treatment numbers. Neither happened in this instance in Uganda. What didn't happen either, however, was any immediate external intervention by the WHO. This is surprising given the undeniably huge epidemiological risks being created by the gap in supply. To anyone unfamiliar with the bureaucratic nature of the WHO such a lack of intervention might also seem an impossibility, particularly given that Uganda is a country on its own special list of 22 High Burden Countries. It really should not have been difficult to have initiated an emergency supply from manufacturers or from a stockpile to address the problem, and the WHO certainly has the powers to act in this way.

With regards to the second line drugs at least, UNITAID, has financed a stockpile so that more expedited shipments can be organised by the GDF in order to overcome the self-imposed restrictions created by piecemeal drug supply. According to MSF, however, this stockpile was used by 60 national tuberculosis programmes during 2011 and served mainly to complement orders for which quantities were already missing. As many as 20 national tuberculosis programmes did place 25 emergency orders in 2011, however, ones which were delivered with a median lead time of just 31 days. "Unfortunately", the MSF report recounts, "25 emergency orders with expedited delivery represent only a small proportion of GDF orders."

MSF offered its own solution:

> "National TB programmes … need to fully pre-pay their orders before they can be processed by GDF. If agreements with donors and consequent disbursements are delayed, the process is blocked. A revolving fund mechanism where money could be advanced to countries before donors funds are made available could alleviate this road-block."

Quite crazily, delays are also sometimes even caused by local regulations. Second line TB drugs are often not actually registered at all for use in the countries where GLC treatment projects are located, since they have never been used there. MSF's hard-earned experience has led them to report "that cumbersome special authorisation is frequently needed to import them."

When it comes to XDR-TB the problems are worse still since some of the drugs that are identified as being needed to treat it fall outside the remit of the GLC completely. Neither linezolid nor clofazimine, for instance, have any approved indication for DR-TB so often are also not be approved for use in national programmes despite the fact that they are often used as drugs of sole resort. Access to clofazimine for the treatment of XDR-TB patients has actually been denied on occasions on the basis of unclear efficacy, while linezolid is sometimes denied simply because of its expense. In South Africa, this single drug currently can cost up to R700 (US$70) a tablet due to current patent protection. The treatment is required daily for a period of two years. What is particularly worrying is that the South African Medical Control Council has not allowed the importation of the drug's generic equivalent (which costs 28 times less than the patented product), rejecting an application for this made by MSF. Meanwhile the South African Department of Health won't pay for the drug itself because of its expense. As a result, MSF itself has resorted to buying the drug as best it can on the open market and adding it to the standard regimen they use in South Africa whenever the see it as being necessary.

Furthermore, while its patent for the drug expires in 2014, a second patent on a crystallised form of the drug may still block cheaper generics from entering the South African marketplace until 2022.

MSF summed these appalling ironies up in a nutshell:

> "These high prices are a reflection of the fact that current market demand is low, due to limited capacity to diagnose and treat DR-TB, which does not provide a sufficient incentive to manufacturers. The global DR-TB market was estimated to be worth US$300 million in 2010, with only US$125 million procured through the public sector."

Keshavjee and Farmer together have made further noise on the subject. In a paper published in the New England Journal of Medicine in 2010[131] they baldly identified that "the rate at which treatment programs are being launched or expanded is inadequate as a response to a global emergency"

[131] Salmaan Keshavjee and Paul Farmer, - "Picking up the pace – scale-up of MDR-Tuberculosis treatment programs", New England Journal of Medicine 363 (2010) 1781-84.

and that "advocacy for scaling up MDR tuberculosis treatment has been inadequate and must increase – exponentially".

"Moreover," they wrote, "there has been limited organized demand for treatment from patients with MDR tuberculosis, their families, or their advocates — a marked difference from the situation with HIV." Given that they know better than most the nature of what it means to be among the most at risk of tuberculosis, that they are more often than not the pathologically disempowered, the voiceless and the impoverished, this hardly seems to have been an extreme observation.

The Beijing meeting

It was their reference, however, to the "the best efforts of the World Health Organization (WHO) to highlight the MDR tuberculosis crisis through a high-level ministerial meeting in Beijing " that suggests that even these fearless advocates can be cautious at times if they have good political reason to be.

Part of the report from this meeting in Beijing in 2009 stated without any sign of reservation that: "In our assessment, it is possible to reverse the spread of MDR-TB with currently available treatment regimens, and by improved case finding, even in settings where MDR-TB is high and increasing." This relatively unqualified assessment, at the very least, might seem to some to have been either naïve or even disingenuous, but it came with a rider which may have seemed hugely important to Farmer and Keshavjee. The report proclaimed that:

> "[The] WHO's future planning aims to achieve universal access which is the diagnosis and treatment, by 2015, of at least 80% of patients with smear-positive MDR-TB in the 27 countries most affected."

We may raise our eyebrows and wonder what is being intended to happen to the patients in all of the other many countries with MDR-TB beyond the borders of this special group of 27 – countries where MDR-TB is being missed or misdiagnosed – but both Farmer and Keshavjee may have been hugging each other at the inclusion of the those two particular words "universal access" in such a statement because of the precedent it implied.

The vision of these two doctors for the proper treatment of tuberculosis has been consistent, as well as being compellingly logical – put patients first, get drugs to them, achieve full compliance with quality assurance, pool SLD orders with malaria and HIV drugs, apply 90 day rules for their supply, and use the strength of the WHO to encourage governments to act on the difficulties of the drug supply. The idea of universal access has been enshrined in each and every endorsement they have made on the matter.

MSF, in their own 2012 report, had other recommendations which they offered to the individual parties concerned:

The Global Drug Facility –

- Should continue to publish prices of medicines on its website in order to improve transparency,
- Should work on the expansion of the existing rotating stockpile to decrease the time it takes for countries to receive medicines for all orders, and not just the emergency ones, and
- Should further develop a strategic revolving fund with international donors to provide manufacturers a financial guarantee to secure the production and supply of second line TB drugs.

The World Health Organization –

- Should promote the use of quality-assured medicines at country level,
- Should keep a balance between stimulating an optimal offer of older second line drugs and the introduction of new compounds, and
- Should support the evaluation of shorter treatment regimens and give timely advice on the use of new compounds.

Donors –

- Should support research to define a better and shorter DR-TB treatment regimen with the inclusion of newer drugs,

- Should promote the use of quality-assured medicines at country level by harmonising quality criteria for medical procurement across donors, and
- Should streamline supply chain mechanism both at country and global levels.

And Governments –

- Should commit to use medicines which meet WHO standards,
- Should ensure patients have free access to a complete course of DR-TB treatment in quality programmes,
- Should regulate DR-TB medicines in order to preserve their efficacy and
  avoid fuelling resistance, and
- Should establish a framework for compassionate-use programmes.

There was another major development at the Beijing conference, however – the creation of what Mario Raviglione described as a "proper basis for discussions among pharma companies". This amounts to the formulation of a panel of interested parties intent on focusing on new combinations of drugs rather than on individual drugs themselves in order to effectively short-cut research programmes. In the language of TB research this in turn means the creation of a "Critical Path for TB Treatment Regimens (the CPTR)". Given the decades-long history of combination therapy such an approach might appear logical, obvious, and a little belated, but to the political spin doctors who continue to script the sluggish global response to MDR-TB it was hailed as being "visionary".[132]

[132] http://www.nbr.org/downloads/pdfs/CHA/NBR_Raviglione_interview.pdf

"Double Trouble" – the Ungodly Twins of HIV and TB

"IF WE ARE TO DO SOMETHING ABOUT AIDS, THEN WE HAVE TO DO SOMETHING ABOUT TB.
IF WE ARE TO DO SOMETHING ABOUT TB, WE ARE GOING TO HAVE TO DO SOMETHING ABOUT AIDS.
AS WE HAVE OVERCOME APARTHEID, SO WE SHALL DEFEAT TB AND HIV/AIDS, THESE UNGODLY TWIN KILLERS."

Archbishop Desmond Tutu

"WE CANNOT WIN THE BATTLE AGAINST AIDS
IF WE DO NOT ALSO FIGHT TB.
TB IS TOO OFTEN A DEATH SENTENCE FOR PEOPLE WITH AIDS.
IT DOES NOT HAVE TO BE THIS WAY."

Nelson Mandela

We know that the mechanisms of both of these diseases work in perniciously different ways, although how this happens is still only partially understood. The HIV virus certainly works by compromising its host's CD4+ T cells, something which in turn stokes the immune deficiency that is the feature of the infection. These particular CD4 immune cells turn out to be the very ones which are essential in the walling off of the granulomas in the tubercles that in turn establish the initial latent stalemate. We already know that tuberculosis bacilli proliferate whenever opportunity presents – most often when the host immune system is compromised, so, as the integrity of the immune system declines as a result of the reduction in CD4 cells, the tuberculosis bacilli appear to seize the moment and break out of their latent containment, often, in HIV cases, as a straightforward roll-over process following on from the primary infection. As such, the 'normal' granulomatous response to TB infection becomes profoundly compromised.

Overall a lot of problems result – and they are evident in a sobering roll call of facts and statistics which may be challenging for the unfamiliar reader to take in in a single reading.

Whilst the 'normal' risk of developing active TB disease is generally accepted as being 5-10% in a lifetime, in circumstances of co-infection the estimated risk is revised to be 5-15% in ***every year*** that the patient might survive their HIV infection if it is untreated. The more regularly quoted likelihood of developing active disease if someone is HIV-positive and already has a latent TB infection is that it is rendered between ***21 and 34 times*** more likely to become active following HIV infection than it was beforehand. Whatever the true probabilities may be (and they may well vary dramatically in different countries), it is clear that the likelihood of developing active TB if you are latently infected and contract HIV (or vice versa) is extremely high.

The two diseases then seem to work both bi-directionally and synergistically, each progressing more quickly in the presence of the other than they generally do when developing on their own. One dramatic estimate has suggested that the life expectancy of a TB/HIV patient is reduced to as little as six weeks following the diagnosis of the second disease, although it is hard to believe or substantiate such a claim. A reference in the Global Plan for TB 2011-2015 presents the risk from the two diseases in a slightly different way, stating that people living with HIV who develop TB but do not receive effective TB and HIV care have only a one-in-ten chance of surviving for three months or more.[133]

Often, with co-infection, the patient's sputum unfortunately fails to show the bacilli when it is stained and examined in the microscope. This leads to delayed diagnosis or complete misdiagnosis. This pauci-bacillary nature of a co-infected patient's sputum is thought to be because of the lowered host immune response to the disease which results in fewer visible bacilli. The resultant diagnostic delays must both further explain and contribute to the massively reduced life expectancy as suggested above. What also seems to occur is that, whilst treating one disease on its own, the other naturally accelerates, meaning that treating either disease when they occur together is difficult and can be very hazardous to the patient.

There is some evidence available to explain this phenomenon. The presence of one particular amino acid (CCR5) can affect immune cells in ways which exert diametrically different impacts upon each of the two diseases, promoting an immune response in one disease whilst negating it in the other.

CCR5 triggers some of the immune cells' response to TB. Without it the mycobacteria are believed to be able to thrive within the host cells as the

---

[133] WHO - "Global Plan for Tuberculosis 2011-2015", page 24.

infected person's immune system never gets the signal from the CCR5 to attack it. Some HIV drugs, however, work by inhibiting these CCR5 receptors because CCR5 cells also act as receptors for the HIV virus. As a result, carelessly administering of these drugs to patients who have TB as well can prove to be disastrous. Such observations go some way to explain why the two diseases are so difficult to treat together, and also why each disease might progress so much more quickly in the presence of the other.

The combination of these two diseases together is simply the deadliest double-whammy of disease of our age. In Africa TB is recognised as being ***the*** AIDS-defining illness, unlike in any other region, and this is why TB has gone rampant in Africa since HIV first emerged there in any epidemic sense. If the drugs to treat HIV are available (and unfortunately they often still are not in Africa) they frequently have to be withheld until the TB is brought under control; but the drugs for TB immediately exacerbate the HIV-provoked immune deficiency and so accelerate its progression. Furthermore, even when the drugs for both diseases can be safely applied together, regimes of reduced efficacy often have to be employed because of the interactions between them, some of which are still to be fully studied and documented.

TB is also known to increase HIV infectivity, as well as reduce HIV treatment efficacy.

TB in co-infected cases also exhibits higher-than-normal rates of extra-pulmonary disease (at a rate of at least 25% instead of a more normal 10% and often much higher still). This means that active disease is far more difficult to recognise in co-infected cases because symptoms may be atypical, and because sputum tests will generally show negative even in cases of active disease.

Co-infection of HIV and TB is also thought to result in more rapid potential development of MDR-TB and XDR-TB if the drugs are at all mismanaged. This in turn poses a huge epidemiological risk wherever high rates of co-infection occur.

What is undeniable, as a result, is that people living with HIV (PLWH) need the earliest diagnosis and the best possiblt treatment of active TB disease if it emerges.

It is estimated that at least one-third of the current 34 million PLWH worldwide are latently infected with TB bacteria, although most are not yet ill with active disease. Looking at the two diseases from the opposite direction, however, about one in every five tested TB patients also turn up to be HIV-positive.

TB is a leading cause of death in people with HIV infection. Overall, almost 25% of deaths among people with HIV are due to TB – in fact in 2011 about 430,000 people died of HIV-associated TB. In Africa, however, TB is ***the*** leading cause of death among PLWH, and most HIV-positive patients die from it.

In 2012 there were an estimated 1.1 million cases of HIV-positive new TB cases. Around 75% of these were in Africa. In 2011, the percentage of TB patients found to be HIV-positive in the 28 African countries in the list of 41 HIV priority countries ranged from 8% in Ethiopia to 77% in Swaziland. Besides Swaziland, the countries with more than 50% of TB patients who were tested HIV-positive were Botswana, Lesotho, Malawi, Mozambique, Namibia, South Africa, Uganda, Zambia and Zimbabwe.

More than two-thirds (69%) of all those people currently living with HIV (an estimated total of 23.5 million people) live in sub-Saharan Africa — a total which includes a terrible 91% of the world's HIV-positive children.

Estimates have suggested that in 2011 1.8 million people in the region became newly infected with HIV, and 1.2 million adults and children died as HIV-positive on the continent. This latter number accounted for 71% of the total world's AIDS deaths in that year. In that same year 330,000 children under 15 contracted HIV and 230,000 HIV-positive children died: most of them would have died from TB, and almost all would have died in Africa.[134]

Clear progress has been being made in this concerted campaign against the co-epidemic. Cambodia, particularly, is identified as having been especially successful. Global estimates of HIV-associated TB deaths have been falling since 2003, and the decreases have been accelerating more recently, but there was still at least 320,000 deaths from HIV-associated TB in 2012. The UNAIDS and Stop TB Partnership's target is to halve TB mortality rates among PLWH by 2015 compared to what it was in 2004. The high point back in 2005-6 was a little over half a million, so, while there is work to do, this target is clearly in sight. There has also been a very encouraging increase in Anti-Retroviral Therapy (ART) among HIV-positive patients,

---

[134] Most of the above comes from the WHO. "Tuberculosis (Fact Sheet no.104)" (2010). http://www.who.int/mediacentre/factsheets/fs104/en/

up to 57% of all estimated patients in 2012, but, given that the WHO's recommendation is that ***all*** HIV-positive TB patients should be automatically eligible for ART (at the earliest possible moment irrespective of their CD4 count), there is still much to do. The earliest possible initiation of ART after the start of TB treatment is now seen to very seriously reduce the risk of morbidity and mortality for PLWH.

By itself, ART is now judged to reduce the risk of re-activated or primary TB disease in PLWH by as much as 65%. In the latest WHO recommendations for HIV the threshold CD4 count at which ART is recommended to be commenced has been raised from less than 350 CD4/mm^3 to anything less than 500. ART is already recommended for all TB patients living with HIV whatever their cell count, but this raising of the threshold for those diagnosed HIV-positive should mean that many more PLWH would be eligible to start treatment and also that, as a result, fewer PLWH will then be seen to develop TB. And as a further result, it is then hoped that all rates should correspondingly continue to improve further still.

There is still little in the way of a real evidence base for the pharmaceutical treatment of both diseases together. Most treatments have been developed by expert opinion only, and much of the work has been done in Europe, where arguably substantially different disease profiles exist, so that what has been developed may not be so universally applicable where the co-epidemic truly thrives. Also, of course, expert opinion often varies between authorities.

Considering that most of the rates in the co-epidemic are moving in the right direction, however, it looks like expert opinion may well have been getting it more right than wrong, stimulated by the activity of HIV advocacy groups who rightly recognise the threats to their concerted campaign against HIV from tuberculosis. It may not be that things will continue to turn out quite as hoped, however, particularly as the impact from MDR- and XDR-TB enters the mix more noticeably. This is because deficiencies of knowledge as regards effective treatment in co-infected cases are most acute with second line drugs, the ones which are used for treating DR-TB since they have yet to be properly tested for interactions with HIV medication. Doing this has simply not been a priority for the developers of HIV drugs since co-infection with TB is still less common in wealthier countries with co-infection with drug-resistant strains even less so.

There remains a gold-standard model for the campaign against HIV/TB, and it is called the 'Three I's for HIV/TB'. These are:

- Intensified case finding for TB,
- Isoniazid preventive therapy, and
- Infection control.

All three together are intended to reduce the burden of TB among PLWH and therefore are intended to be implemented by all HIV services. Reported figures in relation to these 'Three I's' are also moving in the right direction. Encouragingly, the number of PLWH who were screened for TB (an element of the "intensified case finding") almost quadrupled from 600,000 in 2007 to 2,300,000 in 2010. In 2012 this figure shot up to over four million. However, this still represents fewer than 7% of the 34 million people estimated to be living with HIV.[135]

It is particularly being encouraged that, if there is evidence of latent infection but active TB is confirmed as ***not*** being present after screening, then patients should automatically receive Isoniazid preventive therapy (IPT), a treatment is intended to be free of charge and not to be prohibitively expensive for any health system.

The numbers are improving year on year. Of the 1.5 million people reported to have been newly enrolled in HIV care in 2010 just 12% were put on IPT. By 2012, 1.6 million were reported to be newly put on HIV treatment, and 30% of them were put on IPT. Furthermore, 42 countries are now reporting data, where a year earlier only 29 were doing so. There are undoubtedly immense efforts being made to ramp up this part of the Global Plan.

There are worrying complexities to be untangled for this part of the policy, nevertheless. As we have seen, the major risk from using IPT is from the possibility of using it on already active disease because it may then stoke drug-resistance. The WHO recommends a four-symptom algorithm to rule out this risk as a result of which it expects approximately 50% of all PLWH to be eligible for IPT. In 2012 the estimated number of PLWH was 35 million, implying that the current target should be 17.5 million PLWH being swept up and put on IPT. How fool proof is the algorithm? Knowing that TB has such an unfortunate habit of not showing symptoms until sometime after it has re-activated, it's difficult for anyone to be certain. With these sorts of numbers, only a small percentage of 'misses' (i.e. PLWH being put on IPT when they already have asymptomatic re-activated or primary TB) could make for a lot in terms of absolute numbers.

---

[135] WHO - "TB/HIV Facts 2011-2012".

The current rate of increase of implementation of IPT is actually greater than the rate of improving screening for HIV which testifies to the efforts that are being made. Meanwhile, the Global Plan still intends that all of those eligible for IPT should be being put on the treatment by 2015. It is just possible, however, that these herculean efforts might prove to have been worse than doing nothing if it is seen to reduce rates of treatable disease while simultaneously stoking rates of disease that is untreatable.

Certainly where there are already high rates of MDR-TB, despite IPT being indicated for PLWH, it has to be accepted as being an epidemiologically risky treatment. In fact it is arguable that it should not be embarked upon at all as a general policy in such countries. Furthermore, the data on the efficacy of IPT has been harvested mainly in low-incidence countries, ones without high rates of co-infection and without high rates of drug-resistance. If an HIV patient who presents as a candidate for IPT is already Isoniazid-resistant, what will the effects be from being put on a lengthy course of the single drug? It's far from clear that anyone knows. The eight countries which currently have the largest proportion of HIV patients being put on IPT are (in order): South Africa (370,000), Ethiopia (30,000), Malawi (21,000), Mozambique (17,000), Lesotho (16,000), Haiti (15,000), Ukraine (14,000) and Namibia (12,000). Whatever the official figures may say, it's unlikely that any of these countries do not have rates of MDR-TB that are well above the global average (particularly in the pool of latent infection where drug-resistance is so frustratingly undiagnosable). They are almost certainly also already being affected by the insidious threat of XDR-TB, which will already be there in their respective pools of latent disease. South Africa, for instance, the country with the most HIV patients being put on IPT, is reported to carry 71% of the reported global burden of XDR-TB.

There is also the factor of re-infection in any high incidence environment. Without doubt re-infection is common in all high incidence countries although it is also certain that its risk should be reduced with ART if HIV is impacting on the local epidemic. High incidence rates therefore dictate that preventative treatment needs to be rolled out in really big numbers in order to make any impression on the latent pool and then bring down number of cases of re-activating disease as intended. But will it turn out to be a circle of much less than is being expected of it – with the unintended effect of stoking the DR epidemic if only by unwittingly but inevitably treating asymptomatic re-activated disease in a proportion of cases if so many patients are treated?

In the meantime, how is the success or failure of the initiative itself being measured? It can't be measured by skin testing. The only way is by long-term follow-up studies to see whether patients have really avoided re-activated disease.

It seems probable that the progress in the roll-out of IPT has been largely down to the relative strength of the HIV lobby. The concomitant neglect of the associated issues relating to drug-resistance in TB disease strongly suggests that this has been the case – the priority having been more intensely focused on the epidemiology of HIV rather than on the two diseases equally. Archbishop Tutu, at the start of this section, offered his insight on this problem. While Nelson Mandela was rightly seeing the problem of AIDS as being insoluble without confronting TB, Tutu recognised the more complex issue: that looking at one disease through the lens of the other without doing exactly the same in reverse would miss vital clues. Both men suffered from TB themselves, Mandela while in prison, and Tutu in his youth, so they both know the disease first hand. But Tutu's message is unequivocal: neither disease can be resolved on its own, but nor can both diseases be resolved together without each being resolved individually. We can add that the complexities of both diseases must be fully considered and given equal respect in this process. All this can be done, just as it was done with apartheid, but it is an immense challenge and is fraught with further complications and risks, not least that they have to be continuously reviewed together with every possible angle being considered as developments inevitably unfold.

Children

"ZINHLE, SFUNDO, SNETEMBA, ZAKHENI, NTOKOZO, THANDIWE,
STAY STRONG...
BE BRAVE.
I'LL MAKE SURE THIS WORLD KNOWS YOUR NAMES."

Sage Francis (2012)[136]

Children can easily catch TB from the very close contact they need from their mothers and families. There's nothing new in this – it's always been that way.

When there are high rates of HIV in the community, however, the situation becomes a lot more complicated, and, unfortunately, also a lot worse. If a mother herself is co-infected with HIV and TB (as is too often the case in southern Africa) the odds of her child contracting TB become pretty dreadful: maternal TB is associated with a 2.5-fold increased risk of vertical transmission to an unborn child in circumstances of HIV co-infection (a risk which is normally about one in four if the mother is HIV-negative). This computes into a probable risk of transmission of over 60%. Kids who are HIV-positive also unfortunately cannot be vaccinated with BCG so they are at the mercy of TB infection from the moment they first breathe.

What is equally concerning, however, is that the global number of children affected and killed by TB generally has remained unknown and officially unestimated.

The wider epidemic in children is sometimes rather ironically referred to as an "invisible" epidemic. There are very simple reasons for this. Because kids often develop extra-pulmonary TB (possibly nearly 50% of children's disease is extra-pulmonary), and also because, even if they develop TB in the lungs, they are normally pauci-bacillary. With too few infectious bugs in their lungs available to be coughed up into the air around them, they are simply not seen to be dangerously infectious agents who might in any meaningful way contribute to the size of the epidemic. Because their infectious threat is so limited, they have been considered worth the trouble of being counted. Their particular suffering has been ignored simply because they are considered to be "epidemiologically insignificant". In

[136] Sage Francis is an American rap artist. These are the lyrics of a song he released especially for World AIDS Day 2012. The song was entitled, "Ubuntu – What's bad for you is bad for me".

other words, they have been ignored because they don't often transmit the disease.

This fact unfortunately only captures half of the equation, because it is also exactly because they carry such an innocent bacillary load (though lethal enough for the child, of course) that they are so infrequently diagnosed and properly treated, and that so many must invisibly and inevitably die. For the same reasons, the probability exists that any figures that are thrown at infant mortalities are both inaccurate and underestimated. The 2012 WHO's Global Tuberculosis Report did take a stab at this for the first time (nearly 20 years after the organisation first declared TB as a global emergency) devoting one section of its report to children, but it was conservative at best in its tone. An MSF doctor observed at the time that the "sad reality [is] that until just last month, there was little data on the global burden of paediatric TB." Even worse, having made their appearance in the report, it turned out that they were immediately going to be taken off it again, as we will shortly see.

More accurate numbers, however, will only go part of the way to depict the suffering and injustice facing children with TB worldwide because such numbers cannot begin to capture the problems of diagnosis and treatment in kids with TB.

The standard diagnostic method of sputum testing has been recently shown to be dramatically more unreliable in children than in adults. Whilst it took nearly 40 years for the medical authorities to properly wake up to the inadequacies of drug treatments for kids (as we will see), it took well over a century for it to recognise this appalling inadequacy with the standard diagnostic method for detecting the disease.

In November 2012 MSF presented some particular findings at the World Conference on Lung Health in Kuala Lumpur, drawing upon data that had been collected over three years from 2,451 children with TB treated in 13 projects in six countries. They showed first of all, not unexpectedly, that children co-infected with HIV and TB were more than twice as likely to die than children solely infected with TB. But it was the findings' revelation concerning the reliability of the sputum test that was even more shocking. While more than half of the entire tested cohort (56%) had pulmonary TB, ***only a tiny 6.4%*** of them tested 'positive' for the disease with the standard sputum smear microscopy TB test. This percentage would normally be expected to be nearer 50% with adults, possibly higher. Such a tiny proportional percentage is simply because kids carry such insufficient numbers of bacteria in their sputa for them to be detected on a microscope slide.

MSF's Dr Philipp du Cros summed up the findings of their report:

> "When you're only detecting TB in one out of ten children, you can be sure that many are falling through the cracks simply because they're not being diagnosed, resulting in unnecessary deaths."

New diagnostics will surely help, but as yet they do not solve the problem. While the new Xpert®MTB/RIF assay for TB may significantly increase the number of children diagnosed with TB in those countries where it is being rolled out, it will still not confirm diagnosis in a significant number of children with clinical suspicion of TB if they cannot provide a sputum sample. Many, unfortunately, cannot do this.[137] The GeneXpert device may be more reliable, but it still relies on sputum as its raw material.

It is often the case that children are simply unable to cough sputum up at all. In such instances, and if there is good enough cause to think there is active disease, then clinicians have little alternative but to resort to unpleasant techniques to support their suspicions. Dr Martina Casenghi, the Scientific Advisor for MSF's Access Campaign, describes them as follows:

> "In an attempt to get adequate samples, health workers are forced to use invasive and painful measures, involving forcing vapour into their lungs to make them cough up sputum, or sucking out sputum from their stomach."

Understandably, a high index of suspicion is required before doctors are willing to undertake such procedures: plainly a TB test for children that doesn't rely on sputum and which might use samples that are easier to obtain (like blood, urine or stool) is seriously needed.

TB in kids can also be particularly lethal. Tuberculous meningitis, for example, an extra-pulmonary form of the disease (with the infection reaching the membranes surrounding the brain) is more common in children. It can also appear quickly and kill fast, especially so by normal tubercular standards.

---

[137] MSF - "Standard TB test failing to detect the disease in children 93% of the time" (2012).

The overall risk of developing the disease for all ages is actually the highest in the under-threes. It then drops off to kick in again later, so, whilst no data is available, it's reasonable to assume that most kids who die from the disease are less than five years old. It is estimated that between 10-15% of TB cases each year occur in children although in some regions they are thought to carry as much as 20-40% of the burden of disease. The simple fact is that childhood TB has yet to be properly studied and is still not being anywhere near adequately monitored.

According to the WHO's 2012 report, around half a million children became ill with TB in 2011 and an estimated 64,000 children died from it.[138] The estimated death toll in this instance, however, did ***not*** include those kids who were HIV-positive, since these WHO figures were counted elsewhere. Not mentioning these in the report has to have been disingenuous given that MSF recognise that mortality rates are twice as high in these cases. According to other WHO reports, 230,000 children died as a result of being HIV-positive in 2011. If we assume that 50% of them died of TB (which might well be typical of the African syndemic) then that TB death estimate of 64,000 could be as much as tripled at a stroke.

These numbers used in the report are, in any case, acknowledged to be probably underestimated. In order to estimate the incidence of TB among children, for instance, the report assumed that the ratio of 'notified' cases to estimated incident cases was the same for children as it was for adults (which at the global level in 2011 was pegged at 66%). This is unlikely for good reasons as we will see. But on this simplistic assumption the report concluded that TB incidence among children must be "equivalent to about 6% of the total number of 8.7 million incident cases". If 20% of the disease burden is in the under-15s, however, (an estimated percentage which is quoted elsewhere) then actually at least three times the WHO estimate may have become ill in 2011 and three times as many may have died. And if the overall WHO estimate of global incidence is under-estimated as well, then the actual numbers might be higher still. Because of unreliable diagnostic tests it is hardly outrageous to suggest that many more children must simply go undiagnosed (and therefore uncounted and untreated) than ever appear on any lists, whether or not they are notified or otherwise estimated.[139]

[138] WHO - "Global Tuberculosis Report 2012".

[139] MSF – "Uncounted & Untreated: Children with TB", (2012).

Soumya Swaminathan, the director of the Indian National Institute for Research in Tuberculosis sums this anomaly up. In India around 85,000 children are diagnosed each year, and yet:

> "At present, [these] paediatric cases form 7% of the total number of cases under RNTCP [the Revised National TB Control Programme]. But the real figure could be 15 or 20 per cent of the total TB burden."

The WHO in 2012 formally announced its intention to put the lid on the subject, recommending that figures for children should ***not*** be included in its more rigorous future national prevalence surveys and global reports. This decision might have seemed alarming, but there were actually good practical reasons behind it. First of all (and the report candidly acknowledged this) "only a few bacteriologically-confirmed cases would [ever] be found" – so any estimates made would have to be accepted as being hugely uncertain exactly at the time that more certainty was what was being striven for. But there were ethical issues that needed to be considered as well, primarily associated with the necessary mass radiological screening of children as part of any wider survey, most of whom would inevitably have to be assumed to be healthy. While reasonable evidence exists that chest X-ray screening is safe for adults, similar evidence does not currently exist for children.

Unexpectedly, the 2013 report turned out to backtrack on this decision because it ***did*** include further figures for children. It estimated 530,000 new cases in 2012 and 74,000 deaths among children who were HIV-negative. The estimates of TB morbidity and mortality among children were therefore "slightly higher" than those published in the 2012 global TB report, "reflecting new surveillance data that show more TB cases being notified among children globally, and new VR data".

In order to reach this estimate of TB incidence among children, once again "it was assumed that the case detection rate for all ages at the global level in 2012 … was the same for adults and children". This detection rate was once again pegged at 66% for 2012, which again, given what we know about TB in children, was almost certainly still optimistic.

The total number of deaths from TB among HIV-negative children was estimated to be equivalent to about 8% of the total number of 940,000 TB deaths among HIV-negative people in 2012. Any estimate of TB mortality among HIV-positive children was again not included due (the report stated) "to the difficulties arising from the miscoding of HIV deaths as TB deaths". Yet again this suggests the level of relative neglect that has hampered any sort of proper monitoring of childhood tuberculosis, since mortality amongst HIV-positive adults was identified separately in this report as it has been for years.

One piece of good news did appear however – that age disaggregation of HIV-associated TB mortality will be one of the future outcomes of the TB component of Spectrum. This is a software system that is being used to indirectly estimate mortality numbers in HIV-positive TB patients. Whether it will accurately reflect any sort of reality will depend upon not just the data fed into it, but also how the software itself is set up to mathematically extrapolate the final data.

Currently, as well, the number of children affected and killed by drug-resistant TB (as opposed to susceptible disease) is another unknown: it is as yet unestimated and looks likely officially to remain that way. The report explains that "little is known about the burden of MDR-TB in children".[140] The best guess in the 2012 Global Tuberculosis Report came from just 37 countries which offered MDR-TB enrolment data. Based on this, children represented a vague 1–13% of total enrolments on GLC approved programmes. Can GLC approved programmes offer such variable and vague data? The best that appears to have been suggested so far is that any child with TB is as likely as a TB infected adult in the same community to have an MDR strain.

Unfortunately, the true number of children actually infected by drug-resistant disease is quite possibly proportionately higher than for adults, particularly because transmission of the disease to children is almost certainly more common in countries where incidence of drug-resistance is also high. The Sentinel Project for Pediatric Drug-Resistant Tuberculosis has been developed by PIH collaborators at Harvard Medical School, and it is intending to uncover exactly these and other vital gaps in information.[141]

[140] WHO - "Global Tuberculosis Report 2013".

[141] http://sentinel-project.org/

One small scale attempt has already been made.[142] A retrospective study in Peru looked at the rates of development of disease in family members and contacts of patients registered and enrolled on MDR-TB treatments between 1996 and 2003. It concluded that the risk was particularly high in the first two years after the index contact commenced his or her treatment. A total of 87% of the kids they confirmed as having TB were, perhaps unsurprisingly, confirmed to have MDR-TB (and not DS-TB). With the benefit of its data, this study estimated that 20% of the total MDR disease burden was with children (i.e. over three times the WHO estimate) – and it concluded that childhood contact with the disease carried a risk of developing TB that was 30 times higher than other kids in their neighbourhood.

These results highlight a gaping hole in the fight against DR-TB because no-one is yet going out looking for these kids, something which surely should be being done. MSF and PIH, whilst accepting that chemo-prophylaxis of known MDR-TB close contacts is not recommended, still state that they should be being closely monitored for at least two years.[143] A huge proportion of such close contacts, inevitably, are children.

There is, without any doubt, a real and very urgent need to implement contact investigations and establish systems for prompt referral and treatment of paediatric household contacts of MDR-TB patients, regardless of the age of the child, and this should be happening not just wherever MDR-TB is known to exist, but also wherever it ***might*** possibly exist. The Stop TB Strategy launched by the WHO in 2006 included exactly this in its original mandate, including a plan for "case-finding in high-risk or vulnerable groups such as children and prevention of TB in children who live in the same household as newly detected TB cases". The evidence in its own report six years later that this part of its plan is being remotely appropriately implemented is hardly substantial.

Despite this disease having been such a familiar one, this wider business of childhood tuberculosis is only now really gaining the attention it deserves.

---

[142] Becerra M et al. –" Tuberculosis in children exposed at home to multidrug-resistant tuberculosis", Pediatric Infectious Diseases Journal, 32; 2 (2013) 115-19.

[143] PIH & MSF. "Tuberculosis – Practical Guide for clinicians, nurses, laboratory technicians and medical auxillaries" (2014). http://refbooks.msf.org/msf_docs/en/tuberculosis/tuberculosis_en.pdf

It is finally being considered by some not only just as an urgent global public health issue but also (quite correctly) as one of human and humanitarian rights as well.

Two examples of this perplexing neglect can illustrate this.

The first is that there are still no proper paediatric formulations for TB treatment regimens for children – despite the standard first line drug regimen being over 40 years old. In 2010 the WHO recognised that such dosage recommendations as did exist for children were probably being pitched too low – resulting in potentially avoidable poor outcomes and potential drug-resistance. Dosage recommendations have since been revised, but still no first line formulations have appeared. In fact neither fixed dose therapies nor individual drug therapies currently exist. What this means is that adult doses are either divided or ground up in *ad hoc* fashions – pills are cut or crushed, capsules opened, or medications stirred into formula, juice, and food. Nobody can argue with the conclusion that treating children with split or crushed pills might be ineffective as often as it might be effective – but it is also creates another potential recipe for drug-resistance. And such educated guesswork derived from adult doses inevitably also comes with risks to the individual child of overdosage as well.

This applies to paediatric drug-sensitive TB. With MDR- and XDR-TB all of these risks are far worse, not least because of all of the drugs are that much more toxic.

To coincide with World TB Day 2013, Partners in Health published an interview with Carole Mitnick, a TB researcher and assistant professor of global health and social medicine at Harvard Medical School. In it she described how imprecise and time-consuming preparing the medication for MDR-TB really can be, particularly given that there are so many pills being taken for such a long period of time:

> "A TB nurse who works in a public health center that collaborates closely with Socios en Salud, our PIH sister project in Peru, estimated that ***it takes her a full day to create a week's worth of doses for a single paediatric MDR-TB patient*** she is treating."[144]

---

[144] PIH - "World TB Day: A Q&A With Expert Carole Mitnick". http://www.pih.org/blog/world-tb-day-expert-carole-mitnick-on-drug-development-treatment-models-and

Things may just be changing a little, however. In 2012 the WHO added "recommended fixed-dose combinations for treating children with drug-sensitive TB" on to its "Expression of Interest" list. In so doing it was effectively asking pharmaceutical companies to get more involved in the problem,[145] inviting them to submit their products for evaluation, and encouraging them to consider producing paediatric formulations. This is as far as things have gone so far, however, and, given the realities that exist, they may not go much further unless appropriate direct pressures are applied.

UNITAID has also taken on the task of encouraging a healthier market for paediatric TB drugs, acknowledging the challenges that exist but also recognizing the vital importance of getting manufacturers involved in this area. So it is to be hoped that changes will now occur sooner rather than later and that paediatric formulations of both drug-sensitive and drug-resistant TB drugs will finally be developed.[146]

If no drug-susceptibility test (DST) is available (as is statistically predictable given global realities) the child in question may be diagnosed as MDR simply by failing standard first line therapy (defined as sputum smear-positive at two months, but more probably with children simply because of no resolution of symptoms or because of symptoms getting worse with continued weight loss). In such cases, treatment decisions can only properly be based on the prevailing local DST pattern of MDR-TB strains - if they are actually known. Because children with TB frequently never become sputum-positive anyway, a sickening child may even be started on empirical MDR-TB therapy based on the DST pattern of a close contact without any other confirmation of disease beyond symptoms.

As with adults, drugs would generally be chosen using a stepwise selection process working down through the five groups of drugs, with the intention that at least four drugs will simultaneously have some effect on the bacillus. The adverse effects with almost all of these drugs on children are known to be high, particularly so with cycloserine (creating neuropsychiatric problems) and ethionamide (causing acute vomiting and diarrhoea).

This brings us to the second example of neglect because, despite almost all of these drugs being over 50 years old (and most of them older than first

---

[145] http://apps.who.int/prequal/info_applicants/eoi/EOI-Tuberculosis_V11.pdf

[146] MSF – "Children with TB, global interest at last", (2012).

line drugs), only two of them (amikacin and levofloxacin) have ever been developed as paediatric formulations at all – and even these are not widely available.

In fact only three of the drugs which lie outside of the first group are actually licensed today for use in children at all – and one of these (levofloxacin) is only approved for use with children for a maximum of 14 days, when a child with MDR-TB might well need it for two years. Actually no-one even knows how long they should take these drugs for either, because the optimal duration of MDR-TB treatment in children is still not known nor agreed upon either. The WHO's general guidelines recommend treatment until 18 months after the first negative culture is obtained (or 24 months in XDR-TB), but since children often have pauci-bacillary disease, documenting such a culture conversion is in most cases rather difficult to determine as well.

Even with new drugs emerging things may end up in much the same way. In order to comply with current FDA requirements for approval of their new drug bedaquiline, Janssen Therapeutics (the drug's manufacturer) has publicly committed to a formal 'plan to study' its new drug in children. Rarely, however, do such plans ever ultimately get implemented when new drugs are approved – more often than not they amount to being a necessary part of an approval process which then gets quietly ditched because the research required can be so ethically challenging.

Finally we come to what is the secondary impact of TB on children, because they are not only directly affected by TB by being infected by the disease but are also indirectly affected by it. In 2009, the WHO suggested that there were nearly 10 million children who were orphans as a consequence of losing at least one of their parents to TB.

The picture of the disease as regards to children is almost universally gloomy. There is one piece of good news on this front, however. Compliance to drug treatment tends to be far better with kids than with adults because of their regimens being better supervised and observed by concerned adults. At least kids tend to complete their treatments – or at least they do if they survive long enough.

Seed and Soil – the Perplexities of Immunity

"TUBERCULOSIS IS A SOCIAL DISEASE WITH A MEDICAL ASPECT"

Sir William Osler[147]

For centuries it was widely believed that TB ran in families. As a result, such families were readily and regularly ostracised, and diagnosis was often either kept secret for as long as possible or even completely withheld by some physicians in order to protect such families from the resulting stigma.

Such ideas still persist where TB remains rife, and, as with many popular so-called myths or old wives' tales, there may be more than grains of truth contained within them. Apart from the fact that, quite logically, the bacillus can easily transmit between members of the same family, there does appear to be some emerging evidence of potential genetic disposition to the disease. Such an idea does wash clean the racist ideas of the eugenicists, but nevertheless it adds further complexity to our ever-deepening understanding of this disease.

The eugenicists developed their epidemiological theories around ideas of "seed and soil" – the seed being the disease, and the soil being the people infected by it.

In respect of the seed, it is now well known that, even within *M. tuberculosis*, there are strains which are genetically discrete from each other, some of which are probably more infectious or more virulent than others. The W-Beijing family of tuberculosis, for instance, is widely accepted to be a more virulent strain – not just because of the seriousness of the disease it appears to inflict, but also because of its apparent capacity to mutate. Its name identifies where it is believed to have had its origins (in China). It properly emerged into the epidemiological spotlight in New York, however, in 1995, when an outbreak cost millions of dollars to be brought under control. In fact, however, it had already been spread across central Europe, having swept across the former Soviet Union and into former Eastern Bloc countries just at the time that the region's national health infrastructures were collapsing along with their decaying Soviet administrative systems of bureaucracy. By 2010, 13% of all active infections globally were being

[147] Sir William Osler (1849-1919) was co-founder of the Johns Hopkins Medical School. He has sometimes been referred to as 'the father of modern medicine'.

identified as being of the Beijing type, with this strain now being reported to account for as much as 50% of the disease now found in East Asia.

TB 'lineages'

One of the reasons that this strain appears to be so virulent is because it is believed to somehow have the capacity to inhibit the release of a particular part of the cellular immune response to the TB bacillus which otherwise occurs in infected patients.[148]

Different strains of MTBC disease relate to specifically identifiable genetic lineages. There are believed to be seven such major lineages in the complex of *M.tuberculosis*. With the exception of Bovine TB they each originally predominated in specific geographic areas and so have been named according to these geographical distributions. They have also been further differentiated into two basic types – 'ancestral' (older) ones, and 'modern' more recently developed ones.

The three ancestral lineages are *M. africanum* (further differentiated into 'West African 1' (lineage 5) and 'West African 2' (lineage 6), and *M.bovis*. These strains, as we saw in a previous section, are believed to have originally emerged as a human pathogen in Africa and then colonized the world accompanying the 'out-of-Africa' migrations of modern humans.

The four modern lineages are Indo-Oceanic (lineage 1), East-Asian (Lineage 2), East-African-Indian (lineage 3) and Euro-American (lineage 4). These are thought to have developed regionally as a consequence of increases in human population, and then have spread more generally throughout the world through waves of exploration, trade and conquest, and, more recently, through migration and travel.

Three further major sub-lineages exist which are by definition relatively more modern still. These are Beijing (from lineage 2), East-African-Indian (from lineage 1) and Delhi/central-Asian (from lineage 3).

Epidemiological evidence suggests that these different phylogenetic lineages of MTBC initially developed by specifically adapting to different ethnic human populations. The phylogenetically more 'modern' MTBC lineages,

[148] This is confirmed in most, but not all, studies in both humans and animals.

however, are self-evidently more successful at this in terms of their geographical spread when compared with the 'ancient' lineages. Interestingly, the success of the more 'modern' MTBC strains also appears to have been promoted by a correlation with a hypo-inflammatory phenotype in human macrophages, possibly promoting a higher virulence with shorter latency periods in certain individuals. The Beijing strain's advantage, for instance, involves the so-called 'pro-inflammatory cytokines' the tumor necrosis factor TNF, and the interleukins IL-6 and IL-12, all of which are normally released by the host macrophages as part of the immune response. Since it is also a lineage 2 derived strain, it is more prone to mutation than strains from other lineages as well.

These differences between strains are far from insignificant. Lineage 2 strains, for instance, have been shown to replicate to high bacillary loads in the lungs of infected mice.[149] Lineage 4 strains have been seen to grow more rapidly in liquid culture and reach higher plateau levels than other strains. Lineage 2 strains, however, grow faster than lineage 3 strains and induce the lowest levels of pro-inflammatory TNF and IL-12 response when compared to all the other strains.

It turns out that there are further sub-lineages which are now perniciously mixing themselves into the soil as well. One new variant strain of disease (referred to as DRF150) appears to be implicitly resistant to almost all the front-line antibiotics currently used to treat drug-resistant TB, and it has been found in both South and East Africa. It may yet be proved to be more dangerous than any other.

The human factor

So much, for now, for the seed, because just armed with this information, we find ourselves tentatively encroaching on to the soil itself because it has also been found that both mice and humans who are deficient in IL-12 responses are more susceptible to mycobacterial infections. Furthermore, some individuals who inherit defects in their capacity to produce IL-12 or its receptor are also known to be highly susceptible to active TB disease

[149] Rajesh Sarkar et al. - "Modern lineages of *Mycobacterium tuberculosis* exhibit lineage-specific patterns of growth and cytokine induction in human monocyte-derived macrophages", http://www.plosone.org/article/info%3Adoi%2F10.1371%2Fjournal.pone.0043170#pone.0043170-Lopez1

suggesting that this human genetic variation may be involved in susceptibility to TB as well.

But this only seems to be scraping the surface. The normal initial immune response to TB infection comprises a set of 'intruder-fighting' processes in the host which can be described simply as an inflammatory response. This response is a complex one, however, and is known to include changes in levels of interferons (which are immune-signalling chemicals) as well as in the mobilisation of both antibacterial white blood cells and platelets. A recent study has revealed that people of different ethnicity not only respond differently to infection with the same strain of *M. tuberculosis*, but that they also even vary in their responses to the drugs that are administered to treat it.[150]

The study, conducted in London and published in July 2013, involved measuring exactly these inflammatory markers provoked by TB infection. The team from Queen Mary University in London measured 57 of these inflammatory markers in 128 multi-ethnic Londoners who were newly infected with TB. They then compared these markers with the levels seen in healthy people – but they then did something extra, dividing the study's participants into two ethnic categories, either African or Eurasian, and compared these two groups as well. The team found that only four of the 57 markers moved in the same direction in both ethnic groups after infection. They also found that the direction in which ***all*** of those other 53 markers moved could be identifiably split exactly according to whichever ethnic group the participants fell into.

But this was not all, because this differentiation was then seen to continue to maintain itself ***after*** the drugs were begun to be administered. In those people of African descent who were also identified as being slow to respond to anti-TB drugs, for instance, the levels of their anti-bacterial blood cells (or neutrophils) were unchanged, while the levels of the signalling chemical interleukin-4 (IL-4) rose. In a similar group of Eurasian people, on the other hand, the levels of these neutrophils rose, as did interleukin-6 (IL-6) which is another signalling chemical. In fact, the measurable differences in the immune reactions between the Africans and Eurasians became even ***more*** pronounced after they started taking

---

[150] Coussens A et al. – "Ethnic variation in inflammatory profile in tuberculosis" (2013)
http://www.plospathogens.org/article/info%3Adoi%2F10.1371%2Fjournal.ppat.1003468

medication for their TB during the intensive phase of treatment than it was before they started their chemotherapy.

Others have found ethnic differences in the way individuals respond to the disease as well. Ajit Lalvani, the head of TB at the National Heart and Lung Institute in London, has found that more tuberculous infections in Europeans occur in the lungs, for example, while Asians and Africans get proportionately more TB infections in other organs. Such findings have significant prognostic implications, and might also offer insights into how regional epidemics might be better addressed. They must also suggest that regional estimates of EP might be miscalculated and may need to be adjusted.

Further epidemiological reports offer additional ideas about ethnic susceptibilities which deepen this perspective. In one unlikely study, evidence of TB infections (as measured by tuberculin skin tests) was systematically measured in residents in racially integrated nursing homes. Infection was seen to have occurred as much as twice as often in black as in white individuals who were assessed to have been equally exposed to active tuberculosis.[151] It seems that the innate host defence mechanisms of these black residents were simply much less effective against the local strains of disease than those of in the white residents. Such a finding is disturbing, but it is supported by another study which documented how macrophages taken from African-Americans demonstrated what was described as a relative 'permissiveness' for the intracellular growth of virulent mycobacteria.[152] Such data may suggest a compelling but challenging explanation for the terrifyingly high estimated rates of latent disease in Sub-Saharan Africa, one which may be shown to be more independent of the regional HIV epidemic than has been previously thought.

Different strains and different genetic susceptibilities – there is still so much that has yet to be learnt about this baffling interplay between human an mycobacterium. An infecting strain may have a specific influence on infection outcome, for instance, but this outcome may in turn be critically

151 Stead WW et al., - "Racial differences in susceptibility to infection by Mycobacterium tuberculosis", New England Journal of Medicine, 322 (1990) 422-7.

152 Crowle AJ, Elkins N - "Relative permissiveness of macrophages from black and white people for virulent tubercle bacilli", Infection and Immunology, 58 (1990) 632-8.

influenced by the genetic disposition of the host. The most important potential contributory factor of all should not be forgotten, however -that HIV infection, which causes depletion of the CD4 and CD8 T cells (ones which play a vital part in providing post-infection protection against developing active TB) is the most potent risk of all.

Perhaps the most frustrating fundamental paradox of tuberculosis remains, however – that natural infection does not confer protective immunity and yet, despite this, in HIV-negative people, only 5-10% of those infected progress to active disease. We need to unpack this a little more and try to give ourselves a better understanding of what this really means.

Those vital $CD4^+$ T cells, as well as the cytokines IL-12, IFN-γ, and TNF, are now widely agreed to be critical in the control of *Mycobacterium tuberculosis* infection, but the host factors that ultimately determine why some individuals are totally protected from infection in the first place, why some only contract the latent disease, and why others go on to develop re-activated disease remain frustratingly unclear.

This brings us back to the issue of why the BCG vaccine has been so relatively ineffective, because if a dose of the disease does not confer any subsequent immunity to the host, why should anyone seriously expect a tiny dose of attenuated *M. bovis* bacilli to do so? Logically it shouldn't happen, and yet in a certain amount of cases it clearly does, and there ***must*** be a reason for this. This offers us an insight into just how challenging the development of a new reliable vaccine might really be. And finally, it also serves to explain the reality as to why some unfortunate souls who have already been infected by one strain can be subsequently infected by a second one.

To understand this all a little better we have to dip our toes a little deeper into the complexities of the immune system.

A break-down of the immune system

The immune system is classically divided into two components – the 'innate' and the 'acquired' (or 'adaptive'). The 'innate' is accepted to be a system from an older evolutionary age which offers its host what can be best described as an immediate knee-jerk response to an external infectious threat to the host organism. The 'acquired' response, on the other hand, is a more sophisticated system, developed at a later period of evolution by vertebrates in order to counter the more sophisticated infectious threats than those that are easily addressed by the 'innate' system. It particularly uses components of both memory and specificity in its response to a threat once it has been properly assessed and recognised.

This division of the immune response into two parts is both real and useful, but we should remain aware that dissecting the host defence mechanism in such a way is largely an academic artifice. In reality these two individual components of host response normally complement each other and operate synergistically. Discriminating the vertebrate immune system in this way, however, offers us a better view of some of the paradoxical complexities of this particular disease.

Traditionally, the protective immunity to tuberculosis has been ascribed to a response from the acquired immune system – one of T-cell-mediated immunity, with $CD4^+$ T cells playing a crucial role. One unusual characteristic of this acquired immune response to tuberculosis, however, is the long interval required for its development compared with the much faster response which is normal with other infections, or indeed with other vaccinations as well. In humans, for instance, the development of adaptive or acquired immunity to tuberculosis, as measured in response to a tuberculin skin test, only shows itself if there has been a lapse of five to six weeks the infection.

Immunological and genetic studies now support an idea that the clumsier 'innate' immune response is also relevant in any response to tuberculosis, particularly in the early stages, and that this might have a potentially massive effect on the wider epidemic.

Four different developmental stages in an infection of pulmonary tuberculosis were differentiated by Max B. Lurie in his studies in rabbits back in 1964. [153]

1. The first stage begins with the inhalation of the tubercle bacilli. Alveolar macrophages encounter and ingest the bacilli and often destroy them completely. This is an innate response. At

---

153 Lurie MB - "Resistance to tuberculosis: experimental studies in native and acquired defense mechanisms", Harvard University Press, Cambridge, Mass. (1964).

this stage, the final outcome of the disease depends on the balance between the intrinsic bactericidal capacity of these host phagocytes and the virulence factors of these ingested mycobacteria. If this relation proportionately favours the host's innate response, then the infection will have been stopped in its tracks at first base and there will be no further disease – with not even a latent infection. If not, then the next stage will inevitably develop.

2. The second stage depends upon some of the mycobacteria escaping this initial intracellular attack, and then being able to sufficiently multiply to lead in turn to the disruption of the macrophage response. If and when this happens, blood monocytes and other inflammatory cells become drawn attracted to the lung, and these monocytes will in turn differentiate into macrophages which again ingest (but still not destroy) the mycobacteria. During this so-called 'symbiotic' stage, the mycobacteria slowly grow logarithmically, whilst the macrophages will also accumulate, but there will be little real tissue damage. Two to three weeks after first infection, however, T-cell immunity begins to develop, with antigen-specific T lymphocytes arriving on the scene. This is an acquired immune response but it is a relatively delayed one, and these T lymphocytes will now proliferate within the early lesions or tubercles, and then activate macrophages to kill the intracellular mycobacteria that they find.

3. At the end of this phase the bacillary growth of the second stage will be stopped, and a third stage then slowly begins to unravel. The solid necroses at the centres of these primary lesions effectively inhibit any further extracellular growth of mycobacteria, and, as a result, the infection essentially becomes dormant. Disease may still progress but, if it does, it might happen years after the primary infection when the surveillance activities of the acquired immune system are either diminished or otherwise diverted.

4. At this time, cavity formations may lead to the rupture of nearby bronchi, allowing the bacilli to spread through the airways to other parts of the lung and also potentially to the outside environment to potentially infect others.

Seen in this way, the *M. tuberculosis* bacilli have to survive a series of encounters with different host defence mechanisms, the final outcome of which depends upon a fluctuating interplay between the initial outgrowth and killing of *M. tuberculosis* and the extent of surviving tissue necrosis, fibrosis, and regeneration. The total elimination of *M. tuberculosis* infection thus depends on the success of a complex flexible interaction between the infected macrophages and the T lymphocytes – and any immune deficiencies, whether they are innate or acquired, can be predicted to have a dramatic effect on this.

The ultimate functional diversities of these T lymphocytes may also be a highly relevant factor because they, in turn, can be divided into two subsets – existing either as 'Th1 clones' which are characterized by the production of interferon gamma (IFN-γ), or 'Th2 clones' which are differently characterized by the production of interleukin 4 (IL-4).

Both of these subsets themselves develop from what are called 'naive T cells', whose final differentiation is influenced by their immediate environment. Interleukin 12 (IL-12), which is itself produced by activated macrophages and dendritic cells, is the principal Th1-inducing cytokine, for instance, while IL-4 promotes induction of Th2 cells.

It is this Th1 cytokine, in fact, which appears to be most essential for protective immunity in any progression of a mycobacterial disease. Other cytokines and cellular subsets remain implicated in this Th1-Th2 concept, however, and one of these offers us a further window through which to review at the potential susceptibility of the human host to progressive TB – this is interferon gamma, or IFN-γ.

'IFN-γ gene knockout mice' (in other words, mice which have been genetically modified to be unable to produce IFN-γ) are known to be highly susceptible to *M. tuberculosis*, and, similarly, humans lacking receptors for IFN-γ are also known to be prone to potentially suffer from recurrent, sometimes lethal, mycobacterial infections. Those other Th2-type cytokines, furthermore, are unfortunately also known to inhibit the production of IFN-γ (at least they have been shown to *in vitro* in the lab) as well as to inhibit the activation of macrophages. So it might well be that they actually weaken the host's defence against the disease in real life. Higher levels of these Th2-type cytokines have certainly been seen in tuberculosis patients, although this has not been completely consistently found, so the total relevance of this Th1-Th2 concept in both TB disease susceptibility and presentation tantalises but still remains frustratingly uncertain.

In fact, the innate defense mechanisms of those phagocytic cells may be as important in the epidemiological bigger picture – maybe even more important still. Those 1964 studies conducted by Lurie used rabbits which were bred to be either resistant or susceptible to TB. They revealed that, seven days after primary infection through inhalation of tubercle bacilli, the lungs of the mycobacterium-susceptible rabbits contained 20- to 30-times more viable mycobacteria than did the lungs of mycobacterium-resistant rabbits. Obviously, such a difference that was observed during the early part of an infection could not be attributed to differences in T-cell immunity since it is accepted that it kicks in later in the disease process – so it could only be attributed to the initial innate immune response. Other evidence supports this conclusion: an acquired T-cell immunity which is created by vaccinating mice is only seen to effectively protect them from disseminated tuberculosis – it does nothing to prevent an initial pulmonary infection.[154]

In human disease, exactly the same thing appears to hold true, since acquired T-cell immunity as a result of vaccination with BCG is known to be relatively ineffective against pulmonary tuberculosis. But the vaccine ***is*** recognised as being more effective against disseminated infection. If this is the case, such acquired T-cell immunity cannot prevent or protect against exogenous re-infection of the lung, something which is exactly the case most frequently in human disease.

Thus it can be seen how much the innate host defence mechanisms may be involved in the fundamental basic protective response to a pulmonary infection. If there are genetic differences in such an innate response in different ethnicities, then such differences may also have impact on the development of a regional epidemic at first base since they would simultaneously either be promoting or resisting a critical accumulation of latent disease within a community.

Further support for the relevance of this T-cell-independent intrinsic bactericidal activity of the macrophages is found in genetic studies which have shown associations between tuberculosis and functional gene

---

154 Cooper AM, Callahan JE, Keen M, Belisle JT, and Orme IM - "Expression of memory immunity in the lung following re-exposure to Mycobacterium tuberculosis", Tubercle and Lung Disease, 78 (1997) 67-73.

polymorphisms.[155] [156] [157] There appears to be ever more evidence emerging, from both clinical and experimental studies, to support the vital relevance of innate immunity in tuberculosis.

At best, what we can conclude is that our sophisticated human adaptive cellular immune response is at best only partially effective against this disease. More often than not, it certainly can restrict the progressive growth of the mycobacteria and then create the state of dormancy, but it rarely (if ever) eradicates them. What does appear to be able to eradicate them on some occasions, however, is that very first response from the more primitive and far less sophisticated innate immune system.

It turns out that the essential hallmark of *M. tuberculosis* infection in humans is characterised by this fatal inability to generate an otherwise effective acquired immune response to eliminate the pathogen when it is in its re-activated disease state. The mechanisms that account for this handicap are unfortunately still very poorly understood. Indeed, it has to be admitted that the mechanisms which underlie the delayed initiation of our adaptive immune responses to *M. tuberculosis* are ***almost all*** unfortunately still inadequately understood.

As a result, and particularly as a result of the neglect in the research into the disease in the last few decades, there is still a lot of catching up to do, both by pulmonologists and immunologists. What we can logically and reasonably conclude, however, is that the level of risk of that primary infection is the single most important factor affecting the magnitude of the tuberculosis problem in any population being as it determines not only the rates and age patterns of initial infection (and hence the gross rates of incidence of disease), the size of the pool of latent disease, and also the very real risks of re-activation.

---

155 Bellamy R et al. - "Tuberculosis and chronic hepatitis B virus infection in Africans and variation in the vitamin D receptor gene", Journal of Infectious Disease, 179 (1999) 721-4.

156 Bellamy R et al. - "Variations in the NRAMP1 gene and susceptibility to tuberculosis in West Africans", New England Journal of Medicine, 338 (1998) 640-4.

157 Wilkinson R J et al. "Influence of polymorphism in the genes for the interleukin (IL)-1 receptor antagonist and IL-1β on tuberculosis", Journal of Experimental Medicine, 189 (1999)1863-74.

So exactly what might awake the disease from its latent slumbering to re-activate? In this case it appears more likely to be a change in the acquired immune system. Professor Ajit Lalvani, the director of the Tuberculosis Research Unit at Imperial College London, has studied the observable spring peaks in rates of tuberculosis in the UK, particularly those which frequently show in the homeless population. Traditionally, these peaks have been being attributed to lower levels of vitamin D, which might well be part of the problem since low levels of vitamin D are known to compromise immune response. Winter episodes of 'flu, however, may also weaken immune systems, along with the seasonal higher frequency of sleeping in poorly ventilated shelters in close quarters which must also contribute. But Professor Lalvani has been particularly interested in how winter 'flu or other viral infections may be what creates the trigger.

He found that the genes for interferon-beta (IFN-β), a virus-fighting protein, were more frequently expressed in the blood of tuberculosis patients with more severe disease than in milder cases. The same has been observed in patients with more severe leprosy, that other dangerous mycobacterial infection in humans. The professor concludes that there is a reasonable possibility that it is the sequelae of "other viral infections [which] are leading some months down the line to progression from latent to active TB disease".

There is much food for thought that arises from this. Perhaps the most potentially exciting is the idea that a counter mechanism, pharmaceutical or otherwise, might be discovered that could shut off the ability of the mycobacterium to be awoken out of its latent state. If this mechanism could be identified and prevented, it would promise the ultimate eradication of the disease. The dormant infectious material could be trapped within the host of latently infected individuals for their natural lifetimes, and it would ultimately expire with them. Could this be possible? It might be – it might even be much more possible than finding an effective vaccine for this elusive pathogen.

Incidence Rates, and the Obscuring of Severities

"WHEREVER WE LOOK FOR DRUG-RESISTANT TB WE ARE FINDING IT IN ALARMING NUMBERS, SUGGESTING THAT CURRENT STATISTICS MAY ONLY BE SCRATCHING THE SURFACE OF THE PROBLEM."

Dr Unni Karunakara (2012)[158]

This section attempts to make sense of parts of today's pandemic in the light of some of the more frequently quoted figures that are invoked to describe it, as well as to develop possible predictions that might be associable with these analyses.

There are a lot of figures to absorb for the unfamiliar, and we will need to unpack a few of them in order to understand them more fully. We will then scrutinise them a little further and even question some of them in the next few pages. Some make much less coherent sense than might be expected to be the case when they are compared to others – or, more accurately, they make less sense if we try to use them in order to better illustrate another part of the pandemic.

It presents something of a challenge to unpick this part of the overall problem in this way, since, by doing so we risk casting a measure of doubt upon almost everything (which unfortunately is unavoidable). We thus risk making one of the themes that underlie this exposition (that the scale of the pandemic may be far more serious than is currently being suggested) a little weaker. But it seems such a certainty that some of the estimates that are being used to measure the scale of the pandemic are wayward that this risk is unavoidable. My intention is to apply some simple logic to a few of the figures because there seems to be a measure of this missing from the current assessments of the disease.

We will try shining a torch into the future, specifically the next decade or two, in order to anticipate what may happen with the disease as trends develop. There has been little work attempted in this respect – to try and assess where future resources are going to be probably most needed.

I fully recognise the difficulties faced by those involved in making any sort of coherent attempt to collate global figures for TB given the many

[158] President of MSF.

variables at play and the uncertainty of the data, and for this reason alone I am reluctant to challenge the fruits of the efforts of those who have done so. Such experts continue to assemble and re-assemble the statistics in ways that make most sense to them, or otherwise in ways in which they are being directed. These statistics might seem to be the most user friendly as far as those who are entrusted with the immense responsibility of confronting the disease are concerned, but if they are wrong then the most useful strategies with which to contain the disease will simply not be developed. I want to test some of their numbers, assessing whether they ring true – and even asking if they are really that useful.

To put these difficulties in the fairest of contexts, we can do worse than to first refer to the WHO's document entitled "Methods used to estimate the Global Burden of Disease caused by TB" which sidentifies the challenges involved in producing all of the global estimates.

We should focus on first is this word 'estimate', because that is all that ***any*** of these figures are, as definitively as they may be being regularly recycled in both the general and the scientific literature. We risk dangerously misleading ourselves if we think otherwise. "No country has ever undertaken a nationwide survey of TB incidence," the WHO document explicitly tells us. This may seem unbelievable given the scale of the ongoing tuberculosis epidemic, but it is true. This statement is then followed by an explanation: that this is simply because the scale of the task is too challenging, both logistically and financially, for it to be attempted. This may well be true, but the fact that no single country in the world has attempted the task, given the known public health risk from it not being carried out in such a serious pandemic, may still come as a shock.

As a summary, estimates of the burden of disease are gathered through three systems:

- Surveillance systems
- Special studies
- Expert opinion and national consultation

We already know that no nationwide survey has been attempted, but neither is a single surveillance system in place in any low-income country where much of the burden of disease is carried. We also know that expert opinion on this subject is variable depending on regional data and can easily shift for a variety of reasons. In association with these three systems for collecting their data, the authors of the WHO report acknowledge the fact that "there are many potential sources of uncertainty", and go on to identify them as being associated with:

- Estimates of TB incidence
- Estimates of TB prevalence
- Estimates of mortality
- Estimates of the burden of HIV-associated TB
- Estimates of MDR-TB
- Input data
- Parameter values
- Extrapolations to impute missing data
- The actual models used

In other words, there is uncertainty in pretty much everything used to develop the estimates as well as in the estimates themselves. And it is on this shaky ground that the global targets for 2015 were set and that the strategies for post-2015 are being developed.[159]

The current summary statement from the WHO is as follows:[160]

> "The global burden of TB remains enormous. In 2012, there were an estimated 8.6 million incident cases of TB (equivalent to 122 cases per 100,000 population) and 1.3 million people died from the disease (940,000 deaths among people who were HIV-negative and 320,000 among people who were HIV-positive). Among these deaths there were an estimated 170,000 from MDR-TB, a relatively high total compared with 450,000 incident cases of MDR-TB.
>
> "Although the number of TB cases and deaths remains unnecessarily large for a mostly curable disease, there has been major progress towards global targets for reductions in the burden of disease. The 2015 MDG [Millennium Development Goal] target of halting and reversing TB incidence has been achieved, with TB incidence falling globally for several years (2% per year in 2012). Globally, the TB mortality rate has fallen by 45% since 1990 and the Stop TB Partnership target of a 50% reduction by 2015 is within reach. Mortality and incidence rates are falling in all six WHO regions and in most of the 22 HBCs [high burden countries] that account for over 80% of the world's TB cases."

---

[159] These have since been published and Appendix 3 of this book presents a 'stop-press' analysis of them.

[160] WHO - "Global Tuberculosis Report 2013".

Both of these references – to the 'MDG' and to the 'Stop TB Partnership target' – deserve a little more qualification.

The MDG goals of simply "halting and reversing" the spread of TB by 2015 was a patently unambitious one from its inception. The 'Stop TB Partnership targets', on the other hand, were set up in response to this realisation – as part of the development of a more challenging strategy by the Global Partnership itself. As far as both 2015 and drug-susceptible TB were concerned, the principal Stop TB target was to halve both mortality ***and*** prevalence rates in relation to what they were in 1990. It might be noticed that this prevalence target fails to get a mention in the above WHO statement. Might this be because it is still too far adrift to be highlighted, while the mortality rate is at least "within reach"? In other words, is there subtle evidence here of 'spin'?

Furthermore, this assertion that the 50% reduction in the death rate is indeed "within reach" deserves a very substantial *caveat.* If the 2013 Global Tuberculosis Report is examined carefully, the following is actually the case: the TB mortality rate has fallen 45% between 1990 and 2012 according to estimated figures (albeit they contain uncertainties) ***but this particular mortality rate as applied to the target does not include those who are of known HIV-positive status and who die of tuberculosis.***[161]

In fact, if these are properly computed into the figures (which on other occasions they are) then the world is nowhere near the target. And if the sum of the absolute estimated numbers of HIV-positive TB deaths are added to the number of HIV-negative TB deaths, then the total number of estimated deaths from TB (at a little under 1.4 million) is actually only a little lower in 2012 than it was judged to be back in 1990.[162]

Furthermore, the total estimated number of new cases of disease in 2011 compared to what was assessed to be the case in 1990 was nearly two million more in 2011 than in 1990.[163]

---

[161] WHO - "Global Tuberculosis Report 2013", pages 6-20.

[162] Furthermore, we have already suggested that these figures in any case may be underestimated.

[163] WHO - "Global Tuberculosis Report 2011", page 11, figure 2.2.

What is also important to consider is that these figures relate to the overall pandemic, comprising mainly of drug-susceptible, disease – and this situation exists after nearly 20 years of DOTS which was developed to treat it, and after 20 years of a proclaimed global emergency. There seems to be some reason to wonder whether things are being presented quite as coherently as might be desired. It certainly would seem worth the effort of taking a more detailed look at the current situation to find out, using what data we can find.

One immediate problem presents itself in making any attempt at a retrospective assessment as we approach 2015 (the end of the current target period). Given that ***current*** numbers are still so far from being definitive, how much can we rely on the figures that were used for the baselines back in 1990 when the resource allocated to the disease was far less than is allocated today? It was, after all, three years before the global emergency was first declared and efforts were properly re-mobilised. It was also a year in which there were reported to be only two dedicated staff still on the case in the WHO's Geneva based Tuberculosis Unit.[164] It wasn't until 2008 (18 years after their baseline became operational) that the WHO's estimates of TB mortality used what is known as 'vital registration' (VR) data from more than three countries in the whole world. (Vital registration equals reliable and accurate data, incidentally). By 2009 this number had shot up to 89 countries, but even these were only recording an apparent 8% of the world's estimated cases – so it seems safe to assume that few of these 89 countries have much of a disease burden at all.[165] What this really adds up to is that, almost everywhere that TB deaths occur, there has been and still is precious little reliable data on deaths. The 2012 report specifically acknowledged this anomaly, stating:

> "Major challenges in estimating TB mortality include the lack of VR systems of sufficient coverage and quality in many countries, notably in Africa and parts of Asia."

Furthermore, until 2008, the estimates of incidence rates that were being published only included those who were estimated to be sputum-positive

---

[164] Frank Ryan – "The Greatest Story Never Told: The Human Story of the Search for the Cure for Tuberculosis and the New Global Threat", Swift Publishers (1992). (There are more than 90 dedicated staff there today).

[165] WHO - "Global Tuberculosis Report 2012".

pulmonary cases. This was potentially misleading given the known different ways in which the disease presents, particularly so where incidence of extra-pulmonary disease or HIV co-infection was also known, or at least reckoned, to be high. Additionally, this policy must have almost completely excluded children from any of these official incidence estimations of drug-resistant disease because they so rarely show sputum-positive.

This standard estimation of smear-positive TB incidence was discontinued in 2009 and has moved toward estimations of the burden of ***all*** forms of TB disease, and not just sputum smear-positive disease. This was arguably a rather belated decision since it finally reflected the fact that national TB programmes were and are diagnosing, notifying and treating people with all forms of TB, not just smear-positive ones.[166] Nevertheless, this inappropriate estimation is still appearing in the most recent reports, so they continue to have the capacity to potentially mislead or confuse.

So how much can we rely on these figures at all? The answer is that unfortunately we can't rely on any of them as much as we might want to. Given that the figures that are being used for mortality rates do not include those known to be co-infected with HIV/AIDS, and given the known increased risk of death from TB in cases of co-infection, this alone suggests that the annual reports as they are being presented should be treated with circumspection – particularly if we are being expected to accept that we are "within reach" of that target of reducing mortality rates by 2015 by 50%. We must at the least be entitled to raise our eyebrows and ask further questions about what might be the real state of the pandemic.

Another question deserves to be asked as well: if we accept that the figures were shaky at best in 1990, exactly how trustworthy might these figures be today nearly 25 years later? The only true answer will be what time itself will tell us, depending upon the course that the pandemic takes in the next decade or two.

In 2012 (from the most recent published data available in the 2013 report), 6.1 million 'real' cases of TB were notified by national TB control programmes worldwide and reported to the WHO – with India and China accounting for 39% of such cases. Africa accounted for 23%, and the 22 'high burden countries' (HBCs), with China and India included among them, accounted for 82%. From this figure of 6.1 million notified cases, based on the considered opinion of a panel of experts, the figure of 8.6

[166] Based on current estimates this may be as much as half of the pandemic.

million was pegged as the global ***estimated*** incident number of cases of disease (which was 0.1 million less than a year before).

So is this estimate too few or too many? The major problem with relying on numbers of notifications as forming the basis from which to finalise estimates of incidence is that they depend totally upon expert opinion – opinion about the number of cases that are diagnosed but not reported to national surveillance systems, and on the number of cases that never self-present or are never diagnosed at all. How can you ***know*** with any sort of certainty what you know you don't know – even if the numbers are derived from carefully assessed formulae for different regions and countries? Of course you cannot. Everything is hugely variable, even between regions within the countries themselves, and has to be subject to varying and potentially massive amounts of uncertainty. In the case above, however, it appears that expert opinion, gleaned from numbers that have been measured over the past few years appears to believe that 2.5 million or roughly a third of all estimated new TB cases never get notified. It may yet prove to be an optimistic estimate.

The following excerpt from the 2012 WHO Global Tuberculosis Report casts doubt on some of these numbers:

> "The number of TB cases that are not diagnosed is expected to be low in countries with readily accessible and high quality health care."

This may seem to be an innocent enough statement, but it logically implies the opposite – that the number of cases that are not diagnosed is expected to be proportionately higher in countries without readily accessible and high quality health care. And it is in these same countries that most of the epidemics exist; in which case could the global estimated incidence be being under-estimated?

The following are three further statements from the 2012 report which illustrate this possibility a little further:

> "Cases may be missed by routine notification systems because people with TB do not seek care, seek care but remain undiagnosed, or are diagnosed by public and private providers that do not report cases to local or national authorities."

> "In most countries, ***only a small proportion of targeted care providers*** (my italics)collaborate actively with NTPs [national TB programmes] and contribute to TB case notifications."

> "The recent decision by the Government of India to make notification of TB cases mandatory by law is a welcome step in the right direction."

It surely must have been…

India is a country which is known for its TB patients having little trust in their NTPs, with around 50% of them being reported to be resorting to its unregulated private sector. The directl result of this has been the recently reported exploding strains of DR-TB in the country – because of the country's private sector's widespread misuse of antibiotics. To have been relying on its NTP, therefore, to provide the bulk of the data from which to estimate its national incidence rate seems to be disconcerting.

Another problem arising from relying so heavily on expert opinion for the extrapolation of estimates from such limited data is that, as new revelations emerge concerning the rates of disease and its complex mechanisms, and as the data itself improves alongside this, such opinions necessarily have to shift. There is probably no area of TB epidemiology which is more uncertain as a result than that which relates to rates of drug-resistance, particularly in relation to such expert opinion. In fact, given that the estimated numbers remain so relatively stable, it remains far from clear whether any significant re-assessments are being made.

An interesting example of exactly this relates to the '22 high burden countries'.

The 22 'High Burden Countries'

These are the 22 countries that were, in the 1990s, determined by the WHO to be carrying about 80% of the estimated number of cases of TB worldwide, and which still appear to be doing so. These countries have therefore been the focus for the WHO's more intensified efforts to implement its Stop TB Strategy. Logically, therefore, we can assume that they all carry high burdens of disease.

The following is a list of these countries, along with the numbers of their estimated incident cases, and the estimated incidences of disease. It should be noted that the particular figures that are used in this list are those provided by the Stop TB Partnership in 2011 so are a little different from the ones recorded in the most recent report.[167]

A cursory first review of the list will seem to make some coherent and consistent sense becvause 83% of the estimated mortalities from TB appear to occur in these 22 countries; furthermore 81% of the estimated prevalence, 82% of the incidence, and 81% of the estimated HIV co-infected cases also appear to occur in them. In fact, years down the road from the list's original introduction, everything still seems rather neat.

	Country	Number[a]	Incidence[b]	Mortality Data [c]	Region
1	India	2,200,000	180	√	SE Asia
2	China	1,000,000	110	√	West Pacific
3	South Africa	500,000	971	√*	Africa
4	Indonesia	450,000	189		SE Asia
5	Pakistan	410,000	231		E. Mediterranean
6	Bangladesh	340,000	225		SE Asia
7	Philippines	260,000	280	√	West Pacific
8	DR Congo/	220,000	327		Africa
9	Ethiopia	220,000	266		Africa
10	Nigeria	190,000	136		Africa
11	Vietnam	180,000	200		West Pacific
12	Myanmar	180,000	388		SE Asia
13	Russian Fed	140,000	106	√	E. Europe
14	Mozambique	130,000	539	√	Africa
15	Kenya	120,000	314		Africa
16	Thailand	86,000	137	√	SE Asia
17	Brazil	83,000	45	√	Latin America
18	Tanzania	78,000	183		Africa
19	Zimbabwe	77,000	672	√*	Africa
20	Uganda	67,000	226		Africa
21	Cambodia	61,000	442		W. Pacific
22	Afghanistan	61,000	189		E. Mediterranean

Notes from above follow overleaf:

[167] There is good reason to do this. These incidence rates were averaged across three years (2008, 2009 and 2010). It was a method which was being seen at the time to be more accurate since it allowed for fluctuations. The latest numbers do include fluctuations, some of which could not be that well explained. These averages have not been updated since 2011, unfortunately. As of the 2013 WHO report, some of the current incidences are higher (South Africa is now estimated at 1,000/100,000 for instance), while most are lower (China is now 73/100,000) a number that will be questioned in a later section.

[a] These numbers are the absolute best numerical incidence of national disease as provided by the Stop TB Partnership for 2011.
[b] This is the standard incidence rates of disease per 100,000: three year average incidence rate: 2008, 2009 and 2010. It should be noted that some of these are revised in the 2013 report but relate to a single year (2012). Five remain unchanged; 14 report a lower incidence rate compared with their previous three year average; and three reported rises in incidence rate for the last year.
[c] This indicates whether any data for mortalities from TB have been submitted for these high burden countries.

It will be quickly noted, however, that there are hugely variable incidence rates of disease within this list, ranging from as little as 45/100,000 (Brazil – which reported 46 in the 2013 report) to 971/100,000 (South Africa – which reported 1,000 in 2013). And as we will also shortly see, the tiny country with the highest rate of TB on the planet (and the lowest life expectancy as well) is not even in the list at all.

In fact what we are really looking at are estimated numbers of cases by nation – what amounts to a list of 22 nationally ranked absolute numerical estimates of cases of disease rather than a list of the 22 countries which might have the highest internal burdens of disease when measured proportionately to the size of their populations.

In some ways, this approach makes sense. China and India cannot be ignored to any degree because of the relative sizes of their populations. Between them these two countries have 2.6 billion inhabitants (or around 36% of the world's population) and their absolute numbers as estimated add substantially to the total global burden. The inclusion of populous Indonesia, Nigeria, Pakistan, Russia and Brazil nearly adds another one billion people to the list (some of whom also have TB). These seven countries on their own, in fact, add up to around half of humanity.

However, we can also review this table in a different way. The WHO defines any country with an incidence rate above 250/100,000 as having a national TB emergency. Globally, there were 32 countries that fell into that category in 2011 according to the three-year averaged data, and yet 13 out of these 22 listed HBCs (in other words more than half of those listed) don't actually do so. Some even fall rather far short of it: Brazil's lowly incidence rate of just 45 (or 46) per 100,000, in fact, is less than a fifth of it, and even China's is less than half.

To put it more bluntly, most of these 22 so-called 'high burden' countries don't have a TB emergency at all. By looking at absolute numbers, therefore, we may be falling into a trap of looking in a fundamentally mistaken direction.

Any success in numerically meeting the 2015 targets of reduction of disease, however, must hang on the respective performances of India and China, simply because of their numerically huge number of cases (despite their both being beneath the 250/100,000 emergency threshold). Their potential influence on global estimates has already been proved in fact: China's positive contribution in terms of reducing its disease burden has without question made a huge difference to the overall global figures; it has also significantly helped bring down prevalence rates nearer to the 2015 target. Both of these factors must be a welcome relief to the WHO. With this in mind the strategy of selecting countries with the highest ***numerical*** burden of disease relative to the global burden makes some sense, but it offers a strategy from a single perspective – that of numerical burden, and not the real burden that might be being faced by each country in comparison with any other. It remains a curiosity as to how some of these countries ever came to appear on this immutable list (and stayed there) given that some of them have both relatively small populations ***and*** also lower than the emergency incidence rate.

So we come to our first big questions – is this the best framework around which to have developed and focused the most effective possible global strategies? Is there an alternative argument that those countries facing known national TB emergencies and inordinately higher incidence rates might be the more important ones to be focusing efforts on? As yet, it seems hard to say, so we must look for more clues as to whether there might be reasons that would justify an alternative approach.

What may also not make so much sense from this list is the fact that the vital mortality data (as is shown in the table) had only been submitted by eight of the 22 countries that have been focused upon for such special attention. This seems strange given that reduction of rates of mortality has been one of the targets which has been one of the main foci of the global strategy. According to the WHO, data relating to mortality was requested from a total of 217 countries worldwide; only 122 countries responded on the subject, and only eight of these were HBCs. Furthermore, of these eight, two (South Africa and Zimbabwe) had to be discounted because of recognised miscodings. The WHO recognises that improvements to methods and much greater use of directly measured mortality data are needed, and yet this doesn't seem yet to be happening only two years before the goal's deadline ***even in the 22 countries currently attracting the most focused approaches***.

So if the 22 HBC table has been being seen and used as a main component of the most effective strategy of measuring trends in the disease, it doesn't seem to be a strategy that is being well enough implemented nearly 20 years after its initial introduction. In fact, it's far from clear that the HBC strategy is really being adequately implemented at all.

The 2013 WHO Global Tuberculosis Report also identified that the global laboratory capacity to conduct sputum smear microscopy still requires strengthening. Of the notified cases of pulmonary TB accounted for in the report, for instance, around one-third weren't bacteriologically confirmed by a WHO-recommended laboratory method. There may be good reasons for this, but the fact exists that 20 years after a state of emergency was first declared, 15 of the combined total of 36 high burden Counties (HBCs) and high burden MDR-TB countries (HBMDR-TBCs) failed to meet the basic target of having at least one microscopy centre per 100,000 population. Effectively they didn't even make the bottom rung of the ladder of diagnostic requirements.[168]

In other words over 40% of the countries that have been being specifically focused upon because of their known burden of disease are still failing to meet one of the most basic goals of the strategy. This global target, as mentioned above, is one lab per 100,000 population; the global average is now 1.1 – but the average of both HBCs and HBMDR-TB countries are ***both*** below the global average (at 1.0 and 0.9 respectively). Surely they should both be significantly higher.

Furthermore, in 2009 the WHO recommended the use of the more sensitive fluorescent light-emitting diode (LED) microscopy instead of the traditional Ziehl–Neelsen (ZN) sputum smear method. This modification is believed to improve the reliability of the standard sputum test, reportedly from around 50% to 65% (or a relative 30% improvement which is hardly insubstantial) with a relatively small outlay. The roll-out of the LED modification, however, had been reported to have been "slow" according to the WHO's 2012 report. As of 2011, only 2% of microscopy laboratories globally were using LED microscopes. The 2013 report revised this assessment, describing the switch as being "gradual" but at the same time reported exactly this same 2% percentage as it had the year previous.

[168] In fact, South Africa, which clearly has a national emergency, had 0.4 centres per 100,000 population, and China, which is the scheme's current success story, had only 0.2. One has to wonder how their disease burdens are actually being properly bacteriologically measured at all.

Meanwhile the target for 2015 remains a remote 20%. The increase towards this percentage so far has been just over 1% in three years, so without drastic change, this target is unlikely to be close to being met.

When it comes to the capacity to ***definitively*** diagnose TB, to differentiate strains of MTBC, and to diagnose DR-TB, the situation is more worrying still. Of the 36 countries with the official high burden of both TB and MDR-TB (we will come to the list of 27 'high burden countries with drug-resistant disease' shortly) nearly half of them (16) did not even have the WHO's recommended capacity of at least one culture laboratory per five million population in 2012.

And when it comes to DST laboratory provision in the 27 high burden MDR-TB countries (which are the countries where self-evidently they are seen to bemost needed) things are even more alarming still. Again the target is at least one laboratory per five million, but 23 of the 27 countries with the estimated highest burden of drug-resistant disease still could not meet this target (i.e. relating to being able to perform drug-susceptibility testing just of first line drugs). In fact, while the rest of the world has been relatively speaking racing ahead in respect of this target (averaging out at 0.8 of a lab per country in 2011, but rising to 3.8 in 2012), the average for all of the 36 collated HBCs is currently running at less than ***half*** of this global average.

Meanwhile, no figures at all are available for labs that can perform DST beyond first line drugs (in other words it is still impossible to remotely assess how much XDR disease is out there in the countries most likely to have more extensive strains because of existing rates of MDR-TB).

And if these gaps are still so large in the countries with high numerical burdens of disease, what of those countries which have a proportionally higher burden of disease and have rates of TB at emergency levels? These are the ones which failed to make the cut into these tables, almost all of which are African (see the table on the next page). Well, because the statistical strategy has been focusing figures so much on these 'official' HBC's, we are left with very little idea – but we can surely guess.

The possibility is emerging that there may be another fundamental flaw in the HBC strategy which may still be in the process of revealing itself. Focusing on the 22 HBCs looks to have been seen to be the best strategy because these countries were estimated to carry 80% of the total epidemic (in terms of mortality, prevalence, incidence and co-infection). Such a strategy also assumed that these figures were correct. Notwithstanding this, any sort of success in these 22 countries has been intended to result in the quantitative stalling of the rise of disease and the bringing down of the global death rates. So has this actually been the case?

In contrast to the official list in the earlier table, the following is a list of the 22 countries with the actual highest estimated ***rates*** of incidence of infectious disease (as opposed to absolute numbers). It is drawn up from those same figures that were averaged by the Stop TB Partnership across the three years of 2008, 2009 & 2010 and published in 2011.

Ranking	**Country**	**Incidence per 100,000**	**Region**	**High HIV rate**
1	Swaziland	1257	Africa	√
2	South Africa	971	Africa	√
3	Namibia	693	Africa	√
4	Zimbabwe	672	Africa	√
5	Sierra Leone	645	Africa	
6	Lesotho	634	Africa	√
7	Djibouti	620	Africa	
8	Botswana	548	Africa	√
9	Mozambique	539	Africa	√
10	Gabon	502	Africa	√
11	Timor Leste	498	SE Asia	
12	Zambia	481	Africa	√
13	Marshall Islands	471	West Pacific	
14	Togo	446	Africa	
15	Cambodia	442	West Pacific	
16	Kiribati	409	West Pacific	
17	Myanmar	388	SE Asia	
18	Congo	382	Africa	√
19	DR Korea	345	SE Asia	
20	Mauritania	330	Africa	
21	Cntrl African Rep.	327	Africa	√
22	DR Congo	327	Africa	√

It is arguable that these might be far better countries on which to focus attention rather than the previously listed 'official' 22. One good reason for this is that it can be logically predicted that there will be higher incidental densities of active infection circulating in all of their respective national communities, and therefore far more risk of increasing uncontrollable epidemics.

We could call this list the HICs ('high incidence countries') to distinguish them from those HBCs. It may be noticed that ***only six*** of these HICs are also on the HBC list. It should also be noted that all of the first ten countries are African. In fact 16 of the 22 are in the Sub-Sahara.

So have some of the real furnaces of disease been effectively neglected?

Projecting future disease burden

All countries are asked to report their TB figures annually to the WHO, which then uses these notified figures to help produce estimated TB statistics for each country, then both regionally and globally. Globally it is thought that only about 66% of prevalent TB cases are notified. How accurate such an estimate is we can only really guess at. The WHO's figures for the estimated incidence, prevalence and for the numbers of deaths from TB in each of the WHO regions are given below.[169]

The terms 'incidence' and 'prevalence' should be carefully watched for in all of these figures. 'Incidence' relates to new cases during a 12-month period, whilst 'prevalence' relates to those who are estimated to have active disease during the same period but whose disease may have first become active in an earlier year. This is far from always being clear from the way in which the figures are variously presented, particularly in the media. In all instances that can be imagined with TB, however, prevalence rates should register higher than incidence rates. Bizarrely, in some occasional entries in the national WHO registries year on year, the reverse is true.[170]

In the following official table the deaths of people who had both TB and HIV infection at the time of their death were excluded from the number of deaths. This was because they are internationally classified as HIV deaths. If these were added, the death rate jumps to around 1.4 million.

---

[169] WHO - "Global Tuberculosis Report 2013".

[170] Under one conceivable scenario it is possible that prevalence rates could be lower than incidence rates – if the mortality rates were to increase substantially during the same incident period. Thankfully this does not appear to be the case, so it is an unlikely explanation.

Estimated WHO Regional TB statistics for 2012

Region	Incidence	Prevalence	Deaths	Population
Africa	2,300,000	2,700,000	230,000	892,970,000
Americas	280,000	390,000	19,000	961,103,000
Eastern Mediterranean	670,000	1,100,000	100,000	616,591,000
Europe	360,000	510,000	36,000	904,540,000
South-East Asia	3,400,000	4,800,000	450,000	1,833,359,000
Western Pacific	1,600,000	2,400,000	110,000	1,845,562,000
Global Totals	**8,600,000**	**12,000,000**	**940,000**	**7,053,684,000**

It's easy to become quickly confused if approaching this with the innocence of ignorance. Butlet us now develop these figures in the light of another commonly used marker for the state of the TB pandemic: the rates of latent infection. Latent infection is effectively the long term feeder for the pandemic, and it can also be understood to underpin the expected development of disease. It must therefore constitute a fundamental indicator of any future trends.

We have three figures that we can usefully resort to all of which are still being quoted by the WHO and in the scientific literature:

Latent infection globally	32%
Latent infection in India	40%
Latent infection in Africa	80%

Again, how confident can we really be of these percentages? The reality is that we can't be confident, because, even if good population samples were originally used, the numbers will have been assessed on results from positive skin tests which may well show positive from previous BCG vaccinations. Nevertheless, these percentages are regularly quoted in both the general and the scientific literature with some authority, and they are the best we currently have. If we apply these figures to the current populations in each area, some disturbing possibilities emerge.

The current global population figure is around 7.2 billion. Using the 32% figure we can therefore suggest that a total of around 2,250,000,000 (2.25 billion) individuals are currently latently infected today and are therefore at living risk of active disease. But as we have just seen, there is a concurrent estimated global prevalence total of 12,000,000 with TB that is already active – so we need to allow for this, since by definition they must already have developed active disease. If we deduct these 12 million from our global 32%, however, we still find ourselves left with an astonishing 2,238,000,000 current latent infections.

We can also anticipate that 5% of these might go on to develop active disease in their lifetimes (which is the lower end of the usually quoted estimate), so we can predict that over 111 million cases of TB might re-activate in the course of the lifetimes of those people who are already infected by tuberculosis unless something else intervenes.

A proportion of these 111 million possible cases, of course, will actually die from other causes before their disease has had chance enough to re-activate. This has to be a far from accurate way of predicting disease because we know there are far too many variables at play. It can still be a relatively useful one, however, being as it is based on our understandings of disease progression. We can certainly be sure that the totals arrived at this way will be much higher than might be anticipated if we were somehow able to allow for all of these variables, but the principle is nevertheless useful because we can also roughly predict anticipatable proportionate burdens of future disease in different regions. If we apply the same formulaic calculation to India and Africa, for instance, applying their respective estimated percentage rates for latent infection, we can then elicit similarly rough projections for each region.

So let us take a look at India. The population of India is 1.21 billion. The rate of latent disease of 40% in this particular population is 484 million. The prevalence rate for India converts to 3.1 million cases, so if we deduct this from our latent total as we did before we are then left with just under 481 million current latent infections. If we apply a 10% conversion rate to this figure (assuming that rates of poverty and malnutrition in India dictate that the higher end of the 5-10% conversion rate would apply) we can project the possibility that a little over 48 million cases of TB might develop in the country within current lifetimes. Again many will die from other causes, but at least we can be satisfied that this projection falls into some sort of coherent pattern with our other figures.

But let us now take a look at Africa, and try the same thing. The population of the WHO's African region is around 900 million. It is the Sub-Sahara, however, that is of special interest, and the population there is around 800 million, and 80% of them are said to be latently infected – this gives us 640 million people who can be suggested to be latently infected. If we then deduct the estimated existing prevalence for this area (2,800,000) from this figure, we can reasonably suggest that 637 million Sub-Saharan Africans may be currently carrying a latent infection.

With high rates of HIV co-infection across most of the Sub-Sahara, we know that the 5-10% figure for expected conversion to active disease is certainly too low for the region. So what percentage might it be? The likelihood of progression with co-infection with HIV/AIDS has been calculated rather confusingly as being 21-34 times more likely – something which is impossible to compute against the 'normal' base of 5-10% likelihood of progression. Be that as it may, not every latently infected case in Africa is also infected with HIV, and the estimated prevalence rates of HIV vary dramatically across the region from 1% in Somalia to 26% in Swaziland. The UNAIDS report of 2011, however, suggested that it is around 5% of the total adult population, so it seems reasonable to work with this figure.

So 5% of our 637 million latent African cases can be reasonably predicted to be co-infected. That makes for 32 million – and it's also fair to say that, without intervention almost all would be expected to develop re-activated TB. Meanwhile 605 million latent cases are HIV free, so again, we might reasonably apply the 10% conversion rate to this figure as we did in India. This gives us 60,500,000 prospective TB cases amongst those who are HIV-negative.

If we add these two sums together we come up with a figure which is approaching 100 million (actually 92,500,000) who can be reasonably projected to develop re-activated disease in their lifetime unless they die from something else first or unless some sort of effective intervention is provided for them. That is around one in eight of the Sub-Saharan population which seems far too many, but given that Robert Koch reckoned that one in seven deaths in Europe were down to TB at the end of the 19th century (when the TB epidemic was at its height in Europe), that TB is associated with as many as 69% of HIV deaths in Africa, and that the TB epidemic in Africa is in an extreme state, this figure may not be so outrageous after all.

So now we have three totals of anticipated cases of potentially infectious disease:

Anticipated new cases

Global	111,000,000
India	48,000,000
Africa	92,500,000

These calculations appear to make no sense.[171] If we add the individual projections for India and Africa together, for instance, they alone come to considerably more than the anticipated future global burden of unchecked disease.

But what also stands out is that this total of 92.5 million estimated African cases alone is almost as much as our calculated total global estimate for converted disease (which was 112 million). Either one figure relating to Africa must have been estimated too high, or another one related to the global situation must have been estimated too low.

It begins to seem possible that the 80% latent infection rate is too high. It has been derived from population samples that were assessed by TST to carry latent infection and the simplest explanation would be that this figure never adequately allowed for TST tests that should have been accounted as being positive because of BCG vaccination. If this is the case, however, then the figure certainly should have been revised some time ago. But this may not be the case – two early latency sampling of children in Europe in the early 20th century (before vaccines) showed 81% and 82% rates of latent infection respectively. In other words, in a high incidence population with little in the way of disease control this figure may not be extreme at all,

[171] One reason for this is that we have used a 5% new case rate for the global picture, while we have used a 10% rate for India and '10%-plus-HIV' factor for Africa. As there are significant populations infected with TB in both India and Africa these differe3nces in the base figures distort the conclusions. If we applied instead, say,7.5% as the conversion rate for the global figure this might reduce this anomaly – in which case we should be globally anticipating the possibility 168 million new incident lifetime cases (not allowing for relapse cases). The anomaly reduces, but it should be noted that the anticipatable pandemic still remains immense.

and it is a definite possibility that there are 640 million Africans in the Sub-Sahara latently infected with TB today. And if this is true then, unless something is done, a lot of Africans are going to develop re-activated TB.

And yet, as we have already seen, African countries are barely represented in that list of 22 HBCs.

Of course it may be that we have pegged our conversion rates too high. But, if that is the case, then the frequently quoted factor of latent TB being 21-34 times more likely to convert to active TB in cases of HIV co-infection must be way off as well.

We have one useful way of testing some of this, which is to attempt to do so retrospectively. In the above calculations we have used widely accepted figures, i.e. the rates of latent infection respectively for the world, for India and for Africa. We have applied variable rates of conversion from latent to active disease, and added a factored likelihood of disease conversion in cases of co-infection with HIV. So why is it that we aren't already seeing an explosion of TB in Africa? Well to a degree we are: high incidence rates, high prevalence rates and high mortality rates. But might they actually be much higher than is being estimated?

The simple fact is that we have to accept that some of these basic figures may be wrong – but if they are then how many of the other figures which are being used in all of the 'estimates' might be wrong as well?. And if they aren't wrong, then the fact that we aren't already seeing a ***real*** explosion of TB in the Sub-Sahara beyond what is already visible strongly suggests that a lot of the intervention and treatment work that is being done in the region must be having some effect. We can but hope that this is the case.

But might there be much more prevalent TB in this region than is being either notified or estimated – not being notified because the infrastructures are inadequate to the task and/or not being accurately estimated because the models for such estimations are flawed?

This possibility is very well illustrated by the findings of a national TB prevalence survey which was carried out in Nigeria in 2012. It was the country's first-ever national TB prevalence survey, and was only the second that has ever been successfully completed in the African region. When the number of prevalent cases of sputum-smear-positive TB found in the survey was totalled up and compared to the existing notification data for the same age group it showed an extraordinary prevalence/notification ratio of 5:1. The current belief is that 66% of all global cases are notified (which amounts to a prevalence/notification ratio of 3:2, and this also includes all forms of TB, not just sputum-positive disease). The general WHO estimates and strategies have been developed in general accordance with these ratios. If this Nigerian 5:1 factor were to be typical of the African region and applied across it, however, it would suggest a very different picture to the one that is currently being presented in the WHO estimates. If case detection for the African region is nearer 20% (as suggested to be the case in Nigeria) rather than the currently estimated 59% as is suggested in the 2013 Report, instead of a prevalence estimate for the region being 2.7 million active cases, it would instead be a stunning eight million.

These exercises are largely academic and may bear little resemblance to whatever reality will ultimately present. We can hope that this is true, but they do expose a strong possibility that some of the oft-quoted numbers may not be either accurate or useful. And just as importantly, they cast a very serious further shadow of doubt on the integrity and robustness of the HBC strategy.

Adding drug-resistance into the equations

There is an even more worrying question still, however, and it is the one which lurks behind all such calculations: how many of these latent infections might be carrying strains that are already drug-resistant?

The answer is that no-one knows which is worrying enough – but perhaps even more worrying is the fact that so few experts appear to even want to take a look at it. If all of our millions of projected cases were to turn out to be drug-susceptible (as most of them thankfully should do), this is already bad enough, but if only a small proportion is already drug-resistant, then this might well be the largest global health issue facing mankind today.

The problems are that existing estimates of drug-resistant TB are so highly variable and that the official ones may well be being gravely understated.

So let us take a stab at this particular issue in a similar way that we have already done for projection of regional disease. Let us simply apply the current global percentage rates for new drug-resistant MDR-TB to those figures of active disease that we previously calculated might be expected to develop from the estimated pool of latent infection. We may still suspect that our figures were too high, but we have to start somewhere.

A rate of 3.6% is the proportion of new cases that were identified as being MDR-TB in the 2012 WHO Global Tuberculosis Report. So it seems reasonable to suggest that 3.6% of all new cases in these three calculations (Global, African and Indian) might be MDR-TB. It would certainly seem a conservative percentage – even a ***very*** conservative figure for India given that a pilot study with the GeneXpert machine in the country suggested rates of new MDR-TB nationally might be 7%. So since we are looking at future development of active new disease from existing latency, and we know that these figures are continuously playing catch up with the emerging pandemic, then it seems that we can very reasonably suggest that the following numbers of MDR-TB cases might develop from our calculated pool of existing latent disease:

	Anticipated new TB cases		anticipated new MDR-TB cases
Global	112,000,000	x 3.6% ≈	4,030,000
India	48,000,000	x 3.6% ≈	1,730,000
Africa	91,500,000	x 3.6% ≈	3,290,000

(In fact, if the 7% rate of MDR-TB for India from the pilot study turns out to be accurate, we might more realistically potentially project a worrying three million cases in India.)

Once again these figures make no coherent sense for the same reasons as before. They may well be too high[172] and therefore be way off the mark, but they still offer us one telling insight: whichever way we may choose to look at it, there is a risk of an explosion of drug-resistant disease in the Sub-Sahara. We know that this is the very region which has not only been the most neglected, but also has the least resource with which to counter the threat. It is also the region that has been least planned for.

We can try this calculation another way. In one of our calculations above we suggested that an existing global prevalent pool of 12 million active cases might convert to a global total of 112 million lifetime cases of active disease with a latent pool of around 2.2 billion latent infections feeding the

[172] As we will see in more detail later, in this instance there is good reason to suggest that the opposite is true, since the true current rate of DR-TB by definition remains invisible, hidden in the latent epidemic and only emerging in its true numbers as infectious cases as much as a decade later, by which time the latent rate will have moved on as well.

pandemic. The factor between current active disease (12 million) and projected active disease (112 million) is thus about nine.

So if we apply this same factor (relating to prevalence and anticipatable lifetime active disease from an existing pool of latency) to the WHO's current estimate of 650,000 prevalent MDR-TB cases, we come up with a total of just under six million cases of MDR-TB in the existing pipeline of disease (which is 50% above our own estimate of four million).

In other words, every which way in which we work the numbers, we end up looking at a huge emerging problem of drug-resistance which urgently needs better attention.

Two experts of DR-TB who don't appear to have had much influence in the WHO figures themselves have suggested that:

> "..[MDR-TB] killed an estimated 1.5 million people between 2000 and 2009 — an annual rate 10 times that of the H1N1 influenza virus."[173]

If 1.5 million had died by 2009 and five million had become ill, then nearly 3.5 million can be assumed to somehow be still out there since (at least according to this estimate) only a paltry 25,000 were treated and possibly only half of these 25,000 would have had positive outcomes.[174] Only 12,500 successfully treated cases from an estimated five million – that amounts to a quarter-of-one-percent of MDR-TB (0.25%) cases successfully treated in the first decade of the 21st century if these figures are true. Furthermore, more than 3.4 million cases must have remained untreated and infectious spreading drug-resistant TB in their communities. However accurate such speculations might or might not be, one thing that almost no-one disputes (apart from the WHO itself which was suggesting in its 2013 report that rates of MDR-TB were "essentially unchanged" during 2012) is the fact that this number of high risk cases is almost certainly growing year on year. The next table offers the WHO's own more conservative estimate of new MDR-TB cases. It includes its estimated total of new (incident) MDR-TB for 2012, along with an accurate total of those who have actually been notified (almost all of whom are in the 27 high burden countries). Finally it

---

[173] Salmaan Keshavjee and Paul E. Farmer - "Picking up the pace – scale-up of MDR tuberculosis treatment programs", New England Journal of Medicine, 363 (2010) 1781-4.

[174] The current rates for successful outcomes of treating MDR-TB are 48%.

enumerates those who are also known to be on approved treatment. The picture presented from these figures is that globally 16% of all active MDR-TB cases are on treatment. That's quite different from the 0.5% estimated above, so it certainly sounds a lot more encouraging if it's true, although it's still an appallingly small percentage.

Global Totals for MDR-TB	450,000 Estimated	94,000 Notified	77,000 On treatment

The estimated prevalence rate of MDR-TB in 2012 was omitted from the 2013 report[175] – but it must way below the possible prevalence of 3.4 million calculated above. In fact it was estimated in another of its reports from last year that there were an estimated 630,000 cases of MDR TB among the world's 12 million prevalent cases of TB so we can, for the time being, usefully work with this figure.[176]

We have already identified the distinctions between incident and prevalent disease. In this case, however, there is an even finer distinction. In certain instances in global reports a more refined incidence rate for MDR-TB can be seen to be being applied – one which can further mislead or obfuscate: in slightly smaller print it may be seen that these (smaller) rates relate to numbers of new cases of MDR-TB from only "among those cases of ***pulmonary TB*** (my emphasis)that were reported to the WHO". In other words, cases of MDR-TB that were extra-pulmonary are not always being counted.

Is this useful as a way of offering a true picture of what is happening?

According to the most recent estimates, 3.6% of new cases are drug-resistant, and 20.2% of retreatment cases are also resistant. When calculated together, this amounts to 5% of all cases being drug-resistant (or around one-in-20 cases). Elsewhere it's been suggested that in some high incidence countries MDR-TB is not appearing in one-in-20 cases of TB, it's actually appearing in one-in-five (or 20%). This offers another sobering possibility – one which suggests that, if the focus of the global strategy is being developed by using the lower rate, it may be resulting in a strategy that is both inappropriate and ill-designed for higher incidence settings.

---

[175] A figure of 630,000 prevalent cases was used in "Global Tuberculosis Control 2012", WHO, Geneva, 2012, page 20.

[176] WHO - "Global Tuberculosis Control 2012", page 20.

Sven Hoffner of the rather ominously named Department of Preparedness at the Swedish Institute for Communicable Disease Control in Solna, Sweden, thinks that this higher figure may indeed be nearer the mark. He offered a telling observation in this respect in a comment he submitted to the Lancet in response to a report it published on XDR-TB in 2012:[177]

> "International recommendations for tuberculosis control have been developed for [MDR] tuberculosis prevalence of up to around 5%. Yet we now face prevalence up to ten times higher in some places, where almost half of the patients with infectious disease are transmitting MDR strains of *Mycobacterium tuberculosis*... Updated information on MDR tuberculosis and investigation of the trends are urgently needed, especially since the true scale of the burden of MDR and XDR tuberculosis might be underestimated and seem to be rapidly increasing."

Elsewhere we can find this same scenario being presented in an a more muted way:

> "The proportion of TB patients estimated to have MDR-TB that were actually diagnosed was under 20% in almost all of the high MDR-TB countries outside the European Region – including India (6%) and China (3%).[178] The notable exception was South Africa where the numbers [that were] reported exceeded the estimated number of cases."[179]

The anomalous entry from South Africa deserves consideration, one which was not given in the report itself. The total estimated number of MDR-TB cases in South Africa for 2012 was listed at 8,100; yet the total number of notified cases was 15,419. Exactly what can this mean? For once, we seem to have a smoking gun pointing at both the possible inaccuracy of the estimates and how they have been developed because it is illogic and impossible that the number of notified figures could possibly end up being more than the estimated number of cases (which has to include an allowance for patients who are missed from diagnosis treatment). This

---

[177] Sven Hoffner, - "Unexpected high levels of multidrug-resistant tuberculosis present new challenges for tuberculosis control", The Lancet, 380; 9851 (2012) 1367-9.

[178] Another expert report has suggested that this rate is actually as high as 10% in China in new cases.

[179] WHO – "Global Tuberculosis Report 2012" & also in "Global Tuberculosis Report 2013".

cannot be the case ***unless the estimate itself is inaccurate because of flawed methodology or inaccurate data.***

In this case, using the South African number of patients notified and the possible prevalence/notification ratio of 5:1 uncovered in Nigeria, we could anticipate the possible estimated number of MDR-TB cases in South Africa to be 77,095, or nearly ten times more than the estimate that was most recently published. This calculation would give South Africa the highest number of estimated incident cases of MDR-TB disease anywhere in the world as well as putting it at the top of the table. In the 2013 WHO report, however, it actually quite bafflingly suggested that the percentage rate of incident MDR-TB in both new and retreatment cases in South Africa are well below the global average. It is worrying that this particular anomaly relates to South Africa, a country where we know that MDR-TB is being actively sought out.

Be that as it may, given that the WHO's "under 20%" rate only applies to the so-called 'high burden' MDR-TB countries including China and India, it does seem a little more reassuring than Dr Hoffner's dire warning. We can at least hope that the true rate in the lesser burdened rest-of-the-world must be much less than this almost apocalyptic 20%. In fact the 2013 report stuck estimated figures on this: 3.6% of new cases and 20.2% of previously treated cases are estimated to have MDR-TB.

For South Africa specifically these same figures as published in the 2013 report were 1.8% and 6.7% respectively – i.e. half the global average for new cases and a third of the global average for retreatment cases. But if we dig around in the report we can identify how this anomaly arose: they were extrapolated from a survey conducted in 2002, a full ten years earlier than the report in which they are published.[180] So it's effectively impossible to be in any way sure what the real state of the drug-resistant disease is, even in a country with some significant level of resource and where the problem is well recognised as being more acute.

The picture is further confused by figures developed by the Stop TB Partnership's Global Plan in relation to MDR-TB. The Partnership has estimated that between 2011 and 2015 as many as one million MDR-TB patients will need to have been detected and placed on treatment if the plan is to be adhered to. It therefore plainly accepts that more than one million will have been out there and infectious by then, something which flies a

[180] "WHO Global Tuberculosis Report 2013" – page 131.

little in the face of some of the WHO's more conservative suggestions that insufficient evidence is available to even be certain that the drug-resistant epidemic is actually growing, or the reference in the most recent report which states that it is "essentially unchanged".

This same plan also intends that by 2015 at least 75% of MDR-TB patients will have been, or will be being, treated successfully. During 2012, however, just over 77,000 cases were started on treatment, a number which amounted to just 25% of the WHO's own estimated global total of incident MDR-TB cases. In addition, only 48% of cases completed that year were reported to have had successful outcomes, something which suggests that, with just two years to go and using the WHO's own optimistic figures, only around 12% of MDR-TB cases may be being treated successfully – a very long way off from the targeted 75%.

Somehow things aren't adding up – but then, as we will shortly see, the WHO is elsewhere suggesting that 86% of MDR-TB cases are occurring in just 27 countries, only five of which have a TB emergency, which doesn't add up either.

The 27 'High Burden MDR-TB Countries'

In the majority of countries, the diagnosis of TB has relied until very recently almost entirely on the identification of AFB in sputum smears using a conventional light microscope. In other words there has yet to be any credible surveillance of drug-resistance at all. As a result it has to be accepted that it's impossible for anyone to have any confidence in the estimated figures for drug-resistance since sputum smears are unable to identify it. All the available figures are estimated and many are mathematically modelled from existing data much of which is years out of date – and as a result it is reasonable to suggest that they might be significantly underestimated since drug-susceptibility surveillance is either very limited or almost non-existent in most of these countries.

On the following page is another table, this time of the 27 so-called High Burden MDR-TB countries, followed by some further global totals. Once more it ends up making for disturbing reading.

Several interesting statistics emerge from it:

A massive 87% of global MDR-TB cases are estimated to be occurring in these 27 countries, and so, by inference, only 40,000 cases are apparently believed to exist outside of them. The probability that this is the case must be extremely small.

And, almost incredibly, only five of these 27 countries have a TB emergency (as defined by an incidence rate of 250/100,000). Furthermore, only four of these high burden MDR countries are in Africa.

There are many other anomalies, but some are especially worth mentioning.

According to this table, India has 64,000 cases, yet in a report published in 2012 by MSF it was suggested that the MDR-TB burden in India now comprises nearly 100,000 new cases every year – with only 2% of these cases receiving second line drug treatment under the national programme.[181] The figure might well be even higher: by applying a 7% rate of MDR-TB (from the GeneXpert pilot study) to the country's 180/100,000 incidence rate, we could reasonably suggest as many as 150,000 new Indian cases each year.

	Country	Estimated cases	Notified cases	On treatment	TB incidence
1	India	64,000	16,600	14,143	190
2	China	59,000	3,007	1,906	80
3	Russian Fed	46,000	13,612	18,452	106
4	Pakistan	11,000	1,602	1,045	231
5	Philippines	13,000	679	1918	280
6	South Africa	8,100	15,419	6,494	971
7	Kazakhstan	8,800	7,608	7,213	163
8	Indonesia	6,900	428	426	189
9	Ukraine	6,800	6,934	7,672	101
10	Myanmar	6,000	778	442	388
11	Bangladesh	4,200	513	513	225
12	Uzbekistan	4,000	1,728	855	128
13	Vietnam	3,800	273	713	200
14	Nigeria	3,600	107	125	136
15	DR Congo	2,900	65	179	382
16	Azerbaijan	2,800	596	406	110
17	Belarus	2,200	1,604	2478	71
18	Ethiopia	2,100	284	289	266

[181] MSF - "India: struggling to find MDR-TB treatment" (2012).

19	Kyrgyzstan	1,800	958	790	159
20	Moldova	1,700	894	853	178
21	Tajikistan	910	694	535	204
22	Georgia	630	346	665	107
23	Armenia	250	92	101	73
24	Latvia	120	110	110	45
25	Bulgaria	100	49	36	41
26	Estonia	70	62	54	30
27	Lithuania	300	271	271	70
Total	**for High MDR-TBCs**	**261,080**	**75,301**	**69,302**	
	Regions:				
	Africa	38,000	18,129	9,303	
	Americas	7,100	2,967	3,102	
	E. Mediterranean	18,000	2,236	1,602	
	Europe	74,000	36,708	42,399	
	S.E. Asia	90,000	19,202	15,845	
	W. Pacific	74,000	4,473	5,070	
	Global Total	**301,100**	**83,715**	**77,321**	

More alarming still, if 9% of these are XDR, then India may have over 13,000 new cases of untreatable XDR-TB emerging right now within this host. That figure happens to be eight times the total number of currently notified cases in the whole world.

The Chinese incidence estimate of 57,000 is encouragingly 4,000 fewer from the previous year's estimate of 63,000. With the numbers of notified cases and cases on treatment in the country as listed, however, it's unclear as to how it could seriously be estimated that the MDR-TB burden in the country could be reducing because so relatively little is being done to counter it. Notwithstanding this, if the alternative expert assessment of 10% of new cases of TB in the country being MDR-TB in 2007 is correct,[182] then using the DS-TB incidence rate of 80/100,000 there may be more than 110,000 new cases of MDR-TB now emerging in China each year, nearly half of whom are un-estimated, and who amount to a total which would be 36 times higher than the number which has been most recently counted. This in turn would include nearly another 10,000 new

[182] http://www.nejm.org/doi/full/10.1056/NEJMoa1108789

cases of XDR-TB within these ranks as well (this time, six times the total number of currently notified cases in the whole world).

The total figure of 38,000 for the African region is equally confusing. The total estimated incident number of TB cases for this region is quoted as being 2,300,000, which in turn suggests a rate of MDR-TB for the region of 1.6%. It's hard to believe that this could be a remotely credible rate. At the global rate of 3.6% this figure would in fact be 83,000 (or approaching three times the above estimate), and could include nearly 8,000 new cases of XDR-TB each year (or five times the total number of currently notified cases in the whole world).

The figure for South Africa is perhaps the most troubling of all. With a population of 52 million, and an estimated incidence rate of 1,000/100,000, there must have been around 520,000 new cases of TB in 2012. The estimated number of MDR-TB cases as listed above was 8,100, however, which is less than 2% of this total of estimated new TB cases (or a tenth the rate that is being suggested might be current in Russia). The idea that this might be the case in South Africa is ridiculous and is belied by the number of ***notified*** cases which themselves amount to 3% of all new TB incidence cases. Again if we apply the 3.6% standard to this figure (which must be a very conservative rate for this country) we end up with a total of more than twice the estimated figure (18,685) – and again we could equally easily expect it to be twice this figure or more.

If we take one sample case from one of those 22 HBCs (but one which does ***not*** appear on the list above), we run into yet further problems with the figures. Mozambique has around a 60% HIV/TB co-infection rate – not the highest in the region, though it is a rate that is far from being insignificant which can certainly be expected to have had an impact on rates of drug-resistance. A drug-resistance survey (DRS) conducted in 2007/2008 indicated a prevalence of MDR-TB of 3.4% among new cases and of 8.3% among re-treatment cases in the country – a figure which would not be expected to have dropped in the last few years. In spite of this, the country has no place in the 27 High Burden MDR-TB Countries. Mozambique, however, came in at ninth place on our own list of 22 proportional high incident TB countries with an incidence rate of 539/100,000. This country, incidentally, has actually risen ten places in this unofficial league since 2008 – the year when that DRS was conducted because it then had an estimated incident rate of 431/100,000).[183] The most

[183] http://www.afro.who.int/en/mozambique/country-programmes/aids-tuberculosis-and-malaria/tuberculosis.html

recent census for Mozambique records a population of 25.2 million, itself suggesting nearly 136,000 new cases of TB each year. This in turn would compute to nearly 5,000 new cases of MDR-TB each year if we use the current global rate of MDR-TB of 3.6% of all new cases. Such a total might seem of much less consequence than the far higher numbers that were listed above, nevertheless it would peg the country at 11th place on a revised ladder of high burden MDR-TB countries based on simple absolute numbers (at least if we use the figures listed in the table above). Could this be a typical picture for some of the other countries in Africa have found places in our 22 HIC list – especially if they have similarly high proportional burdens of TB, high rates of HIV/AIDS and also weak health infrastructures, all of which are accepted as high risk factors for development of MDR-TB?

The figures listed above were, to be fair, published with a telling rider:

> "It should however be noted that these are only the estimates for the number of cases of MDR-TB [from] amongst those cases of pulmonary TB notified to WHO. There will in addition have been many cases of MDR amongst those cases of TB which were either not detected and/or not notified."[184]

But to be equally fair, it's far from easy to work out what is really meant by such an ambiguous statement. "These are only estimates for the number of cases… [from] amongst those cases of pulmonary TB notified to WHO." If we take this literally, it would seem that all of these estimates fail to include any MDR-TB that may be extra-pulmonary, and EP is known to be much higher in cases of HIV co-infection Once again, we have reason to suspect that these estimates should be treated with caution.

There emerges a very real probability that the drug-resistant disease itself is already far ahead of all the data that has so far been assembled for the purpose of developing a useful response to it as a real global health crisis. There is, in fact, also a very good epidemiological reason why this is almost certainly the case, though it offers no excuse at all for complacency, rather

---

[184] http://www.tbfacts.org/tb-statistics.html#ref07. It should be noted that these tables appear to have been altered since in this access, with absolute estimated numbers of MDR-TB cases no longer shown or readily identifiable, but rather only percentages of estimated new cases with only prevalence rates being listed in the table (leaving the readers to work out numbers for themselves from separate tables).

the opposite, since it should be being allowed for in any proper strategy. In essence, it is believed that it takes around 15 years for what is happening with the development of drug-resistance at the level of latent infection to emerge as visible data in active disease.

This same 15 year pattern has been seen twice since drugs were first developed – once following the introduction of Isoniazid in the 1950s, and a second time with the wider implementation of Rifampicin in the 1970s. This 15 year period has been usefully divided into three periods of five years.

- During the first five years the drug is first introduced, and becomes widely used so that a substantial number of patients are exposed to it and develop some resistance ("substantial" being defined as being enough to make a difference to the epidemic).

- It then takes a further five years for these resistant patients to, in turn, infect a significant further number of patients.

- Finally, it takes another five years for these newly infected patients to develop and present themselves in sufficiently measurable numbers to show in any survey.

Given that this model was observed before the advent of HIV/AIDS, it might well be that the three phases would develop more quickly today in areas of high rates of co-infection. What this pattern strongly suggests is that all of the potentially visible data (even if it were properly being measured) is almost certain to be permanently well behind the invisible picture that will only properly reveal itself as much as 15 years later. To some extent viewing the current state of drug-resistance is like looking at stars in the sky that are 15 light years away – we cannot assume that the star as we see it at the moment of viewing is either brighter or less bright than it looks to us in the sky tonight. In fact we can't even be certain that the star still exists.

If we select certain other statements from within these reports, we can detect particular patterns of explanation which appear to be, not so much based on what the reports explicitly state, but rather on what they omit. Take this important one, for instance (presented as one of the 2012 Report's "Key Facts and Messages"):

> "Despite progress, the number of MDR-TB cases notified in 2011 represented only 19% of the estimated 310,000 cases of MDR-TB among

> reported TB patients with pulmonary TB, and less than 10% in the two countries with the largest number of cases, China and India."[185]

"Progress" in this context, is hardly good news, but it might also be grossly misleading. The authors knew well that there were at the very least an estimated prevalent 640,000 cases out there (since it was the Report's estimate number of prevalent cases) and that there might be many more if some experts are to be believed. Despite this, they elected to use as part of their key messages the far more conservative estimated figure of 310,000 (which we know are estimated cases from those reported patients with pulmonary TB). From this they can offer up the figure of 19%, when in fact the true percentage of notified cases to the overall true drug-resistant burden of disease has to be at least half of this and probably much less still. With the help of some excavation of the other figures contained in the report, the "progress" that was actually being recorded is far from what was being implied.

We can only really assume, in fact, that this "progress" consisted of the number of cases being put on treatment rising. It's obvious, however, that this progress is very limited. The Global Plan to Stop TB 2011-2015, for example, included a target that, by 2015:

> "…all new cases of TB considered at high risk of MDR-TB (estimated at about 20% of all new bacteriologically positive cases globally) and all previously treated cases should undergo DST. Likewise, all patients with MDR-TB need to be tested for XDR-TB."[186]

In fact the report states that coverage of DST has "remained stable in recent years, and is below that envisaged by the Global Plan". A graph shown in the report[187] demonstrates just how "below" the target this really is. The percentage of new cases tested for MDR-TB dropped in 2011 from just under 5% to 4% (when the target for 2015 is 20%), implying the need for an enormous scaling up of resource in the next few years. In fact we learn elsewhere in the same report that the current likelihood is that this target ***will actually be reduced*** because of the roll-out of the GeneXpert device (which tellingly can't spot either pre-XDR-TB or XDR-TB); and

---

[185] WHO - "Global Tuberculosis Report 2012", page 41.

[186] WHO -"Global Tuberculosis Report 2012", page 44.

[187] WHO - "Global Tuberculosis Report 2012", page 45.

that this might happen at the very same time that the report also recognised that "quality-assured DST is critical to ensure accurate detection of drug-resistance for subsequent treatment decisions".[188] The likelihood exists, therefore, that the other target (that all patients with MDR-TB will be tested for XDR-TB) might be rendered a pipedream.

The table below appeared in the 2012 WHO Global Tuberculosis Report and illustrated exactly how astray this all might be. It related to DST coverage in the 27 high MDR-TB countries. This was followed by numbers for the global regions. It gave an idea of just how much (or how little) was actually available or was being used in these countries to detect DR-TB, whether in new cases, repeat cases or even in confirmed MDR-TB cases. By simply picking out such particular countries (all of whom also have a low GDP), we may easily find ourselves starting to worry for them.

Country	**% of new bacteriological confirmed cases with DST result for MDR-TB**	**% of previously treated cases with DST results for MDR-TB**	**% of confirmed MDR-TB cases with DST results for XDR-TB**
Bangladesh	0.1	10	0
DR Congo	<0.1	2.0	0
Ethiopia	0.1	3.0	0
India	-	-	0
Indonesia	<0.1	9.0	23
Myanmar	-	-	0
Philippines	<0.1	17	0
Nigeria	<0.1	-	15
Pakistan	-	-	0
South Africa	-	-	80
Ukraine	-	-	0
Vietnam	-	-	0
All MDR HBC's	2.6	4.5	21
Goal for 2015	20	100	100

('-' indicates values that "could not be calculated")

At the very least, the table indicated two things. One is how haphazard the collection of data relating to DR-TB still appears to be, even in the HBCs and HBMDR-TBCs. The other is how terrifyingly inconsistent such efforts

188 WHO - "Global Tuberculosis Report 2012", page 69.

currently being made to address and apply resources to counter the threat are – even where the threat is supposed to be. And if this is the case in these targeted countries, how limited must it be in other countries which remain outside the sweep of the WHO's HBC radar?

XDR-TB – the much greater threat

"XDR-TB IS PROBABLY THE MOST DANGEROUS THING WE COULD EVER HAVE IMAGINED."

Dr Mario Raviglione[189]

A prevalence rate of just under 650,000 MDR-TB cases suggests that roughly one-in-20 of the estimated 12 million prevalent cases of TB are MDR resistant (or just over 5%). This percentage would, of course, include both new cases and retreatment cases. The general rate of XDR-TB within the MDR-TB pandemic is now estimated by the WHO to be around 9.6%. If both of these are accurate estimates (and they are almost certainly not less than this) a very sobering one-in-every-200 cases of prevalent TB must already be XDR-TB.

This would have made for nearly 58,000 cases of almost untreatable XDR-TB in 2012, although this number wasn't identified in the current report. That number coincidentally equates to 75% of the total number of patients who were enrolled on treatment for MDR-TB (not XDR-TB) last year, while co-incidentally the target for 2015 is still to get 75% of MDR-TB patients on treatment. Could we suggest from this that the world is essentially one degree of drug-resistance out of step in its response to this ever more dangerous public health threat with no apparent strategy yet in place to even begin to catch up?

With 77,321 MDR-TB patients put on treatment in 2012 we did see an impressive 70% rise in the numbers of patients being enrolled for treatment. The projection from the previous year had been that this number would have dropped, so a firm and definite numerical measurement within the pandemic of DR-TB represented extremely good news. It has to be recognised, however, that it's taken far too long for this sort of increase to be implemented. It's certainly still not being anticipated

[189] The Director of the WHO Stop TB Department

by anyone that the targets for treatment of MDR-TB will be being met by 2015 (a target of 270,000 each year); but with XDR-TB we still have no targets at all.

In 2012 the total global notifications of XDR-TB could be found (with a little searching around in the report) to be a specific 1,596.[190] This represents just 3% of the 58,000 estimated cases of XDR-TB that we have extrapolated are probably already out there using WHO numbers. So even using the WHO's numbers, an estimated 97% of the next wave of more extensive drug-resistance is already being missed – and even worse, we can be certain that these strains must also be active, infectious and in circulation.

It should also be noted that reported numbers in South Africa (the country where XDR-TB is probably being most looked for anywhere in the world since it reported 71% of the world's notified cases in 2012) have increased by a factor or 242% in three years. This does not prove that the rates of XDR-TB generally have been rising by this same percentage in the same three years, but it surely says that the tide is rising and the disease is out there if you care to go looking for it.

Furthermore, treatment outcomes for XDR-TB patients in the same country from 2010 revealed that just 18% of patients treated enjoyed successful outcomes. At least 150 other XDR-TB patients were monitored elsewhere in the world and the treatment success was a slightly higher 27% (possibly because of less co-infective disease) – so prognosis with this strain of TB is statistically extremely poor. This can be readily recognised as being a ***very*** big problem.

There is a further curiosity in the way in which these figures relating to XDR-TB are being presented in these reports because they contrast with those relating to MDR-TB. It might be more logically expected that they should be being presented in a similar format. The focus of reporting concerning MDR-TB consistently incorporates incidence rates (albeit they may be being misrepresented here and there), normally followed by the numbers of case notifications and then by the numbers of patients on treatment. These reports also include important percentage measures of the numbers of new TB cases who are MDR, and also the percentage of previously treated cases who are MDR. When it comes to XDR-TB, however, the references generally focus on just two measures only – the

[190] WHO - "Global Tuberculosis Report 2013".

numbers of countries which have so far reported cases, and the averaged global proportion of MDR cases that have been confirmed as XDR. Is this a significant difference? It certainly looks to be. It isn't actually hiding anything, however, because the rate of 9.6% of MDR-TB cases being XDR can hardly be seen by anyone as being insubstantial. At 9.6%, the proportion of MDR-TB cases that are XDR is nearly twice the estimated proportion of TB cases that are MDR: the numbers that are now being published suggest that there is a really dangerous secondary pandemic developing.

The numbers of countries reporting XDR-TB is also shown to be rising year on year.

But does this different style of presentation of numbers with XDR-TB suggest that, just as multi drug-resistance was being relatively speaking ignored until recently (and thus allowed to slip through the fingers of those entrusted with global infectious disease control), exactly the same thing might be happening today for extensive drug-resistance?

In other words, does it mean that the lessons from MDR-TB in the early 1990s have still to be learnt, let alone appropriately applied with ongoing consequences with XDR disease?

The potential impact of the Xpert®MTB/RIF test

The roll-out of the GeneXpert device during the last three years has been described as having been "impressive". Perhaps this needs to be put in proper context.

While over 1,400 GeneXpert machines and nearly 3.2 million Xpert®MTB/RIF cartridges were reported as having been "procured" for use in 88 of the 145 countries eligible for concessional pricing by March 2013, it is far from clear what stage of this procurement process had been reached. In one laboratory seen by the author, for instance, a machine had been standing idle for three months after delivery while the staff (who had received the training) awaited actual delivery of the cartridges.

If it is being seriously intended that the GeneXpert is to supersede the microscopy test, those 1,400 machines need to be put in proper perspective as well, especially as they amount to only around 800 machines outside of South Africa. Globally, the WHO reckons that there are around 72,000 laboratories which are currently approved to carry out sputum tests for TB – so if every one of these is destined to be equipped with a GeneXpert machine, there is a long way still to go in this impressive roll-out programme.

It's also far from certain that Cepheid, the machine's manufacturer, have had things as under control as might have been hoped. Bizarrely Cepheid's stock dropped in the second half of 2012, just when it would have been expected to have been rising. At the same time, rather than recommending that savvy investors would be wise to back the company (as would also be expected to be the case given that it has effectively cornered a highly lucrative market) industry experts were advising investors to back away. Whilst recognising the GeneXpert as being a revolutionary new diagnostic device, stock-watcher Sean Williams noted that the company was reducing its profit forecast. According to Williams this was because of "higher costs associated with rolling out its products in developing countries". He very reasonably recognised that the GeneXpert has "the potential to make the company extremely profitable" but added a rider that this was only "assuming [that] it can stay out of its own way". So does this mean that Cepheid, and therefore the roll-out of the device itself, is being hampered in terms of requisite investment simply because the company is not charging enough for the device – in other words because of the negotiated price reductions of both the device and the cartridges?

South Africa has been the biggest purchaser of the GeneXpert by far having ordered 43% of all modules purchased so far. It clearly sees the device as having the potential to revolutionise its TB systems of care and control, but the country was recorded as experiencing serious shortages of the testing cartridges in the first half of 2013. Cepheid has since planned to increase its production capacity to buffer stocks to avoid future stock-outs, but it's not yet clear whether it has sorted things out.

But has South Africa been right in this policy development anyway? Is the device all that it's being cracked up to be? Actually it may yet prove to be even more so, because, while the WHO has only endorsed the device for pulmonary disease, two pieces of research have also been done into using it as an assay for extra-pulmonary TB as well. The results from these studies are not ideal, they are certainly far superior to standard smear microscopy.

One Italian study revealed an overall sensitivity and specificity of 81.3% and 99.8% for Xpert, while the sensitivity of standard smear microscopy was 48%. In instances in which biopsies, urines, pus or cerebrospinal fluids were tested, the device's sensitivity exceeded 85%, while it was slightly under 80% for gastric aspirates. It was at its lowest (at less than 50%) for cavitary fluids. Of great importance as well (given that EPTB is so much more common in children), high sensitivity and specificity were also obtained for paediatric specimens (at 86.9% and 99.7%, respectively). The ability of the test to effectively rule out tuberculosis with a definitive negative finding, however, remained, according to the study said, at best "suboptimal".[191] Despite this the results from the study have to be seen to be extremely exciting.

In a full evaluation the study was rather more soberly assessed to be "very encouraging".[192] One particular idea that has been mooted as a result is to use it to test fine-needle aspirated biopsies of lymph nodes, potentially providing a vitally important adjunct to testing respiratory samples when screening HIV-infected patients for TB prior to antiretroviral therapy in sub-Saharan Africa. Such an innovation could prove to be really useful.

A second study, carried out in India, was similarly positive. The sensitivity of the GeneXpert assay in this report was almost identical to the other study at 81%, with a specificity of 99.6%. The sensitivity was found to be encouragingly high for the majority of specimen types (though not for cerebrospinal fluid, which ***had*** been found to be high in the Italian study). Whereas in the Italian study it had been found to be above 85%, in this study it was just 29% (from 2/7 specimens). The researchers concluded that the GeneXpert test showed "good potential" for the diagnosis of extra-pulmonary TB and "that its ease of use makes it applicable for countries where TB is endemic".

Altogether this is more than encouraging but, as with almost everything concerning this disease, there are downsides.

---

[191] Tortoli et al. "Clinical validation of Xpert MTB/RIF for the diagnosis of extrapulmonary tuberculosis". European Respiratory Journal (2012). http://www.ncbi.nlm.nih.gov/pubmed/22241741

[192] Stephen Lawn and Alimuddin Zumla - "Diagnosis of extrapulmonary tuberculosis using the Xpert® MTB/RIF assay", Expert Review of Anti-infective Therapy, 10; 6 (2012) 631-5.

One is that, while the test is cheap, it is not cheap enough. TB control in New York, of all places, has being suffering from financial constraints, and one issue identified as having impact on the city's programme costs has been the GeneXpert. Another is that, while the test is fast, a constant supply of electricity is required for the full 100-minute-test duration. This is a major handicap in many of the environments in which it might be put to best use. A sizeable percentage of tests may well end up being aborted because of predictable power cuts with consequent unbudgeted unproductive cost.

Another is that, while it is effective, it might just prove to be ***too*** effective for the resources that will be subsequently needed to satisfy the demand that it may well create. It has been conservatively estimated, for instance, that it might double the number of TB patients needing to enrolled on DOTS.[193] What is more likely, however, is that it will significantly increase the demand for second line drugs for cases which are identified as being proxy-MDR-TB – drugs which are already in short supply. In fact, it has been estimated that it will double and possibly treble the number of estimated drug-resistant cases, changing the face of the pandemic at a stroke.

The human resource for the existing TB burden is already on its knees. Can it cope with a much larger workload, particularly in those countries where DR-TB has so far not been actively looked for and is probably already out there? It hardly seems likely. There are also existing well-calculated shortfalls in anticipated budgets based on the estimates of prevalent TB – given the proportionately higher costs of treating MDR-TB, doubling the global case load (or worse) is not going to make much more budgetarily possible in terms of treatment roll-outs.

In fact, in an MSF project in Zimbabwe, preliminary results showed that its introduction led to a near quadrupling of DR-TB cases being diagnosed. Similar revelations in countries where DR-TB has not previously been properly looked for could cripple health infrastructures. The resources that would be required to attend to such revelations are simply unavailable and, in this sense, a technically impressive cart may be being put before an already emaciated horse.

---

[193] It has to be said that, given that half the pandemic is already being treated as sputum-negative based on clinical judgement, this estimate might well be over-egged.

Similar results have also been found in hotspots in South Africa. In one of these, in KwazaZulu-Natal, again reported by MSF, the rates of total TB diagnosis (all types) after the initial launch of the device in 2011 exploded by an increase of 211% a ***month***, with patients flocking to the clinic in unprecedented numbers. A worrying 13% of those diagnosed were drug-resistant.

The worry, therefore, must be that this device may create as much of a problem as it is intended to solve by exposing the scale of both drug-resistant and drug-susceptible disease in countries which up until now have had no capacity to diagnose drug-resistance and have no spare capacity with which to respond to any sort of increased burden of disease.

Dr Helen Bygrave, an HIV/TB specialist working with MSF in South Africa, says that:

> "This new TB test is helping expose the true size of the drug-resistant TB epidemic and get people on treatment faster."

This superficially sounds like it has to be a good thing, and it will certainly be in those projects in South Africa which have the drug-susceptibility testing on hand and also the second line drugs to treat DR disease, but what about in a country like Zimbabwe to the north?

The fact that South Africa has invested so heavily in the device raises an even more worrying concern as well – particularly if it is focusing on rapid diagnosis for drug-resistance using the GeneXpert, and not ramping up culture testing proportionately at the same time. It's difficult to deny the probability that South Africa has one of the highest burdens of XDR-TB in the world – the 2013 WHO report suggests that it may carry nearly three-quarters of the global burden. Globally, the percentage burden of MDR-TB which is XDR is now 9.6%, so we can assume that it is likely to be more in South Africa – maybe even as much as double. We can also assume that this sort of proportion of infectious extensively drug-resistant disease is circulating in the community.

Again, we can do some speculative calculations here. If we are talking of communities which carry a high burden of MDR-TB (both new and retreatment) in which, say one in five patients are MDR (which is known to be the case in hotspots), and that 18% of these cases are XDR, then we are looking at a burden of XDR-TB that itself may be running at 3.6% of the whole national TB epidemic. This, by very worrying coincidence, happens to be exactly the same as the current estimated percentage of new TB cases globally that are reckoned to be MDR-TB.

So if the Xpert device might be used for diagnosis in such communities ***without*** proper culture follow up of all cases confirmed as proxy-MDR automatically, all of these XDR-TB cases will be missed. Worse, they will be treated with inappropriate protocol drug regimens which will, in some cases, further amplify the degree of drug-resistance. Given that second line drug DOTS-Plus treatments are normally three or four times longer in duration than first line DOTS treatment, the bacilli will have proportionately more opportunity for mutation than they do with basic treatment for DS-TB. There is a possibility that we may be looking not just at turning MDR-TB into XDR-TB, but at turning XDR-TB into XXDR-TB and beyond, because, just as the standard microscopy test is useless for spotting MDR-TB, the GeneXpert is equally useless for spotting XDR-TB.

And this situation won't just affect South Africa: it has to be considered in every neighbouring country as well. In fact, by implication, it should be being considered in every country with a known or suspected problem of MDR-TB. If the GeneXpert is rolled out at any sort of scale, then drug-susceptibility testing must be proportionately ramped up as well, otherwise mis-treatment is almost guaranteed.

This is not an academic concern. The WHO's 2011 report on MDR-TB identified the relative gains that had been made in the fight against drug-resistant TB in terms of improvements in second line drug availability, diagnostic capability, and in better national TB drug-resistance data. National laboratory capabilities, the report recorded, had also improved and all high-burden countries could now conduct drug-susceptibility tests to confirm MDR-TB at least in their larger reference laboratories, although point-of-care diagnostics were still scarce. This optimism (and indeed the summary) may have been a little over-egged in the light of other evidence, however. The WHO was expecting that, by 2012, all 27 high-burdened MDR-TB countries would have representative data on TB drug-resistance to help guide the ongoing response. If this has happened, it has yet to be published.

In fact it must still be impossible for anything but vastly unrepresentative data to have been collated. According to the 2012 Global Report, only seven of the 36 'combined' high-burden countries[194] have any sort of

[194] Those identifiable on both lists as either having high burdens of either TB or MDR-TB, or both.

routine diagnostic DST in place, and this in spite of the launch of the Global Project on Anti-Tuberculous Drug-resistance Surveillance originally kicking off in 1994 – nearly 20 years ago.[195] Furthermore, we must continually remind ourselves that these so-called "high burden" countries are not necessarily those countries that are truly the most burdened by the disease.

There are good reasons for highlighting this concern relating to the growing threat from XDR-TB. Because of the introduction of the Xpert®MTB/RIF assay, the WHO suggested in its 2012 report that it was likely to ***revise downwards*** its own target for culture and DST capacity of one laboratory per five million population in the future.[196] Thankfully it hasn't done this as yet but, in the absence of any better test being developed, culture remains an essential for testing resistance to drugs other than Rifampicin. This is particularly so for testing resistance to the second line drugs in relation to XDR-TB.

India was reported to have been initially refusing to endorse the GeneXpert device with no official reason given. Aside from the possibility that it recognised the risks outlined above (which is somewhat unlikely given the country's institutional denial of the problem) three reasons appear to be possible for the initial refusal.

One could have been financial: the test could have been judged to be too costly for it to be rolled out in the sort of numbers required in India without sending the existing TB budget off the rails.

A second might have been that members of the Indian Health Ministry believed that another better test was in the offing, and so didn't want to commit to this first device because they saw it at best as being temporary and so a wasteful investment. It is certainly generally accepted that a better device is still needed – one that can be used at point-of-care, is cheaper and which can better identify more extensive drug-resistance, so this could well have certainly been the case. If a more promising newer device was indeed under development in India its refusal to endorse the device would certainly have made sense. In fact, a battery powered micro-PCR system

---

[195] The countries concerned were Lithuania, Latvia, Estonia, Moldova, Kazakhstan, Georgia and Armenia.

[196] WHO - "Global Tuberculosis Report 2012".

was launched in India in 2013, but it is still under evaluation, so the explanation remains the most probable.

The third possibility is the most worrying of all, however. MSF has been reporting significant hikes in rates of TB in India, as well as of diagnosed cases that are drug-resistant. It is also no secret that the Indian authorities are thought by many to be in official denial of the scale of drug-resistance in the country, and that the national rates of drug-resistance in the country are believed by some to have been growing exponentially. Dr Shelly Batra, the founder of Operation Asha, an NGO working with TB in India, has unequivocally stated:

> "The world is on the brink of a multi drug-resistant TB epidemic [and] India will be the epicentre."

She has as much reason to know this as anyone and, if she is right, the Indian government must be similarly aware. Was it blocking the device simply because it wanted to stall the inevitable exposure of the problem? We may never know, since the situation has changed now. India has since begun investing in the device, being reported in 2013 to be the second largest national investor in it after South Africa (although still way behind it).

Since the entire epidemiological world may, for these last two years (and for the next several years as well) be having its epidemiological data shuffled and reshuffled by new and more reliable data being produced by the GeneXpert, all of this offers food for thought. Some massive and very challenging mathematical re-modelling will be needed to re-assess the situation given the information that the GeneXpert device must already be making available.

The 2013 WHO Global Tuberculosis Report came out on 23rd October 2013. This was six months later than usual, being as it has been customarily appearing on or before March 24th to coincide with World TB Day. This particular report might have been expected to offer the first clues as to what may be happening in respect of this emerging information. Since the GeneXpert is about 80% reliable, we could have expected two things to be revealing themselves in this report.

- that the number of confirmed sputum-positive cases of TB would rise in some countries (in the ones which have procured the machine in any significant number) – by a factor of as much as 60%.

- that the confirmed numbers of (at least proxy) MDR cases might rise dramatically wherever the device was being rolled out at any scale, particularly wherever there is little or nothing in the way of culture or DST labs.

Both would seem to have been entirely logical expectations given the evidence of the small surveys already conducted by MSF. Of course if this happened then it would also completely foul up some of the existing projected trends in the disease because the extrapolated global burdens of disease should also be shifting around in accordance with such findings as well.

Unfortunately there was really no numerical sign of this in the 2013 report – instead it stated that the estimated rates of MDR-TB were "essentially unchanged" – something which goes against much of expert opinion as well as going against epidemiological logic. Even the numbers of bacteriologically confirmed cases of disease don't really seem to have jumped in the relevant countries as might have been expected to happen.

We shouldn't suspect that the WHO isn't taking MDR-TB seriously, however. But we can suspect that, behind the closed doors of the organisation, there may be less than coherent ideas on how to confront the problem: the overall message on DR-TB is simultaneously both too muted and too mixed to be otherwise.

Far from every country burdened by the disease is using the new device effectively yet anyway. When the report says that 3.2 million Xpert®MTB/RIF have been "procured" we have no way of knowing how many of them have been delivered and put to use. South Africa remains the country to watch, however, because the machine has been rolled out in far bigger numbers there than anywhere else. Although the TB epidemic in this country has grown again, the incidence increases have remained consistent over the past few years: this jump in figures of confirmed disease that we might have been expected from the GeneXpert just hasn't shown up yet. Even more surprisingly, there's no visible jump in their overall estimated figures of MDR-TB either. Bafflingly, it decreased.

The 2013 report, in fact, does go so far as to specifically identify the number of cases that were positively diagnosed for RR-TB with the

GeneXpert (the only evidence of any contribution from the device yet in the figures);

> "In addition, just over 10,000 RR-TB cases were detected using rapid molecular methods, though without results for Isoniazid DST at the time of reporting."

It has to be suggested that just over 10,000 is a suspiciously round figure. And with 3.2 million cartridges so far procured over three years of roll-out, it's either highly unimpressive or a huge relief that only just over 10,000 tests have as yet shown confirmed resistance to Rifampicin. It would be highly unimpressive because it would suggest that a disappointingly small proportion of those 3.2 million cartridges have yet been delivered and used. If it is the latter, however, we should have expected it to have been identified – but it's an unlikely possibility. The greater likelihood is that the production problems with the assays have been holding things up. But least impressive of all is the implication that not one of these 10,000 cases would appear to have been followed up with DST testing to confirm MDR-TB or worse as would have been expected to be the case.

The report contains other clues which may also help explain why these numbers aren't turning up yet. Another section provides a list of definitions of TB disease that are in the process of revision. The reports states that:

> "These updates were necessary to accommodate diagnosis using Xpert®MTB/RIF and other WHO-endorsed molecular tests, as well as offering an opportunity to improve aspects of the existing framework, such as inclusion of more comprehensive reporting of TB cases among children."

This amounts overall to promising future improvements in data, but it does nothing to help validate the most recent statistics if these GeneXpert figures are not really appearing in the current data when they might have been expected to appear. Nor does it help formulate the future policy which is currently under review.

The real picture becomes clearer still with further investigation – the use of those earlier definitions of disease were effectively intended to be stopped at the end of 2012, and the new ones intended to have been put to use from the start of 2013. As such, the report says, they will still be "used in WHO's 2014 round of global TB data". The implication of this is that we are in a state of statistical hiatus, with the full impact of the introduction of these revised definitions (and also therefore the data coming on-stream

from the GeneXpert) appearing properly for the first time only in the WHO global report of 2015, after the post-2015 strategy will have been finalised.
Two other things will be happening in 2015. One is that those targets set by the Stop TB Partnership will be reported as having been either hit or missed, and the other is that a new set of targets (and strategies) will be having their baselines set.

So is it unreasonable to suggest that some of the data that is currently being gathered won't show until 2015 and so may avoid some uncomfortable and inconvenient re-assessing for the WHO as these targets are being passed? At best it looks like the figures will be being used to assess the next set of targets and not measure the success or failure of the existing ones. To be fair, using figures harvested today that are measured by a device that wasn't even dreamed of in 1990 in order to compare numbers from that year would be indisputably unscientific. The only possible solution to this conundrum would have been to recalculate and re-estimate retrospectively to adjust the 1990 baseline figures based on what the device is revealing today (which is probably impossible at this stage).[197] The more practical alternative is to leave the figures pretty much as they are and not to include much about what the GeneXpert is revealing until 2015 when they can be used to establish the new baselines and also (perhaps much more importantly) proper new targets. It very much looks like the WHO has chosen to do the latter.

Dr Ernesto Jaramillo, the WHO medical officer in charge of MDR-TB policy and author of the WHO's 2011 report on MDR-TB, was already resigning the world to the fact that it is far from being on track to meet some of the deadlines, pointing to MDR-TB as the major bug-bear. By way of explanation he stressed that MDR-TB is a consistently complex issue, and he cited lack of funding, diagnostic and treatment capacity and adequate staff in the 27 countries with high MDR-TB burdens as all being contributory factors to the lack of progress. If this remains the case in this relatively small number of targeted countries after a decade of focusing efforts on them, particularly with only four of them being in Africa where

[197] The WHO suggests in the 'Global Tuberculosis Report 2013' that this does happen: "Estimates for all years are recalculated as new information becomes available and techniques are refined, so they may differ from those published in previous reports." It remains unclear, however, whether such revisions are as extensive as they might need to be if they are to be properly fit-for-purpose. Certainly the wider consequence of only a minor revision can be easily seen to be both substantial and very confusing.

some of the worst shortages of all are known to exist, we do have cause to worry about what may be in store for much of the developing world. We also need to be hopeful that what might be being strategically developed by the WHO will at least stop DR-TB from growing.

The epidemiological impact of current drug-susceptibility testing

As we have discussed, with the arrival of the GeneXpert device we may be seeing the first signs of a change in the weather regarding the particular problem of effective point-of-care drug-susceptibility testing. Certainly if a more comprehensive method of rapid diagnosis can be developed and rolled out – one that can also identify the potentially complex strains of drug-resistant disease that present such a threat today – then the particular problem that is entwined within this component of the wider epidemic could yet be wiped out at a stroke.

Meanwhile, the situation remains for the vast majority of those most at risk of drug-resistant disease much as it has been since the first instances of resistance to Streptomycin were identified in 1948: identifying probable infectious TB takes a matter of hours with the help of some spit, a glass slide, some chemicals and a microscope. To provide a definitive diagnosis, however, the sample needs to be cultured for a matter of weeks. And in order to identify drug-resistance the results of the culture need to be tested systematically against each drug that is suspected of being able to act against the active bacillus, with its response to each being evaluated in order for effective treatment to be prescribed.

At the very least, therefore, this process offers the drug-resistant bacilli a space of six weeks in which to infect another human being – although in practice it will take much more than this because the time taken to culture a sample is only the last part of a longer overall period which begins even before the first day of self-referral of a patient.

Epidemiology is a complex science. In order to see a disease decline a measurement known as a 'basic reproductive ratio' (or R_0) of less than 1.0 is looked for. This measurement is also known as a disease's 'transmission number', and basically refers to the number of cases that might expected to be infected by a single primary case of a disease during its natural course. With HIV, for instance, the R_0 is estimated as being between 2.0 and 5.0; for tuberculosis it is estimated at between 3.4 and 4.5 – with a doubling period of between one and three years. With both diseases together these numbers can be assumed to be different again in both cases.

Since it is generally accepted that there are between 10 and 15 cases of re-infection from a single case during every year of infectiousness, these transmission numbers may seem at first glance to be too low. Such cases of infection, however, do not necessarily develop into further active disease, being as re-activation is expected to occur normally only in 5% to 10% of those infected. Such complex factors all need to be fully considered before such measurements are finally arrived at.

It needs to be realised, as well, that this R_0 of between 3.4 and 4.5 applies only to TB without intervention. Once intervention is applied the figure reduces dramatically. From an epidemiological perspective, therefore, the key to successful treatment relates to identifying active disease as soon as possible after it first appears and then rapidly rendering it non-infectious. Without bringing the disease down to the magical 1.0 or below by effective intervention, TB is simply never going to go away. In many parts of the world this has already been achieved; in other parts it has proved so far to be impossible. With drug-resistant disease it has so far globally proved to have been impossible.

If we wish to roughly compare the potential reproductive ratios of drug-resistant TB to susceptible TB, we need to logically consider three separate components to the overall period of opportunity for the bacillus. In fact each of these will vary in length depending geographically and sociologically upon where the disease strikes. By reviewing this as best we can, we should be able to very loosely compare the R_0 of the two types of disease.

In all cases, the first critical period is the one from the moment when the disease re-activates from latency and becomes infectious (with the patient also probably noticing symptoms) up until when he/she presents at a clinic where a preliminary diagnosis is possible (i.e. where the sputum can be taken and examined) and a clinical judgement is made. If the disease is pulmonary, then practically speaking this period might be considered to start from the moment the patient begins coughing, when he will most probably become infectious. This period is completely dependent, of course, on several factors – upon the patient himself, on his capacity to get himself to a clinic, and on the availability and quality of the initial diagnostic resource. In fact in one study this period has actually been estimated in resource-poor settings to be as long as two years, itself very strongly suggesting that the reproductive ratio will be significantly higher in such environments compared to in a well-resourced one.

Since one general guideline concerning presenting symptoms of possible TB is a cough of three weeks' duration, let us settle for now on a simple and very minimal four weeks for this period. Up to the end of this period, the potential for any strain of pulmonary TB to infect another person, whether the strain is susceptible or resistant to locally available drugs, can be assumed to be roughly the same in similar environments. It may be small in a high-income country where the disease will be diagnosed quickly, but it will be much higher in a country where the patient may only take himself to a clinic when he finds himself unable to work and earn a living. In both cases, however, the comparative infectivity of any type of TB in the same environment should be much the same, and we can assume that no one type will have much advantage over another

From here on, however, the possibilities vary.

The best case occurs if the infection happens in an industrialised high-income country. Here, the sputum will be examined, the diagnosis of probable infection will be made, a course of first line drugs prescribed (and directly observed), and some of the sputum-positive sample will be sent immediately for further laboratory testing for more definitive diagnosis and for drug-susceptibility testing (DST).

Any report would be expected in six to eight weeks, and at this point the patient will be scheduled to return to the original prescribing clinician. The patient will have his own story to tell – one that will either relate that his symptoms have improved, or that they haven't. If the symptoms have subsided, the probability is that the patient is already non-infectious by the prescribed first line drug treatment (probably, in fact, in just two or three weeks – so let us settle on three weeks). So we have an initial lead-in period of four weeks to case presentation, plus a further three weeks for the drugs to disable the infectivity, a total of seven weeks.

If the symptoms haven't subsided then there is very good reason to suspect resistance to one, two or even more of the first line drugs. The clinician's response will relate to the contents of the report that will have been returned from the lab. It may well corroborate the patient's story: if the patient's story is positive, the DST report should confirm that there was no evidence of drug-resistance in the sample supplied. If the patient's story is negative and symptoms have persisted, however, the story from the lab may well be equally disappointing – but it should come with an addendum. The lab should have successfully identified which drugs should not be used, and, more importantly, which ones should work.

The most serious downside for the patient is that the treatment period will now be significantly longer (two years instead of six months) but the treatment still has a very good chance of being successful in outcome. At this point the patient will also be very closely managed to avoid possible further infectious opportunities for the bacillus. With a good dedicated health resource this can be confidently relied upon and will be effectively managed.

So, if the first initial period (at the end of which the patient has taken himself to a doctor) is four weeks, and this second period is six weeks, then we have a composite period of a minimum of ten weeks until the first potential definitive diagnosis of poly drug-resistance can possibly be made, at which point the patient infectivity will be effectively controlled. This may take another eight weeks (probably far longer), so we have a composite period of an initial lead-in period of four weeks to case presentation, plus six weeks for DST, plus a further eight weeks for the drugs to disable the infectivity, i.e. a total of 17 weeks.

The second best case might take place in a middle-income country – one which has both second line drugs and an accessible DST facility. We can use as an example what commonly happens in South Africa. In this case, the first period would be the same (four weeks) but the second phase as is currently practised is more extended than in the high-income country. The practice in South Africa is not to start drug-susceptibility testing until there are signs that the patient is failing to respond to first line drugs – at, let us say, five weeks after commencement of treatment. The reason for this is because of both expense and resource. Only at this point will the additional six-week period for culturing and DST kick in.

What this means is that, in a typical case in a middle income country with a known high incidence of MDR-TB, a composite period at the end of which second line treatment will be begun will be four weeks (initial) plus five weeks (first line drugs), plus six weeks (DST) – i.e. minimum 15 weeks, plus at least a further eight weeks for infectivity to be reduced which may not be as well managed, so a total of 23 weeks. It is also possible that the patient may have also had to wait before he can start treatment because of waiting lists.

(All of these periods are the minimal possible periods for each phase of a composite infectious period, so it is very reasonable to assume that in the majority of cases the period may be several weeks longer.)

The third (and worst) case is one occurring in a low-income country, one with neither second line drug provision nor DST facility. In this instance, in the vast majority of cases the patient will remain infectious until a time when she dies or recovers sufficiently through the strength of their own response to be no longer infectious. During all of this period she will invariably also be poorly managed.
For the sake of clarity of comparison, we will now also assume that in both high and middle-income countries the patient's infection is either effectively isolated or infectiously disabled through effective case management upon identification of drug-resistance. Neither should be in any way assumed to be the case.

So we can now roughly summarise as follows:

Type and environment of TB	**Likely minimum infectious period**
Drug-susceptible TB (anywhere)	7 weeks
Drug-resistant in high-income setting	17 weeks
Drug-resistant in middle-income setting	23 weeks or more
Drug-resistant in low-income setting	indefinite

It would be misleading to read too much from such a table, not least because it fails to allow for the first period of all, from the moment the patient becomes infectious until diagnosis beyond the three weeks after symptoms appear. It is generally suggested that this is likely to be much longer in lower-income settings than in higher income ones whether or not the disease is drug-resistant. Whatever the ultimate realities, the purpose of this exercise is to show general relative possibilities, and there are some very serious implications that can be reasonably assumed to arise from all of this.

The first is that, if resistance occurs in a high income country (which is less likely to occur because first line drugs are better managed), then the period of opportunity available to the drug-resistant strain after presentation is only just over twice that offered to a drug-susceptible strain. In other words neither strain would carry any major epidemiologically significant advantage over the other unless it were more infectively virulent. In such a scenario, therefore, the probability is that the drug-resistant epidemic, such as it might be, can still be both contained and controlled, especially with contact tracing and active case finding following on from diagnosis.

In middle- or low-income settings, however, there is good evidence to suggest that the resistant strain is at a measurable advantage in terms of its capacity to infect other human beings. In both such scenarios, in which the incidence rates of drug-resistance is either known to be high or can be suspected of being so, the likelihood of containing the drug-resistant epidemic is therefore smaller and will probably require innovative new solutions in order for it to be contained.

Now let us consider what the comparative probabilities of growth of disease might really be.

An infectious TB patient is, under normal circumstances, anticipated to infect another ten to 15 people in a 12-month period – in other words, in the broadest of terms, approximately one person per month.

Accepting the likelihood that this scenario will be significantly complicated in either direction by a number of additional factors, if we use the above table of figures we can very roughly anticipate that under more normal circumstances:

- A drug-susceptible case anywhere who is put on prompt treatment might be expected to infect at least one further case, and possibly two following diagnosis (although they may not go on to develop active disease). If 10% of infected cases develop re-activated disease, this would almost certainly amount to a basic reproductive ratio of less than one. The overall risk of transmission, therefore, is dependent on the speed of the initial referral.

- A drug-resistant case in a high-income country might similarly be expected to infect at least three further cases and possibly four following diagnosis. If 10% of such subsequent infections were to develop re-activated disease, this would still amount to a reproductive ration of less than one although the total overall risk would again depend on the speed of the initial referral.

- A drug-resistant case in a middle-income country might be expected to infect at least five further cases and possibly six following diagnosis. With a 10% conversion rate of such resultant infections, the reproductive ratio would still be less than one, but it has crept much nearer to this threshold number. Now everything is going to depend on the speed of that initial referral which is likely to be a lot slower.

- A drug-resistant case in a low income country is to conform to the standard accepted figure of between R3.4 and R4.5 as the disease naturally progresses – and this number allows for the 10% who ultimately succumb to re-activated disease. Furthermore the rates of such disease could be predicted to potentially double in between one and three years as happens with untreated TB. The infectivity ratio of a drug-susceptible case, however, could still be less than 1.0 depending on how quickly a patient reports to a clinic if there is any sort of adequate resource.

Epidemiologically speaking this suggests grave consequences for the epidemics in middle- and low-income countries if there is any existing prevalence of drug-resistant disease. Essentially the proportion of drug-resistant compared to drug-susceptible disease can be expected to grow cumulatively year on year. This looks to be an inevitability whatever strategy is put in place to contain it unless diagnostics become available, second line drugs are supplied, the diagnostic periods required for introducing second line drugs are significantly reduced and active case finding is initiated. Furthermore, if there is any existing significant level of drug-resistance in the community, then the local epidemic of drug-resistant disease can be reasonably expected to grow.

This will happen, of course, ***irrespective of how the rates of drug-susceptible disease decline by good DOTS control.***

We can also surmise that this may well already have happened in countries with poor surveillance, or where drug-resistance is not being actively looked for – although this does not seem to be the case in many low-income countries based on the current data. Quite possibly this is simply because this information is not yet being appropriately looked for.

We need to remember, however, that this situation ***is*** now changing with the advent of faster diagnostic solutions. In an MSF project in Swaziland, the delay between the time the patient's sample was collected up until starting DR-TB treatment was reduced from 65.9 days (nine weeks) to 13.9 days (two weeks). These times obviously do not include the variable period before a patient presents when the sample is collected (which would add four weeks to each period using our model). But it does suggest that, even without culture testing, MSF has been operating a system (assuming RR-TB to be MDR-TB) which is believed to be effective in a turn round which suggests that the comparative advantages for MDR-TB would be removed. It would not, however, remove the advantage that would be retained by a more extensively resistant strain, so even with faster diagnostics, unless they can accurately discriminate between poly drug-resistant strains these epidemiological imbalances will persist.

This could be hugely significant in the next five or ten years, depending upon how reliable new diagnostics turn out to be and how widely and how rapidly they can be rolled out. Without improvements of this sort it has to be assumed that the pandemic of drug-resistant disease, which may already be significantly under-estimated, will grow year-on-year not just in absolute numbers, but also in proportion to the drug-susceptible pandemic.

There is even a strong possibility that by 2050, the year when the current Global Plan for 2015 intended to see the disease eradicated, that drug-resistant disease will be the dominant type of tuberculosis, with more extensively drug-resistant strains becoming proportionately more common as well.

Establishing Outcomes – the "Assessment of Inequities"[198]

"YET THE CAPTAIN OF ALL THESE MEN OF DEATH THAT CAME AGAINST HIM TO TAKE HIM AWAY, WAS THE CONSUMPTION, FOR IT WAS THAT THAT BROUGHT HIM DOWN TO THE GRAVE."

John Bunyan (1680)[199]

The challenge of accurately measuring outcomes in the treatment of TB is compounded (and possibly actually confounded) by the difficulties not just of definitively knowing the true condition of the disease, but also in knowing whether it has truly been fully cured.

The methods of assessment have been being reviewed for several years, re-assessed with a view to using new and more accurate methods with which to measure progress towards meeting the next set of global targets for post-2015 – intended to be formally set out in 2014.[200] They are also very sensibly being redesigned to incorporate the new methods for diagnosis. There are two questions which arise from these deliberations. One is whether the assessment methods and the definitions being designed for the future are going to less complex and more transparent than those which have been being used thus far. The second is whether they will make such future assessments more accurate.

Revisions are being necessitated by four factors: the new generation of molecular diagnostics; the ever-developing strains of resistance; the undeniable fact that assessing current disease is a challenging business; and the unfortunate fact that it has not been being done as might well as it should have been. In order to more fully understand the possible bigger

[198] The "assessment of inequities" was a telling phrase used in a 2011 WHO draft report on new definitions that is referred to in the following section.

[199] From "The Life and Death of Mr Badman".

[200] These were announced on May 19th 2014, and an analysis of them has been included in a later section.

picture we need to unpack the cores of these more critical components piece by piece.

Measuring success

Success or failure is currently being measured by a set of parameters all of which are neither fully transparent nor entirely logical. Until recently, for example, successes and failures were being recorded for smear-positive cases only, which effectively meant that around half of the pandemic was being ignored at a stroke. Thankfully efforts have been made more recently to record outcomes for smear-negative cases as well, with the numbers of both notified and estimated cases now being included in the global reports (including sputum-negative and extra-pulmonary cases). This has to have been an improvement, and has certainly provided a more complete picture of the disease than was previously available. But even this has not turned out to have made things as transparent as might have been wished because sometimes these differentiated types of disease have been further disaggregated (with percentage success rates for each being identified), and sometimes they have simply all been collated together as 'all new cases'. Altogether this has been adding up to something that is still unhelpfully muddling.

Any attempt to understand global progress has to make every effort to comprehensively include all categories of cases, but even such an obvious idea turns out to be not that straightforward. In the EU, for instance, diagnosis by smear microscopy is not even considered a confirmatory test of tuberculosis at all (so a category of 'sputum smear-positive' is essentially meaningless as a definition of TB cases in most of Europe). In most of the countries where TB is common, however, (at least until the advent of IGRAs and the GeneXpert device) smear microscopy has been the only confirmatory test available, so it has been the default gold-standard. This sort of two-tiered inconsistency has hardly been making things easy.

In the current reports there are seven different treatment outcomes which have been being monitored – and things will remain that way at least for the Global report in 2014 and probably for 2015 as well.[201] The seven current definitions are as follows:

---

[201] If these measurements were still being used in the field in 2013, as was certainly the case from what was being seen, they should still have to appear in the 2015 outcome figures.

Cured: a patient whose sputum smear or culture was positive at the beginning of treatment, but who was smear-negative in the last month of treatment and on at least one previous occasion.

Completed: A patient who completed treatment but who did not meet the criteria for cure or failure. This definition applies to sputum smear-positive and sputum smear-negative patients with pulmonary TB[202] and to patients with extra-pulmonary disease

Failure: A patient whose sputum smear or culture is positive at five months or later during treatment. Also included in this definition are patients found to harbour a multi drug-resistant strain at any point of time during the treatment whether they are smear-negative or smear-positive.

Default: a patient whose treatment is interrupted for two consecutive months or more.

Died: A patient who dies for any reason during the course of the treatment.

Transfer out: A patient who has been transferred to another recording or reporting unit and whose treatment outcome is unknown.

Not evaluated: treatment outcome is not documented.

(Treatment outcomes for MDR-TB patients have been using these same general criteria, but define them slightly differently to accord with the different longer treatment regimens.)

The overall gross success rate for treatment of both types of disease has been measured by a final category of '**treatment success**' – and this is where things really become confusing, being as this particular category is defined as being "the sum of cure and completed".

No. of treatment successes = no. 'cured' + no. 'completed treatment'.

---

[202] Note the continued inclusion of both diagnostic categories.

This definition of success raises a troubling immediate issue. Whilst 'cured' cases are straightforward in their definition (being that they reflect confirmed successful outcomes), treatments that are 'completed' are not. The current definition for 'completed' has not in any way defined or implied treatment success beyond having completed the prescribed course of treatment – in fact it appears to have deliberately avoided doing more than this for reasons that are unclear.

It is interesting to note that the same definition when used by PIH and MSF is more definitive than when it is used by the WHO. In this case the 'completed' category means "a patient who has completed treatment ***and*** has no sign of continued active disease ***and*** does not meet the bacteriological criteria for cure".[203] 'Cured' for these NGOs (similarly to the WHO definition) means a patient who was initially bacteriologically confirmed (including by microscopy if that is all there is available) who then completed treatment ***and*** who has no continuing signs of active disease ***and*** has at least two negative sputum smears (one at 4-5 months, and the second at end of treatment) ***and*** does not meet the definition of failure.[204] The distinction between these definitions is, in this instance, much clearer.

Treatment defined under this term of 'completed' categorically should ***not*** include ones which give negative sputum smears or cultures at the end of treatment since these should be included as 'failures', so they must amount to patients who inexplicably don't have any bacteriological tests at the end of their treatments as they should do. But there is already another category for such patients, and this is 'not evaluated'. So exactly who are these patients, particularly given that there are a lot of them?

Well we can start by suggesting that patients who have been defined by this definition of 'completion' under the auspices of the WHO definition have not been bacteriologically confirmed as being free of disease, and nor have they necessarily been clinically evaluated as such. The definition certainly implies this. Of course, these patients may well not have had a positive smear in the first place. At first glance, at least, it seems more than probable that this category was originally developed to allow inclusion of both smear-negative and extra-pulmonary cases which were (rather belatedly)

---

[203] Italics are mine.

[204] PIH & MSF - "Tuberculosis – Practical Guide for clinicians, nurses, laboratory technicians and medical auxillaries" (2014) page170. http://refbooks.msf.org/msf_docs/en/tuberculosis/tuberculosis_en.pdf

being seen as being important enough to be included. There are, however, several reasons to wonder whether this was the case. One is because it would then have been logical that a further clause should have been added to the definition for the purpose of final clarification – something similar to the PIH/MSF definition along the lines of "..and who, in the opinion of a clinician, carries no further clinical evidence or suspicion of disease". This would allow cases in which a clinician had originally diagnosed TB and initiated a course of treatment on the basis only of signs and symptoms and perhaps after X-ray analysis to be clinically judged to have been treated successfully at the treatment's conclusion.

But confusingly no such qualifying clause was included in the definition. In fact, when reviewed in then light of the PIH/MSF definition, it looks like it may have been deliberately avoided. Whilst 'cure' is clearly defined in terms of outcome, as indeed are 'failure', 'default', 'died' and 'transferred out', this definition of 'completed' has been left open for interpretation, offering the epidemiologist no proper access to a definite or reliable sense of quantification in terms of the successful outcome for the patient.

There is another more troubling reason to believe that this 'completed' classification was not developed specifically with sputum-negative and EP cases in mind, and this is because sputum-positive cases have not been not definitively excluded from this outcome category as should logically have been expected if this had been the original intention. In fact the disaggregated percentage numbers for both 'cured' and 'completed' have been being applied to cases of sputum-positive disease as if it made perfect sense to do so. In fact the only logical definition for 'success' in any case which was originally diagnosed by bacteriological diagnosis must surely be 'cured' defined bacteriologically by the same method as the original confirmation of disease.

When the reported figures are carefully examined, however, these two definitions ('cured' and 'completed') can be seen to have been ***more*** transparently applied to sputum-positive cases than they have been to sputum-negative. The disaggregated percentages in the published data for the two definitions of 'cured' and 'completed' can actually only be separately identified as such in the data for sputum-positive cases. With this category of patients the two definitions appear separately in the totals of treatment successes for this bacteriologically confirmed category of patient.

With sputum-negative cases, meanwhile, whilst the successful sum total outcome percentage is identifiable, it is not broken down into the two components. But there is naturally no reason that they should be. In the case of these non-bacteriologically confirmed cases (i.e. ones which are not bacteriologically confirmed in the first place) the only possible measurement of successful outcome can be 'completion' of treatment (although such an outcome should surely also be appropriately qualified by clinical judgement).

In fact, in both the 2012 and 2013 Global Reports the category of 'completed' patients was categorically defined to apply to both sputum-negative ***and*** to sputum-positive patients with exactly the same wording accompanying them:

> "This definition applies to sputum smear-positive and sputum smear-negative patients with pulmonary TB and to patients with extra-pulmonary disease."

So the 'completed' definition has unquestionably been intended to include sputum-positive cases who, for indeterminable reasons, have no positive bacteriological confirmation of treatment success at treatment completion and who somehow don't fall into the 'not evaluated' category. If they had fallen into this 'not evaluated' category, then they would have also fallen out of the general 'successful treatment' box and appeared in the box of treatment 'failures or unknowns'. This is the box which includes patients who died, transferred out, bacteriologically failed, defaulted or simply remained unevaluated.

In the proper sense of its WHO definition, 'treatment completion' can measure nothing more for a sputum-positive case than whether or not the treatment was completed. And no further category beyond a bacteriologically confirmed 'cure' can properly be applied to such a case in terms of success – and yet, despite this, one has bafflingly been regularly included and applied.

If we take some examples from the figures published in the 2013 report, the ramifications which arise from this confusion will become a little more evident.

Treatment success rates for 2011 patients (which are the ones which are included in the 2013 report) were differentiated into four different types: 'new smear-positive' (and/or culture positive) cases; 'new smear-negative/extra-pulmonary' cases; 'retreatment' cases; and finally MDR cases (these from the 2010 cohort because of their longer treatment). Generally, as identified above, we are only able to identify differentiated successful treatment outcomes from within the report for the first type of patient, new smear-positive cases – who were further differentiated into these two categories 'cured' and 'completed'. Globally the 'cure' rate for such sputum-positive cases was 80%, and the 'completion' rate was 7%, making a composite success rate of 87% (which meets the global target). So what exactly might have happened to these 7% of sputum-positive cases who weren't bacteriologically assessed at the end of their treatment? If they had been measured and had been found to be negative they would have been defined as 'cured'; but if they were still positive they amounted to treatment 'failure'. Exactly what other options are there? The only one is that, for unknown reasons, they were not measured bacteriologically at the end of treatment, so were not properly evaluated. It's difficult to figure out what reasons there might be for this, unless they were simply not evaluated because they had disappeared. In either case, however, they should have been properly recorded as 'not evaluated'.

Meanwhile overall success rate for 'all new cases' for 2011 (a total which includes sputum-positive, sputum-negative and EP cases) was also measured at 87%. No differentiated breakdown was given for this, which doesn't seem that helpful but, since the successful outcome percentage was exactly the same for 'all new cases' as it was for sputum-positive cases, we can still draw some logical conclusions. We can reasonably assume, for instance, that the sputum-negative/extrapulmonary component of the global pandemic must have 'completed' at the same 87% success rate as the sputum-positive cases: if their 'completion' rate had been higher than those of sputum-positive cases it would have hiked the gross rate for 'all new cases'; if it had been lower it would have lowered it. No alternative is possible.

Global cases	**Cured**	**Completed**	**Successful Outcome**
Smear-positive	80% (2,096,839)	7% (183,473)	87% (2,280,312)
'All new cases'	38% (2,096,839)	48% (2,701,411)	87% (4,798,250)
By deduction, sputum negative and extra-pulmonary cases	?	?	(2701,411-183,473) 87% (2,517,938

There is, however, reason to wonder about this further, although it quickly becomes quite a challenge. The proportion of new incident cases globally that were reported in the 2012 report (i.e. the ones that applied to 2011, the period for which the most recent outcome figures apply) ***was*** indeed broken down between smear-positive and non-smear-positive (comprising sputum-negative, smear-not-done, type-unknown or extra-pulmonary), and this was: 48 % smear-positive, and a composite total of 52% non-smear-positive.[205]

So what does this extra information imply? Well, we definitely know that only 80% of those new sputum-positive cases were subsequently confirmed bacteriologically to have been cured – which amounts to 2,096,839 new cases having evidence of cure (or 38% of 'all new cases'). Meanwhile 7% of those sputum-positive new cases fell into the 'completed' category – amounting to 183,473 cases. Meanwhile 87% of 'all new cases' had successful outcomes as defined above, and 87% of 'all new cases' gives us 4,798,250 'successes'. But this figure also has to include those two million sputum-positive cases who we already know were bacteriologically confirmed to have been cured.

If we deduct the gross total successful 87% of sputum-positive cases (2,280,312) from the total new cases with identified successful outcome (4,798,250) we can further conclude that 2,517,938 non-smear-positive cases completed treatment successfully.

However, 183,473 sputum-positive cases completed treatment without any bacteriological evidence of cure (7% of the bacteriologically confirmed component of the pandemic), and 2,517,938 non-smear-positive new cases similarly completed treatment without evidence of cure (87%), effectively making a total of 2,701,411 new cases in the troublesome 'completed' category (or 48% of all new cases). Meanwhile, 38% of 'all new cases' had evidence of cure. What this means is that, if we look at the big picture, considerably fewer than half of all new cases had any actual evidence of cure. In other words, while the percentage rate of truly confirmed cure (as identified bacteriologically for the sputum-positive cases) is 80%, the overall percentage rate of such cure for 'all new cases' (which is not

[205] The total notifications of new disease in 2011 was 5,515,230: for smear-positive 2,621,049; for smear-negative 1,872,745; smear not done 155,049; extra-pulmonary 813,636; case type unknown 11,784; history unknown 41,702 (total 2,894,916 or 52%) – see Table 3.1 on page 30 of the 2012 WHO Global Tuberculosis Report, which breaks down the numbers used for treatment outcomes.

identified but which we have just worked out) is just half of this. Given the size of the non-smear-positive component within the pandemic, this is hardly surprising, but it's a very sobering figure nonetheless.

This mysterious 7% of global sputum-positive cases may at first seem to be proportionately inconsequential, but this percentage was recorded as being significantly higher than 7% for certain regions. The percentage of sputum-positive 'completed' cases which were included in the gross outcome success rate of 78% for the Americas region, for instance, was actually three times higher, at a very substantial 23%. And in this case, the percentage of sputum-positive cases that were cured was only 55% to start with which is worryingly low. Clearly something quite different was happening in this region – or if it wasn't then the measurements must have been being interpreted substantially differently. Whatever may have been the case, we can run a similar set of numbers and see what this might mean. The total of new cases was 206,827, of which 121,130 were sputum-positive. So 78% of these sputum-positive cases were successfully treated (i.e. 94,481), of which 23% were successfully completed (i.e. 21,731) with the remainder being 'cured' (72,750). In this case 35% of all new cases had evidence of cure. It turns out to be a little less than the global figure, but not substantially so – so it rather looks like the major differences may have been in the way that the definitions were being interpreted.

There was also a total of 85,697 non-smear-positive new patients of whom 71% enjoyed treatment success, adding another 60,845 to our composite 'completed' pot for the Americas. So we have a composite breakdown of 72,750 cured and 82,576 completed treatment, and 82,576 amounts to 40% of all successful new cases.

So we have a rate of cure of 35%, and a total rate of completion without evidence of cure of 40% (making a total composite success rate of 75% which misses the recorded gross outcome rate of 78% by three percentage points for the probable reasons of recording across different years).

Running the same sort of calculation for Africa, we have a cohort of 605,929 smear-positive cases, and 708,981 non-smear positives, making a total cohort of 1,314,910. Smear-positives enjoyed 82% successful treatment, with 72% of these successes being determined by 'cure' (or 436,268). This leaves us with 60,593 sputum-positives in the 'completed' box. Non-smear-positives had a 76% success rate – adding a further 538,826 to our 'completed' box (i.e. a total of completions now of 599,419). So we have a rate of cure of 33% (again around one-in-three of all new cases), and a total rate of completion without evidence of cure of 46% (making a total composite success rate of 79%).

All of these present a fairly consistent picture but they are also substantially different from what is the only visible breakdown between 'cured' and 'completed' in the tables (of 80% and 7% respectively), the one which relates to sputum-positives only.[206]

	Sputum+ 'successful'	Sputum+ 'cured'	Sputum+ 'completed'	All new cases 'cured'	All new cases 'completed'
Global	87%	80%	7%	38%	39%
Americas	78%	55%	23%	35%	40%
Africa	82%	72%	10%	33%	46%

When it comes to individual countries, the numbers relating to sputum-positive cases can seem more confusing still and we need to consult the table below.

For Uganda, for instance, the 'completed' rate for new sputum-positive cases is a considerably more substantial 38%, (while the cure rate was 37% and composite success rate for smear-positive cases arrived at by the sum of 'cured' and 'completed' is 77%). So what happened to those 38% of sputum-positive patients in an HBC that never got bacteriologically evaluated at the end of their treatment? Is a different method of measurement being used here, after nearly 20 years of DOTS implementation in one of the 22 HBCs?

The Ugandan success rate relating to 'all new cases' (which must necessarily include smear-negative and EP cases) was pegged at 73%. The total sputum-positive cases that was notified was 25,614. The 'cured' total of 37% amounts to 9,477 cases. This leaves us with the 38% to go into the 'completed' bucket (or 9,733). The total of all new cases is 45,004, and the combined success rate for all new cases was 73% (making 32,853). If we now deduct the 'cured' sputum-positives from this we are left with 23,376 in the 'completed' bucket. So in Uganda 22% of all new patients were 'cured' (i.e. less than one-in-four of all new cases), and 23,376 successfully completed their treatment (52%).

---

[206] WHO - "Global Tuberculosis Report", page 152.

Uganda was not unique: for Swaziland the 'completed' rate for sputum-positives was 25%, and the 'cure' rate was 48% (making a composite success rate of 73%); for Lesotho, the 'completed' rate for sputum-positives was 11% with a 'cure' rate of just 53% (composite success rate 64%). The success rate for 'all new cases' for these high incident countries, however, is unidentifiable because unfortunately neither is an HBC (as both probably should be). Botswana's sputum-positives had a 'completed' rate of 46% and a 'cure' rate of 36% (composite success rate 82%). As in Uganda, more than half of all sputum-positive cases did not appear to have been bacteriologically evaluated at the end of their treatment. Again, the success rate for all new cases is frustratingly unidentifiable because (unlike Uganda) it is not an HBC.

	Sputum-pos 'successful'	Sputum-pos 'cured'	Sputum-pos 'completed'	All new cases 'cured'	All new cases 'completed'
Africa	82%	72%	10%	33%	46%
Uganda	77%	37%	38%	22%	51%
Swaziland	73%	48%	25%	?	?
Lesotho	64%	53%	11%	?	?
Botswana	46%	36%	46%	?	?

There can be no doubt that this nebulous category of 'completed' has been playing a substantial but troublingly variable part in the measurements of treatment success at least in some countries, but may also have been affecting global outcomes in several different possible ways as well. There can certainly be little doubt that it has been creating confusions. How exactly, for example, has it been being interpreted at ground level by those submitting the data? Is it being interpreted as consistently as it should be, and in the same way as it appears to have been by those experts who finally compile the figures? Might there have been scope as well to have creatively interpreted these categories in some instances in order to improve figures and more nearly match targets?

We can't tell, but we can at least conclude that the measurements which have been (and which still are currently being) taken to assess outcomes of treatment have been far from as well defined as might have been wished for.

So will they improve as the new strategies are unfurled?

The new measurements

Initially it looked like two new options were being considered, one of which was radically different to the one that has been being used until now.[207]

The first option (at least as it was being described within a WHO draft document) still looked very much like the existing one with a couple of amendments. It did include a new disaggregation to accommodate 'WRD-positive' patients – i.e. those cases diagnosed by GeneXpert or other similar 'WHO Recommended Diagnostics' (WRDs) which may be approved in the future. It also intended to incorporate children in the reported numbers for the first time. Because of this version's similarities to the existing definitions, there is no need to list them here item by item. Of note, however, is that those two first definitions ('cured' and 'completed') were still being proposed to be retained ***exactly*** as before, with the intention that they could continue to be amalgamated to calculate a gross treatment success rate.

The second more radical option looked to usefully simplify things, as well as to remove some of the ambiguities in the process. It proposed incorporating the following definitive categories in place of the existing ones:

> **Cured**: Patient with no signs of continued active disease whose treatment was successfully completed and bacteriological success demonstrated.
>
> **Failed**: Patient with clinical and/or bacteriological signs of active disease or deterioration requiring a treatment change.
>
> **Interrupted**: Patient whose treatment was interrupted for two consecutive months or more for any reason without medical approval. (The term 'defaulted' was intended to be dropped and replaced by 'interrupted' implying, wisely, that the problem might be down to the supply of treatment as much as it might be down to the compliance of the patient.)
>
> **Died**: as previous.

---

[207] WHO – "TB Case Definitions" – Revision May 2011(version 6).

Not evaluated: as before but including the former 'transferred out' category within it.

This second option was apparently being carefully considered in order to both clarify and simplify things, since it would result not just in five core categories instead of seven, but also with a maximum of 30 sub-categories (which are not shown in the outline above to avoid further confusions) instead of 58. As significantly as anything, however, it looked as if the erstwhile necessity for the measurement of success to be composed of two separate categories, one of which is so intrinsically vague, might be about to be avoided completely. This possibility certainly promised more transparent and potentially more reliable outcome data for the future. The particular definition of 'cured' under consideration, however, would essentially have excluded all cases who were sputum negative at the start of their treatment, since they would be *de facto* unable to present any bacteriological success as evidence of cure. In fact there could be no bacteriological evidence that could be demonstrated for such patients, so it also looked as if things might be becoming even more confusing still.

(A parallel discussion relating to outcome definitions for MDR-TB cases was also being developed with similar options in the draft document. The optional definitions being suggested for MDR-TB were very much in parallel with those listed above, with the same view of simplifying outcome measurements. In the case of MDR-TB, for instance, the core categories for the second (simpler) option would again be five as opposed to an existing seven, and for the sub-categories would be 30 instead of 42. The details of these proposals are deliberately omitted from our current discussion, however, simply in order to avoid adding confusion to confusion.)

It did look, at least, as if there was reason to be hopeful that things at least were going to be usefully simplified, and that countrywide data might consequentially end up being a lot more reliable. In the end, however, a third option was decided upon and this was announced in the 2013 report. It falls somewhere between the two options, and smacks not just of fundamental differences of opinion amongst those making the decisions, but also of final compromise. The following list provides the definitions which are to be used starting in 2013, supposedly for inclusion in the 2014 report:[208]

> ***Cured:*** A pulmonary TB patient with bacteriologically confirmed TB at the beginning of treatment who was smear- or culture-negative in the last month of treatment and on at least one previous occasion.
>
> ***Completed treatment:*** A TB patient who completed treatment without evidence of failure but with no record to show that sputum smear or culture results in the last month of treatment and on at least one previous occasion were negative, either because tests were not done or because results are unavailable.
>
> ***Died:*** A TB patient who died from any cause during treatment.
>
> ***Failed:*** A TB patient whose sputum smear or culture is positive at month five or later during treatment.
>
> ***Lost to follow-up:*** A TB patient who did not start treatment or whose treatment was interrupted for two consecutive months or more.
>
> ***Not evaluated:*** A TB patient for whom no treatment outcome is assigned. This includes cases 'transferred out' to another treatment unit as well as cases for whom the treatment outcome is unknown to the reporting unit.
>
> ***Successfully treated:*** A TB patient who was cured or who completed treatment.

There are certain aspects that deserve further elucidation.

The category of 'cured' can still only possibly be applied to bacteriologically confirmed cases (as was also previously the case). 'Completed' cases could also still include all cases defined as having TB of any type, but extremely importantly, they can at least now only include patients who show no "evidence of failure" at the end of treatment. This clearly addresses a part of the previous anomaly and serves to clarify matters, but the definition

[208] It should be noted that it is far from clear that these new definitions have been rolled out in the field as at the end of 2013 in the HBCs, so whether they will even be applicable to outcome statistics, even in 2015, is unclear.

technically still could include patients who were, at the start of treatment, bacteriologically confirmed to have the disease, and remains too troublingly vague. It offers a low grade negative assurance of successful completion rather than a more positive one. If patients had bacteriological evidence of disease at the outset, but had no bacteriological evidence of cure at the end of treatment they can still fall into a difficult category. Is "without evidence of failure" good enough for them if "tests were not done or because results are unavialable"? In some sense they must also be essentially 'not evaluated', since, at least in terms of their original diagnosis, this would be the case. So the thorny question remains: under what circumstances is it possible for more than a very few of such bacteriologically defined patients to be "without evidence of failure" other than by a negative sputum test or other WRD? In other words, what is really being looked for within this category of successful outcome? A real treatment success, or a hoped-for one?

Meanwhile, patients that were up until now defined as 'defaulted' will now more simply be included as 'lost to follow up'.

There are now effectively six core categories instead of seven so there has at least been a degree of simplification. Are these definitions more user-friendly and appropriate than the second option that appeared in the first draft of the alternatives up for consideration? Will they effectively measure the burdens of disease in the coming decades? We will have to see.

But the 2013 report didn't leave it there – it had other new definitions identified within it as well.

New definitions of disease

There currently exists a set of definitions of tuberculosis disease that has recently been partially outmoded by diagnostic developments. In fact these definitions have always been slightly problematic, in that they have never been universally applicable and are therefore necessarily two-tiered. The current definition of a 'definite case of TB', for instance, has been defined as:

> "A patient with Mycobacterium tuberculosis complex identified from a clinical specimen, either by culture or by a newer method such as molecular line probe assay (LPA). In countries lacking laboratory capacity to routinely identify *M. tuberculosis*, a pulmonary case with one or more initial sputum specimens positive for acid-fast bacilli (AFB) is also considered to be a

> 'definite' case, provided that there is functional external quality assurance with blind rechecking."

Two issues have been arising from this definition. One is that diagnosis of tuberculosis was necessarily reduced to being a diagnosis of MTBC, simply because the sputum test cannot diagnose beyond this – in fact it cannot definitively diagnose the disease beyond identifying the presence of acid-fast bacilli. The second bugbear has been that appropriate levels of "functional external quality assurance" (EQA), which is the fundamental prerequisite for including AFB smear microscopy within this definition at all, is sadly still widely deficient even today and this doesn't look likely to change much before 2015. Only three of the 22 HBCs, for instance, could report the existence of an EQA that covered all of their national centres in 2012, and only 14 could report EQA coverage for 80% of their centres. Levels of EQA coverage are recognised to predetermine the definitive quality of bacteriological confirmation of disease by smear microscopy so the overall quality of global diagnosis has to be seen to still be uncomfortably questionable – even in the 22 HBCs.

Things clearly needed changing and the development of the new strategy for post-2015 has at least offered an opportunity to clear things up a little. An option that was initially being explored in 2011 seemed intent on boldly addressing these issues.[209] As far as both first and recurrent episodes of disease were concerned it was being suggested that there might need to be just three distinct categories:

> **Confirmed** – diagnosed by culture or other WHO approved molecular assay
>
> **Probable** – diagnosed by smear microscopy, and
>
> **Possible** – who are patient put on treatment in the basis of clinical judgement (who we know to amount to around 50% of notified patients).

This third 'possible' optional category would effectively address the second part of the current definition, which has just been known as a '**case of TB**'. Up until now such a case has been defined as:

---

[209] WHO - "TB Case Definitions" – Revision May 2011 (version 6).

> "A definite case of TB [i.e. bacteriologically confirmed by the 'definite case' definition above] or one in which a health worker (clinician or other medical practitioner) has diagnosed TB and decided to treat the patient with a full course of anti-TB treatment."

In other words, a 'case' of TB currently includes all three of the new definitions which were under consideration – confirmed, probable and possible. In the 2013 report, however, official notification was given of a different set of definitions again – ones which are clearly intended to get around some of the existing problems as well as address the consequences of the approval of new molecular methods of diagnosis. In the end it looks very much like the three-tiered idea of 'confirmed', 'probable' and 'possible' was finally considered a step too far because, regrettably, they weren't included. In an earlier section entitled "Confirming Active Disease" we discussed exactly these issues – that without culture (and now WRD assay as well) tuberculosis could at best be only described as 'probable' or 'presumed'. In fact, as we previously noted, this same thorny issue was struggled over back in 1929 by the British Joint Tuberculosis Council, which proposed then that diagnosis could only be either "beyond all doubt" or "probably tuberculous", though the august members of the Council at the time felt unable to acknowledge such uncertainties in order to preserve the reputations of themselves and their profession if they were to openly accept that things really were so uncertain. A full 85 years later, and acknowledgement of such vagueness and uncertainty still appears to be institutionally unwelcome even if it is essentially accurate, because the new official definitions are to be as follows:

1. ***A bacteriologically confirmed case of TB:*** A patient from whom a biological specimen is positive by smear microscopy, culture or WHO-approved rapid diagnostic test (such as Xpert MTB/RIF). All such cases should be notified, regardless of whether TB treatment is started.

2. ***A case of pulmonary TB:*** Any bacteriologically confirmed or clinically diagnosed case of TB involving the lung parenchyma or the tracheobronchial tree. Miliary TB is classified as pulmonary TB because there are lesions in the lungs. Tuberculous intra-thoracic lymphadenopathy (mediastinal and/or hilar) or tuberculous pleural effusion, without radiographic abnormalities in the lungs, constitute a case of extra-pulmonary TB. A patient with both pulmonary and extra-pulmonary TB should be classified as a case of pulmonary TB.

3. ***A clinically diagnosed case of TB:*** A patient who does not fulfil the criteria for bacteriologically confirmed TB but has been diagnosed with active TB by a clinician or other medical practitioner who has decided to give the patient a full course of TB treatment. This definition includes cases diagnosed on the basis of X-ray abnormalities or suggestive histology and extra-pulmonary cases without laboratory confirmation. Clinically diagnosed cases subsequently found to be bacteriologically positive (before or after starting treatment) should be reclassified as bacteriologically confirmed.

There are several implications from the above.

One is that the issue of actual identification of *M. tuberculosis* (as opposed, for instance, to bovine TB, another mycobacterium, or even the possible spontaneous shedding of non-tuberculosis acid-fast bacilli which sometimes occurs with HIV-infected individuals) remains uncertain, so a bacteriological confirmation under such a definition cannot be considered definitive of TB.

It will also be noted that these three different definitions allow pulmonary disease to be only included within category (2), whilst extra-pulmonary cases could be either in (1) or (3) depending upon whether or not there is any either bacteriological or clinical confirmation of disease.

Curiously, only bacteriologically confirmed cases specifically require notification.

As well as this, those diagnostic differentiations of sputum-positive and sputum-negative disease will no longer apply. We can assume that these terms are now considered not that useful, although they could reasonably still be considered to be of epidemiological significance in that sputum-positive cases are also the most infectious and therefore must constitute a higher priority from any public health perspective.

Dropping these two classifications certainly gets around all of the confusions relating to treatment success rates which were discussed above, since we have seen that cure rates (which have to be fundamentally predetermined by cases at least being sputum-positive) are not currently being used as the only judge of success in sputum-positive cases. It also gets around the undeniable fact that cure rates simply cannot be measured in around half of all cases which are smear-negative or at least are non-sputum-positive. It certainly also does away with one anomaly under the current definitions – that a patient with positive culture but with negative AFB sputum examinations should be counted as a smear-negative case of pulmonary TB. Under these definitions, such patients would be bacteriologically confirmed, end-of-story (as they certainly should be).

It also can be expected that, in all settings where definite cases have previously been mostly smear-positive, the addition of WRD-positive cases within the definite case category will result in increases in the number of such diagnoses. If only bacteriologically-confirmed cases end up being notified, however, the number of notifications of disease may drop dramatically.

The definition of an extra-pulmonary case has also been marginally simplified with no anticipatable consequence:

> ***A case of extra-pulmonary TB:*** Any bacteriologically confirmed or clinically diagnosed case of TB involving organs other than the lungs, e.g. pleura, lymph nodes, abdomen, genitourinary tract, skin, joints and bones, meninges.

New cases are defined almost exactly as they were previously:

> ***A new case of TB:*** A patient who has never been treated for TB or has taken anti-TB drugs for less than one month.

When it comes to retreatment cases, however, things become a little more complex again. It is openly recognised within the ranks of TB epidemiologists that "mis-classification of treatment history is extremely common",[210] so a lot of care has been taken to try to simplify things but to maintain or improve usefulness at the same time. Up until now there have been three types of retreatment case:

(i) a patient previously treated for TB who is started on a retreatment regimen after previous treatment has failed (treatment after failure);

(ii) a patient previously treated for TB who returns to treatment (having previously defaulted);

[210] WHO - "TB Case Definitions" – Revision May 2011, page 23.

(iii) a patient who was previously declared cured or treatment completed and is diagnosed with bacteriologically-positive (by sputum smear or culture) TB (relapse).

Instead of these, we are now faced with four new categories:

i) ***Relapse:*** patients who have previously been treated for TB, were declared cured or treatment completed at the end of their most recent course of treatment, and are now diagnosed with a recurrent episode of TB (either a true relapse or a new episode of TB caused by reinfection).

ii) ***Treatment after failure:*** patients have previously been treated for TB and their most recent course of treatment failed.

iii) ***Treatment after loss to follow-up:*** patients have previously been treated for TB and were declared 'lost to follow-up' at the end of their most recent course of treatment (this category corresponds to the 'defaulted' category.

iv) ***Other previously treated:*** patients are those who have previously been treated for TB but whose outcome after their most recent course of treatment is unknown or undocumented.

Similarly to one of the changes with the new definitions for treatment outcomes, the specific troublesome term of 'default' has been dropped completely.

Multi drug-resistant TB is defined as it was previously with no change, but a new category of drug-resistance has been necessarily introduced to accommodate the GeneXpert device:

A case of Rifampicin -resistant TB (RR-TB): A patient with TB that is resistant to Rifampicin detected using phenotypic or genotypic methods, with or without resistance to other anti-TB drugs. It includes any resistance to Rifampicin, whether mono drug-resistance, multi drug-resistance, poly drug-resistance or extensive drug-resistance.

This classification, of course, makes complete sense.

One last issue is worth identifying however. Given that these definitions are looking to better address the epidemic post-2015, it seems surprising that no further definition of drug-resistance beyond XDR-TB has been attempted, despite ones regularly being unofficially applied. Whilst rates of drug-susceptible TB will hopefully continue to reduce, the probability remains that levels of drug-resistant disease will continue to rise and become more extensive and more complex in the next decades, so this may prove to be a major oversight at an important strategic juncture. Rates of XDR-TB certainly appear to be currently rising faster than those of MDR-TB. Would it have been clinically expeditious to differentiate further at this stage? It could well be so. Would it be useful from a public health perspective? Almost certainly it would be.

Again we are left with having to wait and see what happens, and the next moment at which we will be able to review these definitions will be when the post-2015 global strategy begins to be implemented and reported upon.[211]

[211] See the later discussion on the post-2015 strategy for 2015-2035. As far as information on this is so far available, the comments above still stand.

Pharma, Neglected Disease and Orphan Drugs

"I KNOW OF NO WONDER-CURE FOR TB THAT HAS RECENTLY BEEN LAUNCHED – OR IS ABOUT TO BE...
BUT I CAN TELL YOU THIS. AS MY JOURNEY THROUGH THE PHARMACEUTICAL JUNGLE PROGRESSED, I CAME TO REALISE THAT, BY COMPARISON WITH THE REALITY, MY STORY WAS AS TAME AS A HOLIDAY POSTCARD."

John le Carré (2001) [212]

There is a curious term that is used in the pharmaceutical world. It is that of the 'orphan drug'. Orphan drugs are ones for rare diseases which would not be considered worthy of investment by drug companies because they hold out so little prospect for profitability. Such profitability is viewed (under the regrettably termed US 'Orphan Drug Act'[213]) in terms of the drugs' marketability in the American domestic market and the wider developed world where people who might be able to most afford them live. The developing world is viewed as being a poor marketplace in which to tout modern drugs. As a result of the Act, in both the US and EU (where similar legislation was introduced in 2000) it is much easier and cheaper to gain marketing approval for an orphan drug because smaller scale clinical trials are generally required – but there may be other financial incentives as well, all intended to encourage the development of drugs which might otherwise lack a sufficient profit motive. The assignment of orphan status to a specific disease has certainly resulted in medical breakthroughs that may not have otherwise been achieved due to the modern economic realities of drug research and development, but the picture is still far from being

[212] The Constant Gardener – "Author's Notes". The plot of the book hung around a fictitious new drug cure for TB which le Carré called Dyspraxia.

[213] The US Orphan Drug Act (ODA) of January 1983 is meant to encourage pharmaceutical companies to develop drugs for diseases that have a small marketplace. Under this law, companies that develop such a drug (i.e. a drug for a disorder affecting fewer than 20,000 people in the United States) may sell it without competition for seven years after FDA approval, and may also receive clinical trial tax incentives. It also allows some pharmaceutical companies to make a proportionately larger profit off drugs that have a small market but still sell for a high price.

completely as intended. Only 14 new drugs were approved in the first five years of the EU's legislation, and none is relevant to TB or similar neglected diseases.

The assignment of orphan status to drug-resistant tuberculosis, for instance, offers us perhaps yet another perplexing paradox to this disease. Tuberculosis is the second most common cause of adult deaths worldwide and the disease is officially responsible for 3,800 deaths per day worldwide, but almost certainly more. The number of these that are MDR can hardly be insignificant. In the United States, however, TB is an orphan disease, with approximately 100 to 130 MDR-TB patients annually. As bizarre as this may seem, reducing TB to such orphan status probably offers the greatest possibility of new drugs being developed. The thousand dollar question, however, concerns not how many new drugs might be developed, but how they may be put to use once they have been developed and approved.

Sleeping Sickness (or trypanosomiasis) is a diminutive problem in comparison to the scale of devastation caused by TB with perhaps six million people living in regions which put them in constant risk of the disease, but the story of one particular drug which treats it typifies the problem of actual implementation of orphan drugs. It provides what amounts to an imperfect example, however, because the manufacture of this particular drug that could effectively treat this relatively rare disease was actually ***terminated*** because of commercial considerations.

In 1975, the drug company Merrell Dow synthesized a compound which was found to kill cells apparently without causing major side effects. It called its new drug eflornithine. Initially it was envisaged that it might be a safe new treatment for cancer (a highly profitable potential market), but unfortunately this failed to be the case, and the drug was shelved.

In 1980, however, a parasite biologist unexpectedly found it to be an effective, nontoxic cure for trypanosomiasis with the worst reported side effects being some hair loss and mild anemia. Merrell Dow donated small amounts of eflornithine to clinics in Africa for further testing, and the compound's effectiveness proved to be so remarkable that it was quickly dubbed the "resurrection drug" because of the way it reversed the effects of the disease. Despite this revelation, eflornithine was neither further developed nor was it marketed as a drug for the treatment of sleeping sickness simply because no profit could be seen to be made from something that would be effective only for people who would be unable to afford it. All further development of the drug was thus ditched.

Eflornithine effectively still qualified for orphan drug status, so exactly what had happened?

In the 1990s, the only treatment which MSF had to offer their patients who were suffering from sleeping sickness was Melarsoprol, a drug based on arsenic – at best it was incredibly painful, at worst fatal. It was so caustic that it was reported even to corrode the plastic syringes used for injecting the drug into the veins of patients. It failed patients 50% of the time and was reported to kill one in 20 of those who were treated by it. There was no doubt that a better drug was needed.

The sorry tale of eflornithine took an unexpected twist in 2000 (17 years after the Orphan Drug Act had been passed) when two other companies reconsidered and reviewed the drug's reported side effect of mild hair loss and restarted production of the compound, now marketing it as a potentially profitable treatment for unwanted facial hair in women in the US. It was finally only then, ***27 years*** after the drug was initially developed, that the World Health Organization and Médecins Sans Frontières managed to persuade these same companies to donate eflornithine to help save the lives of thousands of sleeping sickness patients in Africa. Clearly the fundamental idea behind the Act had failed to work in this case: it was only after the drug was being profitably sold in the USA that it became beneficial to those people who could be saved by it.

A second story, and one which affected a much larger number of people, relates to the research and reluctant development of Artemisininin. This drug was first being identified outside China in 1979 as being a viable treatment for malaria. More than a decade earlier in 1967 Chinese researchers had been examining their traditional literature, and had identified that *Qinghao, Artemisia annua*, or Sweet Wormwood had been being used as a tea to reduce malaria symptoms right into the modern era. Its chemical derivative, Artemisinin was then found by the same Chinese researchers to be even more powerful in its effects.

In 1979, Dr Keith Arnold, a malaria researcher based in Hong Kong, heard about the drug. He wangled his way into the PRC to attempt to investigate whether mefloquine, the drug which he had helped develop with the US army and which had been used in Vietnam, could outperform the artemisinin variants which he had learnt were being developed within China. His efforts on behalf of mefloquine failed, with artemisininin proving far more effective in all of the laboratory tests, but the Chinese remained coy about revealing any more about their drug with Arnold remaining uncertain even as to exactly what plant the drug had been derived from.

By 1982, however, not only had Sweet Wormwood been positively identified as the principal component for the drug's synthesis but it had been found to be an endemic plant in the US, even growing on the banks of the Potomac in Washington DC. But, in spite of this discovery, yet another sorry story proceeded to unfold – with a desperately needed drug ending up languishing on shelves because of conscious institutional neglect. The WHO failed to endorse the drug until 2000, and even then it remained generally unavailable until 2006. Once again, a full 27 year period went by – between Arnold's first encounter with it and its full availability.

The reasons for this delay may well have been complex, but they can hardly be excused. With nearly a million children a year being estimated to have been dying from malaria in Africa, Arnold himself branded the delay (whether caused by overcaution, negligent indecision or simple incompetence) "genocidal". Given both the dreadful statistics (with perhaps as many as 25 million children dying in the hiatus period) and the fact that the drug has since been hailed as having been the most important development in the treatment of malaria since the introduction of quinine, his anger was understandable.

In 2000 the Global Forum for Health Research released a landmark report estimating that less than 10 per cent of global spending on health research is devoted to diseases of conditions that account for 90 per cent of the global disease burden. Ten years later, two doctors from Médecins Sans Frontières starkly summed up the general situation concerning the lack of development of drugs which might help those most at risk of particular tropical diseases, ones which were clearly 'orphan' according to the definitions of the Act:

> "Research and development into tropical diseases have come to a virtual standstill due to low profits. Of 1,223 drugs globally licensed between 1975 and 1997, only 13 were for treatment of tropical diseases. Two of these were an outcome of military research (halofantrine, mefloquine), six resulted from veterinary research (albendazole, benznidazole, ivermectin, oxamniquine, praziquantel and nifurtimox) and two were merely modifications of existing drugs (pentamidine and amphotericin B). Thus, over more than 20 years only three drugs were developed specifically for the tropics (artemether, atovaquone and eflornithine). Artemether[214] was a

[214] Artemether is a variant of artemisinin.

> Chinese Academy discovery; the development of atovaquone for malaria would have been endangered had it not turned out that it is effective against AIDS-related opportunistic infections; and eflornithine is no longer produced. Apparently it is more profitable to develop and market Viagra than to research a new drug to treat patients with visceral leishmaniasis, a fatal disease if left untreated. Such a drug is more likely to be developed through veterinary research if it has economic potential on the pet market."

Dr Unni Karunakara, MSF's International President, elsewhere identified that these same diseases account for 11.4% of the global burden of disease burden. It amounted to an uncompromising and deliberate exposure by an NGO of un-ethical practice closeted away within the otherwise apparently ethical framework of pharmaceutical research and development.

When it comes to marketing its drugs, unfortunately the same story runs on. The pharmaceutical industry spends more on advertising its products in the United States than it does on its own research and development of new medicine – the annual cost of which is itself outstripped by the sum of its net profits.[215] Such R&D as does exist is so manifestly focused on diseases affecting the wealthier countries that it is frightening to wonder how the future historians of humanitarian medicine may view our era since this dearth of research so negatively affects such a large part of mankind.

Some researchers in 2002 were suggesting that the pharmaceutical industry was the most profitable industry of any – more than oil, mining, armaments, even more at the time than banking. It was then returning 16% profit. Despite a widely reported 'crisis' in the pharmaceutical industry since, this figure actually rose to 19.3% by 2010 with the industry still ranked as the third most profitable of all. There has been plenty of opportunities to have ploughed more of these profits back into research for much needed new drugs.

Unfortunately, it is not just in the field of tropical disease that progress in research and development has been so sluggish: it has equally occurred in the field of general antibiotic research, and it is in this particular field as well that the problems concerning new drugs for TB are also evident.

Similarly to the stories of eflornithine and artemisinin, until recently there has been literally no investment into any development of new drugs to treat

---

[215] Pollock R & O'Rourke L - "Off the charts: pay, profits and spending by drug companies", Washington DC: Familes USA (2001).

TB. This was not because there was no recognisable need for them (because there most certainly was), but it was simply because there was no perceived market place from which such investment could be profitably recouped (Orphan Drug Act or no Orphan Drug Act). Some existing antibiotic drugs have only reluctantly been looked at for TB quite recently. This was because the companies with the patent rights to them were fearful that their existing profitability for use on other diseases would be decimated at a stroke if they were given any sort of indication for TB. Astonishingly, the last new drug developed and fully approved for TB is now 50 years old, whilst the vaccine is nearly twice this age. Meanwhile the threat from TB had never gone away. For most of this last 50 years, in fact, TB has remained the most lethal infectious disease wreaking the highest number of fatalities on humanity, but most particularly so by stalking the poor.

So given the persistent prevalence of tuberculosis throughout the 20th century, it is almost inconceivable that the disease could have ever been included within any possible category of 'neglected disease'. It has been, however, and furthermore it is often referred to as such.

Between 1945 and 1968, drug companies invented 13 new categories of antibiotics. Between 1968 and today, just two new categories of antibiotics have appeared. Brad Spellberg, the head of the Microbial Resistance Task Force for the Infectious Diseases Society of America has put on record:

> "What kept us out of trouble for the last 60 years is that every time drug-resistance caught up to us, the pharmaceutical companies would go back to the drawing board and develop the next generation of drugs to keep us ahead of the game. That's the part of the equation that's changed. Drug companies are no longer trying to get one step ahead."

Three reasons are regularly trotted out as to why pharmaceutical companies have been so reluctant to commit to antibiotic research despite at least two decades of screaming alarms being made by the public health community.

The first is that the industry thinks that there is just not enough money in it for them. The argument offered is that, while a new antibiotic may bring in a billion dollars of profit over its lifetime, a new drug for heart disease or cancer might net as much as ten billion. Anti-depressive, anti-hypertensive or erectile dysfunction drugs – which are typically, unlike antibiotics, taken daily for years or even lifetimes – are also similarly seen to be far more profitable than new antibiotics.

The second is that inventing and developing new antibiotics has become technically increasingly challenging, especially for antibiotics that are effective against either gram-negative or acid-fast bacteria, the ones with impermeability built into their cell walls. There are also challenging trial requirements for new antibiotics which are both more extensive and expensive than with many other new drugs. Separate trials, for instance, are normally required for an antibiotic for each potentially instance of treatable infection (i.e. for urine, skin or lungs etc.). In contrast, a heart drug needs to be tested for just one indication in just one location.

The third is that, following deaths linked to the recently approved new drug Ketek in 2006, the Federal Drug Administration has become much more reluctant to approve new antibiotics than it has been to approve other drugs. "They've basically made it impossible for companies to develop and market antibiotics in the US," bemoans David Shlaes, the author of "Antibiotics: the Perfect Storm".

As a result, only four of the world's 12 largest pharmaceutical companies are currently researching new antibiotics at all. In 2012, Pfizer, the world's biggest drug company, was reported to have closed its Connecticut antibiotics research centre completely, laying off its 1,200 strong worksforce.

Rather perversely, this situation has been described as being nothing more than a 'market failure', with the blame for the situation being laid on society and not on the biomedical industry itself, since it is suggested that society would benefit most from a steady pipeline of new effective antibiotics.[216] Society, in other words, gets the blame whilst governments, institutions, and the pharmaceutical industry all seem to somehow get let off the hook.

One of the most extraordinary aspects of almost all such discussions on this lack of new antibiotics, however, is that global tuberculosis almost never seems to get any mention at all. Here is one typical example. It is from the Infectious Diseases Society of America (IDSA):

> "The antibiotic pipeline problem may change the practice of medicine as we know it. Advanced interventions currently taken for granted – for example, surgery, cancer treatment, transplantation, and care of premature babies – could become impossible as

[216] https://www.gov.uk/government/publications/chief-medical-officer-annual-report-volume-2

> antibiotic options become fewer. Resistance to the current library of antibacterial drugs is a serious problem in all parts of the world including the Asia-Pacific region, Latin America, Europe, and North America. Accordingly, the regulatory, financial, and scientific challenges/impediments to antibacterial drug development are a global problem."

In March 2013, Dame Sally Davies, the UK's Chief Medical Officer, made a premeditated and concerted media attempt to alert G8 leaders to the problem before they gathered together for their conference in the UK that June. She emotively described the increasing resistance of gram-negative bacteria to existing drugs as being a "ticking time bomb", equivalent in scale of threat to that posed by global terrorism – but yet again no mention was made of global TB. In a separate press release she said:

> "We haven't as a society globally incentivised making antibiotics. It's quite simple – if they make something to treat high blood pressure or diabetes and it works, we will use it on our patients every day. Whereas antibiotics will only be used for a week or two when they're needed, and then they have a limited life span because of resistance developing anyway.
>
> "Antimicrobial resistance poses a catastrophic threat. If we don't act now, any one of us could go into hospital in 20 years for minor surgery and die because of an ordinary infection that can't be treated by antibiotics.

So where is the mention of global tuberculosis today, when at least 1.3 million are dying each year, and when the drug-resistant threat is already current and rapidly growing out of control? Is it also worth noting that, if none of the existing second line drugs are available in environments where DR-TB exists, then patients infected there by drug-resistant disease are effectively already living in the 19th Century environment which she frequently refers to in her announcements in relation to this issue.

The solution she suggests is one of 'incentivising' antibiotic research, although there is little public elaboration about this. Does this mean public subsidy of one of the most profitable industries of our era? Or does it mean lowering the goal posts of approval, or just sharing public liability with the pharmaceutical sector if things go wrong?

Exactly what might interest these huge multi-national companies to gear up their research into new antibiotics? It will certainly have to be substantial. It turns out that there are four categories of incentives which are being proposed to foster antibiotic R&D. They are termed 'push', 'pull', 'lego-regulatory' and 'hybrid push-pull'.[217, 218]

"Push" incentives intend to reduce the marginal cost of R&D. They would comprise public funding and tax incentives which would both have to be funded by the tax payer.

"Pull" incentives would foster R&D via financial rewards, which might include monetary prizes for delivering specific results, advance market commitments and/or offering patent buyouts, again funded by the public purse.

"Lego-regulatory" incentives are also sometimes more clumsily referred to as 'outcome-based market determined rewards'. They can include adjusting prices and re-imbursements, extending patent periods or even expediting regulatory reviews. Examples of this already exist, including the US 'Generating Antibiotic Incentives Now' (GAIN) Act and the US 'Limited Population Antibacterial Drug' (LPAD) Approval Mechanism, whereby a limited licence can be granted based on safety and effectiveness data from smaller-than-usual clinical trials.

Finally, "hybrid push-pull" incentives include product development partnerships with public bodies.

In short, there appear to be some innovative ideas which are already quite well-developed which intend to align the interests of both researchers and producers with the risks of the various different stakeholders. The challenge that is being confronted is to appropriately balance these approaches by ensuring that what is done is not just cost-effective and attractive to the developers but is also broadly available to all, sustainable and safe.[219]

---

[217] Mossialos E et al. - "Policies and incentives for promoting innovation in antibiotic research", London: London School of Economics and Political Science (2009).
www.euro.who.int/__data/assets/pdf_file/0011/120143/E94241.pdf

[218] Towse A and Sharma P - "Incentives for R&D for new antimicrobial drugs", International Journal of the Economics of Business, 18; 2 (2011) 331–50.

[219] https://www.gov.uk/government/publications/chief-medical-officer-annual-report-volume-2.

Paul Stoffels, the chairman of Janssen, the Belgian pharmaceutical company which developed Bedaquiline (the recently developed new last-resort TB drug which we will shortly be discussing more fully), suggests a further idea of 'incentivising-with-trade-offs' – with tax reductions and a 'priority review voucher' systems which might allow the regulators to fast-track any parallel scrutiny of other drugs which might be being developed by the same company as a 'reward'. The problem then may be establishing exactly who is liable if such fast tracking proves to create subsequent safety problems.

The suggestion is that research into new antibiotics should, at least partly, be publicly funded may well seem a reasonable solution but, given the larger picture, it rings shamefully hollow. The story is being spun that major blockbuster drugs (like the anti-cholesterol statin drug Lipitor which is manufactured by Pfizer) are now coming out of patent, and that it has been these drugs that have been keeping the pharmaceutical sector financially so healthy for the last decades. With so little new in the pipeline, profitability is stagnating, and so the sector now has no choice but to lobby for public assistance.

The online journal Knowledge@Wharton (from the University of Pennsylvania's Wharton School of Business) released a special report in 2011 entitled "In Search of Faster Cures" suggesting that:

> "No fewer than nine of the industry's ten biggest blockbusters will go off-patent and face low-cost generic competition within five years ... There is little in the pipeline to replace these top sellers. The number of new drugs has been steadily falling despite rising public and private spending for research and development."

Somehow not everything adds up. Paradoxically, in the very decades when the sector was most profitable it seems to have been least focused on forward-looking antibiotic research and remained most intent on rewarding its shareholders with the profits from its block-buster drugs. In fact, given its focus on drugs for longer-term treatment rather than on desperately needed short-term ones, the industry itself has come to resemble the corner drug-pusher. It only wants to get his vulnerable potential customers dependent on its long-term pharmaceuticals.

What is equally concerning is that the public purse may end up paying twice over for the benefit of the drug – once by subsidizing its development and a second time for its purchase. Furthermore tax incentives in the UK have not been seen to have been in any way successful. Under current UK tax law, 175% of qualifying expenditure on R&D activities is deducted for small and medium size enterprises when calculating profit for tax purposes, and 130% is allowed for large companies. The criteria for qualifying for these tax credits remain relatively loose with companies simply being required to be seen to be attempting to "advance science and technology".

Meanwhile the cost of the scheme has spiralled from just £89 million pounds in 2001 to £1.1 billion pounds in 2011 with the majority of this money going to large companies – and yet in spite of all this extra resource, the number of innovative medicines coming to the market has been.

Even the argument that short-term drugs are *de facto* unprofitable rings hollow given that the industry has the habit of dictating the prices of its products directly as a result of patenting them – and even of hiking them when it suits. How could a new antibiotic possibly be so unprofitable, given the probable immediate global demand for it?

In an interview in 2011, Mario Raviglione, the head of the Global TB Programme at the WHO, attempted to explain the problem relating not just to the lack of interest in developing new drugs, but even in the manufacture of existing ones. He was explaining in the interview that, even if all MDR-TB cases had been identified that year, there would have been nowhere near enough drugs available for them all to be treated. He said:

> "I think we have not yet succeeded in convincing manufacturers to produce them in sufficiently large quantity. This is a vicious cycle, as the manufacturers' response is that today there is no market, in view of the insufficient detection of MDR-TB cases. Thus, we truly need to diagnose more patients, create the market, and insist on the increased production of quality drugs."

There are key issues here that need identifying. The profitability of the sector seems to have come to a halt; and the number of manufacturers engaged in second line drugs has been falling in spite of the increases in spending on the part of both public and private sectors. A market does most definitely exist, meanwhile, whatever the manufacturers may claim, and the industry appears to be playing a close game of poker with the appropriate authorities in order to try to maintain its percentage profitability.

There can only be one real reason why companies do not want to manufacture second line drugs when no-one can deny that there will be an ongoing demand for them for the foreseeable future: such profits that might be expected are simply not seen by these companies to be enough to satisfy their dividend-expectant share-holders.

In his keynote address made while accepting the William Fulbright Prize for International Understanding on behalf of MSF, Dr Unni Karunakara, its International President spoke out on this topic:

> "The lack of safe and effective medicines for these neglected diseases is completely unacceptable. Resorting to drugs or diagnostic tools that have not evolved in half a century is nothing less than denying that millions are affected.
>
> "Why don't we have better tools available to combat neglected diseases? It is precisely because they are poor that the patients who are affected by these diseases are neglected … It does not have to be this way."

The WHO and the WTO

"FROM SNAIL TO ... SOMETHING FASTER THAN A SNAIL."

Shawn Harmon (2009)[220]

Do we all have any sort of real right to health? Well, of course, technically we can't do since some of us are born healthier than others, but might we under current understandings of human rights nevertheless expect equal rights to decent health care? The answer to this second question – at least from a moral perspective – must be "yes."[221]

What is immediately obvious, is that an uncomfortably large proportion of humanity comprehensively lacks access to such care, and that inadequate efforts have been made so far to resolve this inequality. These same people also happen to be the host who is most afflicted with tuberculosis today because TB and deficiencies in health care walk hand in hand. The fact that there is so much less TB in the industrialised nations is exactly because of their more sophisticated medical resources and their fundamentally healthier and better nourished populations. It is also why these parts of the world have so much less cause to fear DR-TB than those parts of the world which already suffers from the disease.

So if people everywhere do have a right to decent health care, whose duty should it be to confer it on them?

---

[220] Shawn HE Harmon - "International Public Health Law: Not so much WHO as why, and not enough WHO and why not?", Medicine Health Care & Philosophy, 12;3 (2009) 245-55.

[221] There is a wealth of international covenants that can be used to support this claim: the Universal Declaration of Human Rights (1948), European Convention for the Protection of Human Rights and Fundamental Freedoms (1950), the International Covenant on Economic, Social & Cultural Rights (1966) the Declaration of Alma-Ata on Primary Health Care (1978), the Ottawa Charter for Health Promotion (1986), UN Convention on the Rights of the Child (1989), UN's Agenda 21 (1993), the Rio Declaration (1992), the Jakarta Declaration on Leading Health Promotion into the 21st Century (1997), UNESCO's Universal Declaration on the Human Genome and Human Rights (1997), and the Council of Europe's Convention on Human Rights and Biomedicine (1997).

Well, at least at first base, it must be down to the nation state, based on its particular citizen-state contract. In fact, if any state has signed up to the basic fundamental idea of human rights then it must be down to the state itself to act as the primary provider of health care and it should be doing all in its power to provide it. The fact is, however, that such provision remains beyond the means and capabilities of most low-income countries without additional help and even of some middle-income ones as well. In these instances the responsibilities default to a wider constitution, one which has to include those wealthier nations who remain so little troubled today by infectious disease.

Dr L.O. Gostin has published strong views on the wider subject:[222]

> "There is a growing recognition that wealthy nations have roles and responsibilities in raising the health status of poor nations."

Elsewhere he explains the importance of such an idea in the context of a fairer world:

> "Health, among all the other forms of disadvantage, is special and foundational, in that its effects on human capacities impact one's opportunities in the world and, therefore, health must be preserved to ensure equality of opportunity."[223]

Such an idea is difficult to dispute, at least if we seriously want disadvantaged countries to develop. Health has been described by Amartya Sen, the Nobel Prize winning economist, as being a "fundamental freedom" which enables us to define our identity and do the things we value.[224] But it is also more even than this. The WHO's own constitution (in its Preamble) describes health as being a right which is "fundamental to the attainment of peace and security". We can certainly see these ideas tragically illustrated in a negative sense in the case of Swaziland where widespread ill-health arising from TB and HIV/AIDS is creating not just human tragedy, but also national non-viability.

---

[222] Gostin LO - "Meeting the survival needs of the world's least healthy people. A proposed model for global health governance", Journal of the American Medical Association (2007) 225-8.

[223] Ibid.

[224] Amartya Sen - "Development as Freedom", Oxford: OUP (1999)

But Gostin then puts his finger on the major stumbling block:

> "States that have the wherewithal are deeply resistant to expending the political capital and economic resources necessary to truly make a difference to improve health outside their borders."

So it becomes the responsibility of someone or something else to orchestrate this activity – and, in the case of global health this job has so far been entrusted to the WHO whose guiding imperatives include promoting development, fostering health security, strengthening health systems, harnessing research, information and evidence, enhancing partnerships, and improving performances in health care.

Article 1 of the WHO's constitution unequivocally states that the objective given to it by its member states includes the attainment by all peoples of the highest possible level of health. Article 20 adds that it can even direct its members to "take action" relative to the acceptance of any convention adopted by the World Health Assembly, and then to notify the Director General of the action taken or the reasons for their non-acceptance. In the case of DR-TB, this call to action was made in Beijing in 2009 and it related to "universal access" of treatment, not that much appears to have been able to have been done internationally to enforce the idea. So while the WHO has definitely been granted extensive law-making or normative powers it remains visibly reluctant to use them, even in the face of a global crisis with millions at risk.[225]

So exactly what has the WHO done to date with the powers it has been given? In a penetrative essay, Shawn Harmon has suggested that it amounts "to put it bluntly, [to] very little", and he puts this down to its institutional culture, its self-image as being more of a scientific and technical agency, along with the weakness of international law in general. He was not talking specifically about tuberculosis in his essay, but it does seem that it is in relation to TB that the capacities of the WHO to enforce change do seem to be the most challenged.

What is of real concern is that there appear to be some morally unhealthy reasons for this inertia. With both SARS and the H1N1 'flu virus the WHO could be seen to be able to mobilise itself both rapidly and at great expense. We have already compared the differences in death toll between these two

---

[225] The word "normative" is used here and in the following discussion in the sense of enabling things to be done according to standards that can make the world essentially a better place.

pandemics and TB, with TB standing infinitely taller in terms of deaths in comparison with either, but there may be a further anomaly at work here as well. In a 'worst case' future 'flu pandemic it has been predicted that 50% of the whole world's population might be affected by it – a percentage which is assumed to include everyone, not just the world's poor or the more normally sick. We should take note that this still only relates to a percentage of the world's population being 'affected' – not being killed or maimed by the disease. But isn't 32% of the world's population already chronically being 'affected' by TB in exactly such terms? Or 40% of the population of India, or 80% of Africans? Do such numbers not add up to a compelling case for a similar mobilisation of resources as was used for SARS and H1N1? Well of course it should do, particularly if the WHO was to match up to its own articles.

Harmon also identified exactly how the WHO has so far advanced international health law under its designated powers – identifying only four instances so far in its 57-year history.

The first was the Codex Alimentarius of 1963. Broadly speaking, the Codex established food standards and guidelines with the aim of both protecting the health of consumers and promoting fair trade practices in food.

The second was the International Classification of Diseases (ICD-10) of 1990, which we have already encountered in reviewing the way that deaths from TB are being omitted from global targets when they occur in people who are known to be HIV-positive. Generally, the ICD-10 provides standard diagnostic classifications which facilitate international comparisons of morbidity and mortality data. In the case of tuberculosis, however, it hardly seems to have been helping the cause of properly monitoring the disease, and could even be argued to be working against the WHO's own aims of TB eradication because of the way its implementation has confused the figures.

The third was the International Health Regulations (IHR) of 2005. Its origins can be traced back to a series of European-based sanitary conferences which were held back in the 19th century1800s directed at preventing the importation of cholera, plague and yellow fever into Europe. The WHO's IHR represents an attempt to harmonise conduct and response more globally, however, both preventing the outbreak and spread of disease and prompting its containment. The Regulations' intentions are to facilitate a co-ordinated global public health response to an international spread of disease, but they are qualified as being ones which simultaneously should "avoid unnecessary interference with international traffic and trade whilst conforming to individual dignity, human rights and fundamental freedoms, and the UN Charter". This, as we will see, is a revealing rider, but nevertheless the WHO has thus generally adopted all the powers it needs to properly respond to a public health emergency. Gostin has gone so far as to suggest that the IHR has been the high-water mark so far for the WHO regarding its designating itself with any normative powers.

The fourth was the Framework Convention on Tobacco Control (FCTC) of 2005. The FCTC did represent the first WHO-initiated normative instrument and was interesting in that it had direct impact on a previously lawful activity which itself was a part of that "international traffic and trade". As such, it appears to be a promising example of the WHO flexing its muscles. Harmon, however, suggests that it was only made possible "by the reputational nadir plumbed by the tobacco industry as a result of its persistent denials of the harms of smoking, its deceptive advertising, and its engineering of its products to be highly addictive".

So we have four instances, with only one having any major impact on what might be considered a part of the international *status quo.*

That third instance, the International Health Regulations of 2005, bears some further consideration, not only because they relate directly to the business of TB management, but also because they relate to the issue of access by the poor to decent health care. Perhaps this single factor of not interfering with "international traffic and trade" might help explain how sluggish the WHO's response has been to its own unprecented self-proclaimed global emergency in 1993. Gostin has stated that the WHO has been "historically, politically and structurally inadequate to do what is needed", while Harmon adds that it has also been hampered by being fragmented, unco-ordinated, unplanned and inconsistent in its actions. There is a saying in some NGO circles that the UN "knows everything but does nothing". If we consider the story of the Green Light Committee as reviewed in an earlier section it would be hard to disagree with this analysis. But is it this conflict of interest between the WHO's activities and international trade - and particularly with the parallel activities of the World Trade Organisation (the WTO) - that has been the biggest bugbear of all?

The WTO deals with the regulation of trade between participating countries; it provides a framework for negotiating and formalizing trade agreements, and offers a dispute resolution process to help enforce participants' adherence to WTO agreements.

In both its current and earlier incarnations it has facilitated a proliferation of trade agreements which have all been intended to increase economic, political and social interdependence by promoting the movement of capital and traded goods. This process of globalisation, however, implies other integrations at the same time, ones which sometimes conflict with the interests of the traders themselves. They inevitably include, for instance, the mobilisation, merging or diffusing of peoples, along with a necessary universal acceptance of concepts, ideas and values across national boundaries. Globalised free trade should not be allowed to develop properly, however, if it does not also come accompanied by decent ethical and moral standards – and these should definitely include ones which impact positively on public health. Although some of the WTO agreements have included provisions intended to help protect life and health, they have been observed in the longer run to have generally tended to force such standards down around the world rather than raise them up as they should have done. This is simply because such uniform high standards are seen to be simultaneously so restrictive to trade. In other words, to put it in a nutshell, the interests of trade tend to trump interests of public health.

Harmon has queried whether international public health should be managed in such a trade-dominated manner. He has even suggested that it amounts to "pure folly" to leave public health direction to the sorts of interests that also direct both the WTO and the world's economic status quo.[11] He developed his argument by suggesting that relying on market-driven economic policies and/or the organisations that are driven by them is unlikely to achieve any of the sorts of social goals which include public health. As such he sees the whole venture ending up being founded on fundamentally unresolvable tensions which are unlikely to be of benefit to the poor as they should be.

A current impasse within the WTO itself usefully illustrates how such tensions play out. This relates to the so-called 'Doha Round' which was initially launched in 2001, and which remains unresolved 12 years later. It was originally intended to make globalization more inclusive and help the world's poor by slashing the barriers and subsidies in farming being used by richer countries to protect their own interests, but it remains a sorry story of unresolved self-interest on the part of the wealthier nations. The US first blamed the impasse on Brazil and India for being "inflexible", then it blamed the EU for impeding agricultural imports. Brazil's response argued that progress could only logically be achieved if the richest countries (especially the US and countries within the EU) made deeper cuts in their national agricultural subsidies than they were prepared to make and so further opened their markets for agricultural goods. The impasse is still maintained only because the few with the most power to make the necessary changes that could be of benefit to the many are continuing to choose to wield their power to protect their own interests.

Within this sphere of globalised trade and self-interest is the pharmaceutical industry, with its own history of self-interest, part of which relates to its hanging on to its intellectual property rights (IPR), particularly those relating to patents for its drugs.

In 1995 the WTO formally adopted an agreement known as the "Trade-Related Aspects of Intellectual Property Rights" (TRIPS). TRIPS required that all signatories to ensure minimum standards of IPR protection. These were standards that were much more stringent than those that previously existed in poorer countries. Prior to the TRIPS agreement, the Indian government did not award product patents for pharmaceutical inventions, for instance, which meant that Indian pharmaceutical manufacturers could freely produce medicines created by foreign companies at a fraction of their normal cost. The Indian government had, however, awarded process patents – protecting ***how*** a product is created, though not the product itself, intending to give Indian manufacturers incentives to find their own cheaper ways to manufacture otherwise expensive and unaffordable products.

These laws had made India what was described as the 'pharmacy of the developing world'. They generated an industry which, despite what then happened with TRIPS, is still the second leading provider of medicines distributed by UNICEF in the developing world.

In January 2005, however, India had to become compliant with the TRIPS agreement, having to abide by the WTO's "minimum standards for intellectual property protection" which mandated the awarding of patents for pharmaceutical product (not processes) for a period of twenty years.

Treatments that were developed before 2004 could still be manufactured generically, but from 2005 onwards any new drugs would be globally protected by patent for 20 years. Countries which had been previously buying new drugs from generic Indian manufacturers now had no other option but to have to buy all new drugs at brand price, often at significantly greater cost, or not to purchase them at all.

Anand Grover, an Indian activist lawyer who is also the UN Special Rapporteur in the United Nations Human Rights Council on the "Right of Everyone to the Enjoyment of the Highest Attainable Standard of Physical and Mental Health", has stated:

> "TRIPS and FTAs [Free Trade Agreements] have had an adverse impact on prices and availability of medicines, making it difficult for countries to comply with their obligations to respect, protect, and fulfil the right to health."

It may even be worse than that. They seem to have given all of the deciding power on the matter to the wealthier nations. Patents have a long and illustrious history going right back to Europe's middle-ages. A 1474 Venetian law granted the patent-holder the sort of monopoly rights that all today's developers of new drugs defend fiercely. The principal deterrent was a steep fine. The canny Venetians incorporated an important clause within its law that still lies at the heart of modern-day patent law in the form of what is today called a 'compulsory license':

> "But our government will be free, at its complete discretion, to take and use for its needs any of the said contrivances and instruments."

Such a compulsory license allows the issuing government itself to break the patent if they see fit – in the case of the Venetian Republic this was in order to maintain its regional supremacy and its technological and trading dominance. It certainly wasn't conceived at all as a way of protecting the public good, but the mechanism for this to happen is there in the legislation. Such legal mechanisms have been used frequently since, having been used consistently over hundreds of years, right up to the present day. Between 1969 and 1992, for instance, the Canadian government issued 613 compulsory licenses to keep the cost of medicines down in the country, so it can be done. In 2001 the US government even threatened to issue a compulsory license against Bayer in order to assist in stockpiling anti-anthrax medication in the face of a terror scare.

It seems that the citizens of the whole developing world hold less sway in terms of their rights to affordable medicine than citizens in North America.

Recently, the South African government has been making its own attempts at weakening such industrial protections of drug patents for the benefit of its people. In September 2013 it published the draft of a novel policy on intellectual property (IP) rights in the country – one which included intentions to weaken patents over life-saving drugs. The industry itself responded almost immediately by launching its own campaign which is currently still trying to create even tighter protection of its patent interests.

South Africa's draft document (to the delight of organisations like Médecins Sans Frontières) revealed an instinctive suspicion not just of multi-national companies but also of the multilateral bodies which operate sympathetically with them. It even endorsed a general principle of only seeking advice from NGOs rather than accepting any from developed countries as would more normally be expected. This idea was explained as being because such advice would be expected to be unduly influenced by such countries' own controlling commercial interests. Furthermore, the document urged South African policymakers to put the interests of consumers first rather than continuing to kowtow to those of the intellectual property "producers".

The document's intentions surely align with the general aims of the WHO, at least if they are unhitched from those of global trade. The response of those multi-national drug companies with local operations and interests in South Africa, however, was instinctive. It revealed a reactionary campaign intended to force the country's government into a complete reversal of direction.

The industry's first visible response may have appeared innocuous enough – it was entitled the 'Campaign to Prevent Damage to Innovation from the Proposed Draft National IP Policy in South Africa". It contained some curious initiatives. One of these was the setting up of a supposedly locally run "coalition" (with the equally innocuous name proposed to be "Forward South Africa"). This coalition, however, was really intending that its campaign be directed from outside the country, from Washington DC in fact, however, because the drug companies' umbrella body had already approached the Washington-based lobbying firm Public Affairs Engagement' to lead its campaign. This campaign was also intending to involve countries like Rwanda and Tanzania to convince South Africa that it could lose its leadership role on the continent if it should continue pushing ahead with its radical initiative. The net intention of the coalition, at least as far as South African Health Minister Aaron Motsoaledi was concerned, amounted to nothing more than putting corporate profits before health – not just in South Africa, but also all around the globe.[226] In

226 Different segments of the document spelt out these intentions: "Mobilise voices inside and outside South Africa to send the message that the proposed IP policy threatens continued investment and thus economic and social wellbeing";

other words it revealed exactly those tensions elsewhere identified by Shawn Harmon. Motsoaledi quickly became outspoken in his announcements on the matter, seeing it as an attack by the developed world on both low- and middle-income countries:

> "This is using South Africa as an entry point, but this is an attack on Brazil, an attack on India … an attack on China, Russia and the whole developing world."

When he first learnt of the coalition's plan Motsoaledi had been so incensed that he publicly claimed that it amounted to "genocide" and to a conspiracy of "satanic magnitude". "They are not hoping to influence government," he stated, "they are hoping to influence society to turn against government. If you read carefully what they are saying, they want to prove to patients that the lack of access to medicine has nothing to do with IP but everything to do with the incompetence of the government."

Perhaps Motsoaledi has become over sensitive himself as a result of the fact that the South African health service is still failing to get to grips with its drug-resistant epidemic, but if he has he isn't alone. MSF has also described the planned campaign as a "covert attempt by the multi-national pharmaceutical companies to spend extraordinary amounts of money to interfere in South Africa's legislative process". MSF, even with the support of the manufacturers of generic medicines, can certainly never match up to the financial resources of the pharmaceutical industry so it has little muscle that to usefully add to such arguments, but Motsoaledi himself has pledged to throw the weight of the whole South African government behind a counter-campaign of its own. "We will resort to public engagement," he said. "We will say in public: 'These are the conspirators.'"

But will the WHO consider joining them in the fight? It seems unlikely since it will mean going head to head with the WTO, despite the legal

---

"This mobilisation will occur through an energetic campaign, which will feel like a political campaign."; and the FSA should be led by "a visible South African, most likely a respected former government official, business leader or academic", but at the same time would be "directed by staff from Public Affairs Engagement and PAE's South African partner". PAE itself is headed by former US ambassador James Glassman, who held several high-ranking government positions before spending four years as the executive director of the George W Bush Institute. The "visible South African" set up to front the campaign was said to be the lobbyist Abdul Waheed Patel from a Cape Town political consulting firm opportunities afforded it to do so by those Venetians back in the fifteenth century. Article 15 of the International Covenant on Economic, Social and Cultural Rights does state that anyone has the right to profit from an inventions – but what if applying this right in the form of monopoly deprives others of their rights to decent health care? It is clear that any nation states' obligations to its citizens in respect of issues of public health and the well-being of its population ***must*** take precedence over any obligation to ensure the material interests resulting from scientific innovation by other parties. Such obligations should be fought for as ferociously as the pharmaceutical industry can be seen to continue to protect its own already privileged position.

In fact what real chance does the WHO have to change things in accordance with its mandate unless it takes better normative control not just of the field of public health, but also of the industry it depends upon?

The other players and the 'Grand Challenges'

One response to this apparent gridlock of disparate interests was the creation in 2003 of a multidisciplinary panel of experts from 13 countries, convened in order to articulate the so-called 'Grand Challenges' for modern public health research. It particularly looked towards helping to solve the key health problems in the developing world. As such, the 'Grand Challenges in Global Health' comprise a family of grant programmes which are largely funded by the Bill & Melinda Gates Foundation focusing on one unifying purpose – to overcome the persistent bottlenecks in the creation of new tools that might radically improve health in the developing world.

Many of the projects have featured the insights of leaders in their fields many of whom have ever before focused any real attentions on issues of global health. It is an exciting innovation.

The 'Grand Challenge for Infection' is an excellent example as an example, particularly as it included three specific aims, all of which (for once) can be seen to acutely relate to drug-resistant TB:

1. to discover drugs that minimise the occurrence of drug-resistant micro-organisms;
2. to create therapies that can cure latent infections;
3. to create immunological methods that can cure chronic infections.

These all look to be encouraging aspirations, but a critique of the fundamental idea behind the Grand Challenges was published in the Lancet in 2005. Anne-Emanuelle Birn, an associate professor of Public Health Sciences at the University of Toronto, has described the initiative's role as being "weak" if only because of its fundamental focus on the power of science to solve such problems whilst ignoring the simultaneous importance of allowing for the contribution of economic, social, and political factors both to the problems and their ultimate solutions.

Such a criticism certainly must also apply to much of the current global strategy to contain tuberculosis.

Professor Birn cited the developed world's continuing obsession with technological advancement as promoting the ducking of any consideration of the redistribution of resources within the impoverished communities most affected by the challenges themselves. She argued that, rather than putting most effort into trying to finance and develop new vaccines (and also, in the case of TB, new drugs), a more sustainable effort should be focusing first on engendering global public support for a universal, accessible public health system.

She specifically referenced Grand Challenge Number 4 to support her argument, one which relates to improving nutrition, and she explained how shortsighted it remains since it "overlooks key distributional questions". In her eyes these questions don't amount to being technical obstacles that can be solved by science or technological innovation, but remain straightforward political and economic ones. Avoiding confronting them, she argued, merely serves to perpetuate the problem rather than ever solve it. In her opinion, in other words, it is poor income distribution and market shifts which lead to populations being unable to afford food and become malnourished, and this is what lies at the heart of the problem. Many might consider that the same sort of ideas apply to the fight against TB.[227]

[227] Anne-Emanuelle Birn - "Gates's Grandest Challenge: Transcending Technology as Public Health Ideology", The Lancet (2005) 514–9.

The Doctor's Dilemma

"THERE ARE SO MANY FIRES BURNING ON OUR EARTH, HOW DO YOU DECIDE WHERE TO DIRECT THE LIMITED ENERGY AND RESOURCES?"

Dr Michael Iseman[228]

"The Doctor's Dilemma" is a play by George Bernard Shaw and was first performed in 1906. The eponymous dilemma of the play involves a fictitious British doctor, Sir Colenso Ridgeon, who develops a revolutionary cure for tuberculosis. His private medical practice with its limited staff and resources, however, only allows him to treat ten patients at a time.

From an initial selection of 50 patients he selects ten whom he not only believes he can cure but whom he also believes are most worthy of being saved. The plot then takes a dramatic twist after he is approached by a young woman with a dangerously ill husband. He decides that he can, at a stretch, treat one more patient beyond the chosen ten, but he feels more convinced than ever that the individual in question must be demonstrably the especially worthy of being saved.

The situation becomes more complicated when an old friend and colleague reveals that he too needs the same treatment, leaving Sir Colenso having to decide which patient he will save: the kindly, altruistic but poor medical colleague whom Sir Colenso is also very fond of, or an extremely gifted but also very unpleasant womaniser, bigamist and amoral young artist (who is the dying husband of the young woman). To make matters worse, Dr Ridgeon then finds himself falling in love with the young and vivacious wife of the womaniser, making it even harder for him to differentiate his motives for the decision as to who should live and who should die.

This central dilemma of the play has been reincarnated today, and not just in relation to TB, as medicine becomes ever more expensive and treatments becoming either so scarce or costly that only a few can access or afford them. Under such circumstances who should decide who should get what, and on what grounds are such decisions to be taken? The truth is that such

[228] World-renowned TB expert, previously Chief of the Division of Mycobacterial and Respiratory Infections, Dr Iseman was also a member of the Advisory Board of Partners in Health.

decisions are already being made, not just by individual doctors (like the hapless Sir Colenso Ridgeon in the play), but also by national policy makers, NGOs, committees of experts, and the World Health Oganisation.

So, as a pipeline of new TB drugs begins to emerge (as is looking increasingly likely) the issue at the heart of this play from over a hundred years ago becomes the fundamental dilemma for those developing the global strategies for the future management of the disease.

New drugs

"IT'S NOT JUST ONE OR TWO DRUGS.
WE NEED FOUR OR FIVE IMMEDIATELY."

Dr Jim Yong Kim[229]

New TB drugs are finally now in both preclinical and clinical development. They are the first to be developed for the disease in almost 50 years. One (bedaquiline) was approved as a treatment of last resort by the FDA in late 2012, and another (delamanid) was undergoing registration by the European Medicines Agency and was expected to be more widely approved for use in 2013. Both have been found to be active against drug-resistant forms of the disease.

Carole Mitnick of Harvard Medical School and PIH describes the prospects:

> "The approval of the first new anti-TB drug in nearly 50 years is a huge breakthrough, demonstrating that at least one profit-driven company saw value in pursuing a TB indication. Second, it created a regulatory precedent for approval of MDR-TB drugs. Last, and most important, it means that there is an alternative to the current regimens that have high toxicity and inadequate efficacy. There is even the potential that this new drug, and others in the pipeline, could shorten treatment.
>
> "Their introduction represents a critical opportunity to improve DR-TB treatment and every effort will need to be made to ensure, not just that they

[229] Co-founder of Partners in Health, former Director of the WHO HIV/AIDS Department and
currently President of the World Bank.

> are used in a way that allows treatment to be shortened and made more tolerable for patients, but that they can be made affordable and accessible to patients in developing countries. At the same time, given the lessons of history that resistances to new drugs can be expected to reveal themselves in as little as a year if they are not used with extreme care, their wider distribution must be managed with extreme care."

Dr Manica Balasegaram, the Executive Director of MSF's Access Campaign, endorses this with a similar general view:

> "With new medicines for drug-resistant TB at the doorstep for the first time in half a century, the global health community can't afford not to seize the opportunity of a lifetime by stopping drug-resistant TB from spiralling out of control."

Their language is unequivocal. No-one can afford to get this wrong.

Currently there are also some ten new or re-purposed further compounds in the later stages of clinical development (in Phase II or Phase III trials), and the intention is that some of them will be part of a future single treatment regimen active against both drug-sensitive as well as all forms of drug-resistant TB.[230]

Examples of the classes of compounds that are being investigated include the macrolides, pleuromutilins, quinolones and 2-pyridones, and oxazolidinones.

A list of some of the specific candidate drugs and their manufacturers includes:

- Oxazolidinones – a group of antibiotics most of which were developed in the 1990s for use against gram-positive drug-resistant bacteria, though normally only as a treatment of last resort
- Delamanid (OPC-67683), developed by Otsuka Novel Products GMBH
- Pyrrole (LL3858) which is being developed by Lupin
- Diarylquinoline (TMC 207, Bedaquiline), developed by Janssen and Johnson & Johnson

[230] Zhenkun M et al. - "Global tuberculosis drug development pipeline: the need and the reality", The Lancet, 375; 9731 (2010) 2100 – 09.

- Diamine (a macrolide) SQ 109 which is being developed by Sequella Inc.
- PA 824 (a Nitroimidazole) which is being developed by the TB Alliance & Chiron.

Pfizer and Astrazeneca are also both said to have new TB drugs in experimental stages of development. Additionally some existing antimicrobials (including moxifloxacin and gatifloxacin) are being tested for use in combination with some of the new drugs for TB. Moxifloxacin, although still not currently licensed for treatment of TB, is sometimes already being used as a treatment of last resort for cases of XDR-TB, having been seen to have sometimes rendered cases bacteriologically negative. The experimental application of a drug which is unapproved and used outside of a clinical trial is often referred to as "compassionate use".

The story of bedaquiline is an interesting and compassionate one in its own right. Janssen, the Belgian company that developed it, began working on the drug because of both a corporate and personal interest in tuberculosis: the sister of Paul Janssen (1926-2003), the company's founder, had died of TB. Janssen (the company) was subsequently bought up by Johnson and Johnson, and the initial development of the drug by what was by now a Belgian subsidiary was reported to have been continued discretely because it was accepted by those working on the drug that there would be little or no support from the parent company. It is said that their investigations continued quietly, with those working on the drug recognising the potential humanitarian aspect of continuing the work, and with Paul Stoffels, the company's chairman, personally supporting the project. He has since stated:

> "All together, we came to the conclusion that, even if we don't earn a lot of money we won't lose a lot and it will make a huge difference."

As refreshing as such an observation might be, TB expert Carole Mitnick still remains a little cautious about the new drug:

> "The primary issue that dampens my enthusiasm is safety. We know that Bedaquiline has potential heart toxicity. And too few patients have been evaluated to really know how safe the drug is, across populations. It should be noted that, in the small clinical trials, more patients who received Bedaquiline died when compared with patients who received the placebo. This does not mean people shouldn't get the drug; it merely reinforces that all people who receive this drug as part of an MDR-TB treatment regimen need to be assured the highest standard of care and vigilance while receiving it."

Certainly these are causes for concerns. That the drug appears to be effective is one thing, but the fact that more patients died on the drug than on the placebo (which is what was reported in the study's published results) certainly makes the results of the trial unusual. Toxicities from TB drugs are nothing new, but heart toxicity is unusual. The way things stand it looks like it can only be practically lining up as a treatment of last resort for use in both extremely well-managed and well-resourced facilities.

The 2013 WHO Global Tuberculosis Report offered "interim guidance" on its use, identifying five conditions that need to be fulfilled for the drug to be used on adults:

> 1. Effective treatment and monitoring. Treatment must be closely monitored for effectiveness and safety.
>
> 2. Proper patient inclusion. Special caution is required when bedaquiline is used in people aged 65 and over, and in adults living with HIV. Its use among pregnant women and children is not advised.
>
> 3. Informed consent. Patients must be fully aware of the potential benefits and risks of the new drug, and give informed consent before embarking on treatment.
>
> 4. Adherence to WHO recommendations. In particular, four effective second line drugs must be part of the regimen … bedaquiline should not be introduced into a regimen in which the companion drugs are failing to show effectiveness.
>
> 5. Active pharmaco-vigilance and management of adverse events. Active pharmaco-vigilance measures must be in place to ensure early detection and proper management of adverse drug reactions and potential interactions with other drugs."

The WHO also strongly recommended the acceleration of Phase III trials of the drug to generate more comprehensive evidence that can inform future policy guidance on the new drug. So far it has been tested only using a Phase II Randomised Control Trial (RCT). Normally new drugs have to go through larger Phase III RCTs before final approval so there is already some urgency being applied towards approving this drug in line with orphan drug policies. Janssen has started a phase III trial of 600 subjects with sputum smear-positive pulmonary MDR- or pre-XDR-TB (confirmed rather surprisingly by a rapid diagnostic test). Participants in the first arm will receive nine months of bedaquiline and a background regimen. Those in the control arm will receive a placebo and the same background regimen. A third rollover arm will capture the expected failures from the first two arms, with participants receiving an individualized salvage regimen. The primary endpoint will be relapse-free cures at 15 months for those in the first two arms with the final analysis looking at relapse-free cures after 21 months. It will be some time before full results are publishable and we can learn more about how this drug performs. It is also unclear exactly what the intentions may yet be concerning investigating the drug with HIV co-infection as well as investigating its possible application for children.

Bedaquiline certainly looks to be a useful start, but if more new drugs aren't quickly developed alongside it, the fear is that TB may develop resistance to this drug as it has to so many others.

With any new TB drug there is far more at stake than just this single new drug from the very outset, because they must ultimately be tested not just on their own, but also in combinations. It is only in combination that they can ever be expected to be administered safely and not to be exposed to risks of rapid resistance themselves. Bedaquiline, for instance, is being tested with a background regimen which itself could potentially interact negatively with its intended outcomes. Because of this, entire new regimens of drugs will need to be considered and tested together, something which is an immense challenge to the development of any new treatment.

Janssen has set up a partnership with non-profit TB Alliance regarding the further development of the drug. In doing so the Alliance has been granted a global, royalty-free license to use the drug for drug-sensitive TB regimens, and is including bedaquiline in one of its trial regimens. Janssen meanwhile, has retained the rights to market and sell the drug for multi drug-resistant TB (where it is truthfully most needed). It's a compromise because Janssen will still have control of the price of the drug when used for treating drug-resistant disease, but it has to be better than no compromise and no drug.

Other innovations are also being developed. As long ago as February 2002, the Chiron Corporation (the company which owns the patent on PA-824) entered into an agreement with what was then the Global Alliance for TB Drug Development to support the continued research into what they believed was their own potential new drug. This had significance far beyond the sharing of the costs of development: it implied that the final price of the drug, if finally approved, could be much lower than would otherwise be the case.

In 2010 the TB Alliance launched the first trial of the drug, testing multiple compounds with PA-824 in differing combinations hoping to find for the combination with maximum safety and efficacy. The favoured combination (initially called NC-001, or 'New Combination 1') has now been shortened to 'PaMZ'. It consists of PA-824 (Pa – the new compound), moxifloxacin (M – an existing antibiotic not previously approved for use for TB), and Pyrazinamide (Z – an existing first line drug).[231] The composition of the combination itself has to be seen as confusing, since the WHO guidelines recommend that four effective drugs should always be used, and this combination only uses three. The sizes of each group which was tested was also very small, with fewer than 15 patients in each group.

This multi-combination study was developed in partnership with Bayer Healthcare AG and was funded by the Bill & Melinda Gates Foundation, the United States Agency for International Development, UK Aid, and Irish Aid. It certainly promised an exciting new approach, summed up as such by Mario Raviglione, the Director of the Stop TB Department:

> "Because of testing drugs in [such] combination, we have already saved several years in the research process to find new, effective regimens to treat TB. The results look strongly promising from this early trial. If further testing holds up these results and the regimen is affordable in poor countries, it is huge progress. We could shorten drug regimens substantially for everyone, regardless of whether the form of TB is sensitive or multi drug-resistant. That would be a dramatic step forward."

A second study, NC-002, has been developed from this first study and it has been testing the same combination in a two-month trial in both South Africa and Tanzania. It is a landmark study because it is the first that has tested a new treatment using both drug-susceptible and drug-resistant patients with the same regimen (although obviously excluding any patients who are resistant to any of the individual drugs in the combination).

---

[231] Bovine TB is resistant to Pyrazinamide. Whilst there may have been no prevalence of *M. bovis* in the cohort being tested, it may comprise a substantial proportion (possibly 10% or more) of the rural populations in some countries most afflicted with TB today. As such, this regimen would be a non-starter in such countries without diligent DST.

There have been other recent developments. In November 2013 the European Medicines Agency's (EMA) Committee for Medicinal Products for Human Use (CHMP) adopted a "positive opinion" and recommended the granting of a conditional marketing authorisation for Deltyba (or Delamanid) for the treatment of MDR-TB. Deltyba had been designated an orphan medicinal product in February 2008.

In November 2013, the Committee for Medicinal Products for Human Use (CHMP) also "adopted a positive opinion" on another product, and recommended the granting of a marketing authorisation for Para-aminosalicylic acid Lucane for the treatment of MDR-TB. Para-aminosalicylic acid Lucane was designated as an orphan medicinal product in December 2010. The applicant for the medicinal product was Lucane Pharma SA.

New drugs are also being tested for the treatment of LTBI. One in particular, a combination regimen called TBTC 26, is currently being tested on children aged between two and 11 as well as on PLWH. The trial was scheduled to be completed in September 2013. Preliminary results were said to be showing "substantial advantages" compared with the current treatment with Isoniazid.

But four fundamental questions remain, whatever the results of these studies:

- Will they be affordable to those most in need of them?
- Will they be safe for use with co-infected patients?
- Can they be used on children?
- And how will each one be used?

The possible cost

It's impossible to properly predicte the price that any new TB drug will be sold at because of so many existing uncertainties. At least we can be sure that any developer will be looking to recoup the cost of research and also to make a reasonable (or unreasonable) profit. Much could depend on how the drug is sold, and how much of it is ordered at a time. A recent estimate has suggested that it costs as much as US$1.2 billion to get a new drug through to full approval (and can take six-11 years).[232] It's unlikely, in fact, that either will be the case for a new TB drug because of the genuine efforts that are being made both to short-cut and to short-change the more usual processes. Nonetheless, it's questionable whether there is sufficient motivation (or indeed time) to support this process for developing new drugs for TB unless drug-resistance spreads significantly into the developed world. If it does so, it will be sure to sharpen focus and promote motivation for investment. There are some signs that the existing drug development movement is already struggling for funding since new developments at Phase II stage are possibly being overhyped, probably in order to stoke interest in funding for the requisite larger studies in which the responses of as many as 1,000 patients would be expected to be studied.

A single new drug (even if it is 'shorter course' of just a couple of months) is highly unlikely to roll in at less than US$500 per patient and probably will cost a lot more. Some new antibiotics, for example, cost more than US$100 per pill, and on the open marketplace in the developed world Bedaquiline already costs more than this.[233] To keep costs down, the drug's bulk production would have to be guaranteed and it would have to be manufactured in massive quantities. But would this ever be affordable in Africa or in India?

Furthermore, since a single new drug can never be contemplated as being safe for use on its own, it will also still have to be used with at least two other drugs (and more properly with three to guarantee safety from drug-resistance) so there will be the costs for these to be added into the equation as well. On top of that, the cost of closer management of treatment (which will be vital) has to be anticipated to be far more for a new combination regimen than the current cost of managing DOTS.

Such a new combination could come in one of three possible varieties. The first would be in combination with two or more of the mass-produced first line drugs. This would be by far the cheapest option, but it would be unlikely to be a successful one because all of these drugs are already tainted with existing widespread incidence of resistance. A second variety of combination would be one which includes some of the far more expensive second line drugs. This alternative would be far more expensive. There

---

[232] Joseph Di Masi et al. - "The price of innovation: new estimates of drug development costs", Journal of Health Economics 22 (2003) 151–85.

[233] A course of bedaquiline for one patient in New York has been reported to have cost US$20,000.

could be expected to be significantly less global resistance to the drugs used – though it could still be substantial enough to doom the combination to failure. These drugs are also less effective and so might render the package weaker, possibly needing longer treatment regimens. The third would be in combination with other newly developed or as yet unapproved drugs. This last possibility would be desirable not just because of an automatic lack of existing resistance but also because they might well also have faster action. Their combined expense, however, may even be too much even for developed countries to contemplate except as a treatment of last resort.

Seen this way, the design of a new and effective treatment regimen for those patients who already desperately need one can be seen to be a challenging affair. The possible consequence of failing to meet this challenge, however, remains a grave concern. If the MDR-TB and XDR-TB pandemics continue to grow the stranglehold which this disease now has on high incidence lower-income countries may well become effectively complete, with the result that these affected countries might remain unable to address their drug-resistant epidemics at all.

So how will new drugs be used?

This remains a very sensitive question because no-one should be in any doubt that they will have to be extremely carefully managed. Three issues will need to be considered before any new regime is widely implemented in any environment – the calculated risk of fresh resistance, the consequential risks if the drug is inadequately or incorrectly prescribed, and the drug's potential applicability in the real-world of limited diagnostic infrastructure and management resource wherever the disease is most common and where the new drug might best be used.

The WHO calculates any intervention not just in terms of its cost, but also by awarding it a value assessed by its potential positive economic benefit. This is technically referred to as a treatment's 'cost-effectiveness ratio'. In the simplest of terms the gross cost of an intervention that comes in at less than the per-capita gross domestic product (GDP) of the country in which it is being applied is regarded as being highly cost-effective.

The gross cost of such an intervention should include diagnosis, treatment administraition and cost of the drug itself. With first line drugs using DOTS, this gross cost of treatment can come in between US$100 and US$500 in a low-income country, the actual cost of the drugs comprising just US$20 of this total. With DOTS-Plus this adds up to much more. The 2012 WHO Global Tuberculosis Report reckoned that national programmes were spending between US$1,200 and US$3,800 per MDR patient on drugs alone. MSF has reckoned on even more than this – between US$4,500 and US$9,000. Certainly the WHO appeared to be already budgeting for increases in 2013 – up to around US$2,600 per patient in low-income countries to around US$4,700 per patient in upper middle-income ones but these figures weren't developed any further in its most recent report.

Calculated against all of these costs when grossed up to include the costs of diagnosis and treatment management is the potential economic benefit which might become available to a country from a proportionate predicted reduction in deaths from a disease, bearing in mind the known economic costs of the disease. So will these new drugs be seen as being economically affordable in the countries where they are most needed?

According the TB Alliance the disease will rob the world's poorest countries of an estimated US$1 to US$3 trillion over the next ten years - a massive sum of money which they can ill-afford to lose. The economic burden incurred on developing countries because of TB has long been recognised to be serious if only because three-quarters of all infections are estimated to develop during the most productive adult working years (i.e. between the ages of 15 and 45).

But in much of Africa, this positive computation needs to be offset further by another negative one – the anticipated costs of ongoing anti-retroviral therapy for TB/HIV cases who might then survive their TB co-infection which would otherwise have killed them. Rates of co-infection vary dramatically across the continent. In Lesotho, for instance, rates of co-infection are claimed to be as high as 90%; in Sierra Leone it is just 10%. Both have high incidence of tuberculosis, but the roll-out of a new treatment could be seen to be far more economically beneficial in Sierra Leone, as a result, and might be introduced there much more readily. Such calculations make for a grizzly balancing of cost against each 'disability-adjusted life year' (or DALY) which might be expected to be averted.

A DALY is defined by the WHO as "the sum of years of potential life lost due to premature mortality and the years of productive life lost due to disability".

In 2010, the per-capita GDP in Africa ranged from US$7,000 in South Africa and Botswana to US$982 in Lesotho. In one of the modelled scenarios which compared the standard sputum smear diagnostic with the new GeneXpert device, it was suggested that the GeneXpert could avert an estimated 132,000 TB cases and 182,000 TB deaths in southern Africa over the ten years following its full introduction, and that it could simultaneously reduce the proportion of the population with TB by 28%. But this would also have come at a price, since it would also increase health service costs by US$460 million.[234] Much of these calculated costs include increased long-term antiretroviral therapy for those TB/HIV-infected individuals who might now survive TB infection because of better case-finding and treatment. After further comprehensive computation, the estimated final gross cost of a ten year roll-out of GeneXpert across southern Africa was suggested to be as much as US$959 for every DALY averted – in other words the gross cost of the new diagnostic alone could be just US$23 less than the per-capita GDP of Lesotho for every DALY averted in the country because of additional long-term drug costs for another illness. And this cost unfortunately doesn't even allow for the cost of the treatment of TB itself.

There are further complexities to be factored in as well.

The TB Alliance has estimated that over five years as many as four million women may die of TB leaving as many as 10 million children motherless or orphaned (quite possibly with the children themselves left infected as well).

The World Bank has estimated that some countries' GDP is negatively affected by between 4% and 7% because of this disease – and this figure doesn't include any of the economic burden of caring for those that are infected (and affected).

The WHO has also estimated that, while treatment itself may be free, the average TB patient loses on average three to four months' worth of income as a result of being ill with the disease.

There can be no doubt that the cost of TB to both patients and their families is, relatively speaking, very considerable. Direct costs include

---

[234] Menzies NA et al. - "Population Health Impact and Cost-Effectiveness of Tuberculosis Diagnosis with Xpert MTB/RIF: A Dynamic Simulation and Economic Evaluation" (2012), http://www.plosmedicine.org/article/info%3Adoi%2F10.1371%2Fjournal.pmed.1001347

transportation, and (if the patient resorts to the private sector) both diagnosis and the medical treatment itself. Indirect costs include income lost, and often jobs lost as well with some TB patients are estimated to have to spend between 20% and 40% of their annual family income while they are being treated.

As many as 2.7 billion people are estimated to live on less than US$2 a day. Meanwhile, around 2.3 billion are suggested as being latently infected with TB. It's probable that in many of these cases they are the same individuals: they are the people who are most at risk from TB, but they are also the people who, literally, can least afford to be infected by it.

"Invest now or pay forever."[235]

"PUBLIC HEALTH IS PURCHASABLE."

Hermann M. Briggs (1911) [236]

In terms of absolute numbers, TB affects the 15-45 age group more than any other. This age range more often than not also constitutes the wage-earner or the principal carer of any family, so this particular phenomenon can have complex consequences.

In 2012 the WHO suggested that there were as many as 10 million children who were struggling to survive because of being orphaned as a result of tuberculosis. This is an enormous number of children whose lives have been blighted by the disease without even having directly suffered from any of its symptoms. An Indian survey has suggested that 11% of children in families in which a parent became infected had to drop out of school to look after the parent, whilst a further 20% did the same in order to take on the responsibilities of earning a wage to support the family.[237] Neither

[235] Dr Mark Dybul, the Executive Head of the Global Fund.

[236] Hermann M Briggs (1859-1923) was an American physician and pioneer in the field of public health.

[237] Minuyandi M, Ramachandran R, Balasubramian R, Narayan PR - "Socio-economic dimensions of tuberculosis control: review of studies over two decades from the Tuberculosis Research Centre", Journal of Communicable Diseases, 38; 3 (2006) 204-15.

percentage may sound so huge until one considers the incidence rates of TB in India and considers how many children must be being affected in this way by the disease. Roughly 2.3 million Indians are estimated to go down with TB each year. If half of them are parents, then 125,000 kids may drop out of school each year to look after a parent, and 230,000 may drop out to start earning to support their family. Operation Asha (an Indian NGO) estimates this drop out figure a little higher still, at 300,000.[238]

Operation Asha also suggests that in India as many as 100,000 TB-infected women are thrown out by their families each year to die of the disease or to die of starvation, whichever takes them first.

These are some of the many consequences of the disease that would not even begin to be tolerated in a high-income country.

Research has also shown that, with every 10% increase in rates of tuberculosis, a country's economic growth falls between 0.2 and 0.4%. In connection with such ideas, it was being estimated in 1999 that implementing DOTS properly in India could generate economic benefits equivalent to between 0.9% and 3.3% of GDP as rates of disease began to fall.[239]

These estimates, amongst many others, led the World Bank to pronounce that the benefits of TB control were worth at least 10 times their investment. Dr Marcos Espinal, the executive secretary of the Stop TB Partnership, has reported that a survey of 134 countries where TB incidence had fallen quickly showed that these countries also scored well on the Human Development Index as well as in terms of improved child mortality rates and sanitation. Progress in TB control would appear to equate with progress in other departments of public health as well.

Back in 1993 the Word Bank calculated that treating the disease cost between just US$1 to US$4 per year of healthy life saved in a low-income country, and between US$5 and US$7 in a middle-income one.[240] In most

---

[238] http://www.opasha.org/our-work/quick-facts/

[239] Dholakia R, Almeida JR - "The potential economic benefits of the DOTS strategy against TB in India", Geneva, World Health Organization (1997).

[240] World Development Report. "Investing in Health". World Bank (1993) Oxford University Press.

high burden countries, the gross cost for ambulatory first line treatment (including costs of diagnostics, health workers etc.) was then being suggested to be US$400 or less per patient. In 2006, Dye and Floyd suggested that treating MDR-TB costs just US$90 per DALY and was therefore "good value" – and that this could also be much lower in a low-income country.[241]

The 2012 WHO report had slightly different ideas concerning costs per DALY. The cost of first line treatment in the 22 high burden countries (HBCs) generally lies in the range US$100–500 per patient successfully treated (all-in including diagnosis, treatment management, administration, and disease surveillance). The exceptions were Bangladesh, India and Myanmar (at less than US$100); Brazil (at a little over US$500); and the Russian Federation and South Africa (both above US$1,000). It's far from clear how or why such variability exists although additional investments in treatment may be warranted and included in the two last figures. Such variabilities might include high rates of alcohol dependency and unemployment among TB patients, some inclusion of costs for treating drug-resistant disease, as well as a comparatively high proportion of ex-prisoners in the Russian patients, or a high level of HIV co-infection in South Africa). Still, any computation in which the cost per patient treated amounts to less than GDP per capita is considered to be "good value".

The report provided some further enlightening costings, split into the costs of treating smear-positive susceptible TB, and of treating smear-negative susceptible TB (which costs more) and also of treating MDR-TB.

Type of TB	**Cost per year of life saved**
Smear-positive drug-sensitive pulmonary TB	US$5–50
Smear-negative (all other forms of drug-sensitive TB)	US$60–200
TB resistant to both Isoniazid and Rifampicin (MDR-TB)	US$200–800
People living with HIV/TB with TB IPT	US$15–300
PLW HIV/TB: FLDs under DOTS plus ART	US$100–365

(In the case of those in whom TB is suspected and diagnosis of TB is made using the Xpert®MTB/RIF rather than by smear microscopy alone an add-on to the cost of the smear was assessed to be US$40–200 per test).

[241] Dye C & Floyd K - "Tuberculosis" in "Disease Control Priorities in Developing Countries", Oxford University Press (2006) pages 289-309.

From this we can begin to see why the World Bank has considered DOTS to be such an incredibly cost-effective treatment and why such store has been set by it. It can also be seen that confronting MDR-TB is such a very different economic ball game.

The general high cost-effectiveness of DOTS TB care and control was recognized by the Disease Control Priorities Project in 2006, identifying TB treatment as one of its 'best buys' in its so-called shopping mall of public health. In similar fashion, a group of august Nobel laureates more recently published the "Copenhagen Consensus", a document which identified the expansion of TB treatment among its top five investments (among some 40 other proposals).[242] In December 2007 a World Bank report also concluded that high burden TB countries could all earn significantly more than they spend on TB diagnosis and treatment as a consequence of the productive lives saved through effective and well-managed treatment. This study made it clear that the economic benefits of TB control are far greater than the costs of the treatment, something which was intended to enable extra funding. The report even suggested that most highly affected countries could recoup nine times or even more of their investments in DOTS TB control.

An in-depth economic analysis developed by the WHO in collaboration with the Indian RNTCP showed that TB caused a loss of a massive 7.9 million DALYs in 2006 alone, and a consequent reduction of US$23.7 billion in national economic well-being (equivalent to US$21 per capita). In contrast, the cost of TB control was averaged at just US$26 per DALY gained over 1997–2006 and was calculated to generate a staggering return of US$115 per dollar spent.

Some governments have significantly increased their domestic funding for TB care and control as a result of such numbers. The BRICS (Brazil, Russia, India, China and South Africa) countries in particular have mobilized significant domestic funding for TB control (covering up to 96% of gross treatment costs). In other high burden TB countries, however, external donor funding in TB control is only running at about 50% of the gross cost of programme management which, certainly according to some

[242] "Nobel laureates: more should be spent on hunger, health: top economists identify the smartest investments for policy-makers and philanthropists" - Denmark, Copenhagen Consensus (2012) www.copenhagenconsensus.com/Projects/CC12/Outcome.aspx

commentators, warrants much more domestic allocation of money towards TB control than is currently happening in most of them.

Overall, the differences in costs in treating this disease vary dramatically between different environments as defined by their being either high-, medium- or low-income countries. Also it depends massively upon whether the disease is either susceptible or resistant to first line drugs. In the United States, the cost of hospitalization and treatment for one XDR-TB patient, for instance, has been estimated to average US$483,000. Meanwhile the cost of hospitalisation and treatment of an MDR-TB patient in the US has been reported as being US$275,000. In middle-income countries such costs may be significantly lower, but the costs of addressing drug-resistant TB remain relatively speaking massive, and hospitalisation is being increasingly realised to be an economically unrealistic response to the growing problem.

The cost of second line drugs alone in countries with little resource may be disabling from the start. Such costs have massive impact on TB budgets. In South Africa in 2008, just 2.5% of all cases treated were diagnosed as being drug-resistant; the cost of treating them with second line drugs, however, took 68% of the total national Tuberculosis Budget. Meanwhile treating the 97.5% susceptible cases with first line drugs took just 4% of the budget. This begins to suggest a very different and more worrying picture than the one suggested by some of the figures listed above.

It is drug-resistance that knocks the figures sideways. It's clear that treating TB with DOTS has been highly cost-effective, and most of the time it has been patient-effective as well. (With MDR-TB creeping up behind it, however, DOTS can no longer be seen to have been quite as effective as had been intended, since incidence of MDR-TB is also widely accepted as being a good marker for a failing DOTS regime.) Notwithstanding this, the issue of cost-effectiveness and DALYs for treatment of MDR-TB is not yet being properly discussed, addressed or accounted for. Focusing on the positive economic costs, on the DALYs in relation to DOTS and the returns on investment while simultaneously ignoring the underlying trends in the disease may prove to comprise a failure to properly confront the shifting disease patterns in an appropriate fashion.

Once again we can find it easy to be judgemental in, but with all of these facts and figures in view we are left having no option but to ask – why was DOTS not effectively implemented well enough in the first place to stifle the secondary epidemic of drug-resistance given that DOTS was and still is so incredibly cost-effective whilst treating DR disease is looking to be so costly?

The Health Worker Crisis and the Funding Gaps

"THE WELFARE OF EACH OF US IS DEPENDENT FUNDAMENTALLY UPON THE WELFARE OF ALL OF US."

Theodore Roosevelt (1903)

The WHO began monitoring its funding for TB in 2002, so the existing global TB database holds data from 2002 up to 2013. Its principal published focus, however, in line with so much of the WHO's campaign against TB, has been particularly directed towards the 22 HBCs.

A long-term study which is being used by the WHO suggests that TB funding in low- and middle-income countries grew substantially between 2002 and 2011, but so too did the number of patients being treated – from 2.8 million in 2002 to five million in 2011. This patient number is intended to rise further to 6.9 million by 2015. Meanwhile, the gaps between the available funding and the estimated budget to satisfy all global TB programmes have been widening.

The current estimate is that, between 2013 and 2015, up to US$8 billion per year is needed in low- and middle-income countries in order to implement existing interventions. Of this 65% is budgeted for detection and treatment of drug-susceptible TB, 20% is for treatment of MDR-TB, 10% is pegged for rapid diagnostic tests and laboratory strengthening, and 5% for collaborative HIV activities. The current estimated funding gap for this US$8 billion budget is calculated as being US$3 billion a year or around 40%.

In addition to this, the funding gap for research and development of drugs and new diagnostics, which is also recognised as being so vital, is pegged at a further US$1.4 billion.

International donor funding for TB care and control has increased from US$0.2 billion in 2006 to almost US$0.5 billion in 2013, but this still falls far short of funding for malaria (US$1.8 billion in 2011) and HIV (a massive US$8.2 billion in 2011).[243] This may in some ways be improving,

[243] WHO - "Global Tuberculosis Report 2013".

however. The percentage proportion of the Global Fund to Fight AIDS, Tuberculosis and Malaria that is being specifically directed to TB (as against HIV or malaria) has risen from a measly 16% to a more realistic but still disproportionate 25%.

In March 2013 Dr Margaret Chan, the Director General of the WHO, gave a press briefing in Geneva. She identified the gaps in funding as being one of three key constraints that are putting the 2015 Millennium Goals and Stop TB Partnership targets at risk. She reported that the WHO and the Global Fund were identifying an anticipated funding gap of US$1.6 billion in the annual international support for the fight against tuberculosis in 118 low- and middle-income countries, and that this funding gap was still rising. She was leasving little room for doubt:

> "The final dimension is financial. The funding gap for TB care and control is substantial."

These shortfalls don't just relate to donor funding. Within the overall budget there is an estimated US$3.2 billion that is thought could or should be provided by the countries themselves. According to the WHO list national contributions already provide the bulk of financing for TB care and control in middle-income countries like Brazil, the Russian Federation, India, China and South Africa (i.e. all the so-called BRICS economies) and also in some other HBCs. The BRICS alone are estimated to carry as much as 60% of the global burden of TB and (with the exceptionof India) they have been becoming increasingly self-sufficient in respect of their national TB programmes – to the extent that they were branded a "success story" in this respect in the 2013 report. In India, however, the domestic funding budget was disappointingly showing itelf up to be less in 2013 than it had been in 2012.

Similar national contributions from lower-income countries are harder to develop. Currently international donor funding accounts for 54% of the funding for TB programmes in the African region, for instance, if South Africa is excluded; for the 17 HBCs which aren't BRICS countries it accounts for even less at 34%.

It is suggested that filling all of these gaps would enable full treatment for 17 million TB and MDR-TB patients and so could potentially save an estimated six million lives between 2014 and 2016. It's unclear exactly what the proportional breakdown of these figures is between 'ordinary' TB patients and MDR-TB patients in the calculations, but the targets for 2015 are that 6.9 million new patients should be enrolled on DOTS and that 300,000 will be newly enrolled on DOTS-Plus. Variations in this proportional mix (which is set by these numbers at 23:1) could significantly alter both budgets and forecasts. Even in the BRICS countries domestic contributions, as substantial as they now are, are still not reckoned to be sufficient for any serious scaling up of the response to MDR-TB.[244]

Furthermore 60% of this funding gap (around $US1 billion a year) is identified as being directly needed in Africa. Current projections for the region are not encouraging. Furthermore, the proportional gap between available funding and necessary funding is predicted to widen most in those 17 of the 22 HBCs (excluding the five BRICS countries) as well as in those other low-income countries many of which have higher estimated proportional burdens of TB than the HBCs themselves. In other words, in line with almost everything else in the pandemic, the problem is probably going to get much worse where it is already the worst already.

The WHO believes that there is still potential to mobilise a larger share of the funding from domestic resources. Domestic sources of funding in 2013, for instance, are forecast to be US$5.3 billion, whilst funding being required from international donors is estimated at US$1.6-2.3 billion. The latter portion is only expected to amount to US$0.8 billion in 2013, projecting a shortfall of US$0.8-1.5 billion for the current year.

In addition to this annual gap in international financing for critical implementation interventions, the WHO and its partners also estimate that there is a US$1.4 billion annual gap for TB research and development for the period 2014-2016, research which includes the costs of clinical trials for new TB drugs, diagnostics and for new vaccines. These don't come cheap as we have already identified. Dr Mark Dybul, the Head of the Global Fund, spelt it out at Dr Chan's side at the March 2013 briefing:

> "It is critical that we raise the funding that is urgently needed to control this disease. If we don't act now, our costs could skyrocket. It is invest now or pay forever."

TB is already calculated to cost the global economy US$13 billion a year through lost productivity. If this is so, then a budget of US$8 billion a year still makes solid economic sense, and it should be possible for it to be picked up if the world were to work coherently using the agencies it has

244 WHO - "Global Tuberculosis Report 2012".

created for such purposes, ones like the UN, the WHO, the G8, the World Bank etc. The evidence so far suggests that this isn't happening yet, however, and that critical points may be being passed as a result. Some may, in fact, have already ***been*** passed.

Experts like Dr Dybul are anxious to highlight how much this problem may cost the world in the longer run, particularly reminding donor nations that treating drug-resistant TB can easily cost 100 times what it costs to treat drug-sensitive disease. The example that is most frequently quoted is what it cost the city of New York in the late 1980s when a relatively small early outbreak of multi drug-resistant TB was estimated to cost over US$1 billion to be brought under control. The problem with the pandemic today, of course, is that, if the proportion of drug-resistant disease continues to increase (or is already larger than what is currently estimated), the cost of containing this disease could easily skyrocket. No-one really argues that treating a case of drug-resistant disease can end up costing anywhere between 100 and 250 times as much as a drug-susceptible one. If the global percentage of drug-resistant disease is actually higher than currently reckoned, then there are problems ahead indeed.

Already, the figures are not adding up too well. The relative proportions in the numbers of patients intended by 2015 to be treated for drug-sensitive TB (DS-TB) as opposed to MDR-TB implies a ratio of 23:1 for 2015 (6.9 million DST: 300,000 MDR-TB). Current rates of MDR are suggested to be around 5% overall including retreatment cases – so things at first don't look too far adrift but it's hard to be certain. If we try and break things down a little further we can attempt to see whether adequate resources are being either anticipated or allowed for in order to meet the existing estimated MDR-TB epidemic let alone an underestimated one.

If it costs 100 times the amount to treat an MDR-TB patient than a DS-TB one, with this numerical ratio of 23:1, it suggests that roughly four times the amount of money will need to be being allocated to treating MDR-TB than to DS-TB by 2015. If the cost of treating MDR-TB is in fact 250 times higher than treating DST, however, it will need a budget for MDR-TB that is as much as 10 times higher than that budgeted for DS-TB.

The current available funding for MDR-TB and DS-TB respectively in the 36 combined high burden countries[245] is US$0.46 million (for MDR-TB) and US$2.47 billion (for DS-TB). The budget for dealing with drug-resistant TB is therefore about one fifth the size of that for the susceptible pandemic. It begins to look like the proportion of funds that are proportionally available to the two parts of the pandemic in 2013 may be out by at least a factor of 20 compared to what may be needed in 2015. This uses the lower (100 times more expensive) estimate of treating MDR-TB as listed above.

Furthermore, the possibility that drug-resistant TB is being underestimated is not insignificant. In the current 2013 report, there is a perplexing explanation for the low share of funding which is being allocated for MDR-TB in the Western Pacific region. The explanation given for this apparent anomaly is that "most of the estimated cases of MDR-TB [for this region] are in China". The report explains that this is "consistent with the small number of cases reported to have been detected and started on treatment in China in 2012 (just over 3,000)". The idea that this number could possibly be so low has already been discussed and is troubling enough. The discrepancies in the estimations of drug-resistant disease in China will reveal themselves in starker detail still in the next section. The fact that such low numbers might be being used as a base for regional budgeting is very troubling indeed.

The resource on the ground

"ALL MANKIND IS TIED TOGETHER; ALL LIFE IS INTERRELATED, AND WE ARE ALL CAUGHT IN AN INESCAPABLE NETWORK OF MUTUALITY, TIED IN A SINGLE GARMENT OF DESTINY. WHATEVER AFFECTS ONE DIRECTLY, AFFECTS ALL INDIRECTLY."

Dr Martin Luther King (1965)

In November 2011, the Global Fund cancelled "Round 11" of its grant because of lack of funds. In so doing it stated its intention to maintain funding to existing projects, but remained unable to fund any new projects until 2014.

[245] The 36 'combined high burden countries' comprise the 22 HBC's (with drug-susceptible TB) and the 27 HBMDR-TBCs (with MDR-TB). Some countries are on both lists.

The general decline in Global Funding for both HIV/AIDS and TB has been put down to the behaviour of the donors to the Global Fund. Some have cut back on the amount they committed to pay – countries which include Denmark and the Netherlands. Others, including Ireland, Spain, and Italy, have stopped contributing entirely because of their domestic economic crises. As a rule, what is amassed in the pot from all such donor nations is then match funded by the US. So if these smaller donor nations give less, then so does the US and the fund effectively suffers twice over from the same cause.

MSF described the cancellation of Round 11 as having provided only the "thinnest of lifelines to help countries whose treatment programmes would otherwise face disruption between now and the beginning of 2014". The organisation accused the Global Fund board members of effectively sending the message that countries needed to stop accepting patients on their treatment programmes.

Notwithstanding funding issues of this sort, the other key constraint which has been delaying any further proper roll-out TB treatment is the chronic shortage of health staff, particularly in Africa. A Canadian study of 2013 suggested that Sub-Saharan countries that invest in training doctors have lost as much as US$2 billion of investment in their human resource as their clinicians leave home to find work in more prosperous developed nations. The study also suggested that these governments spend between US$21,000 (the figure for Uganda) and US$59,000 (for South Africa) in order to train a doctor, only to see him or her then migrate. (In Uganda, they even simply cross the border into Rwanda where doctors are paid more and from where they manage to get home to see their families on weekends). These researchers also tell us that:

> "Among the nine sub-Saharan African countries most affected by HIV/AIDS, more than US$2 billion of investment was lost through the emigration of trained doctors. Our results indicate that South Africa incurs the highest costs for medical education and the greatest lost returns on investment."

Their findings further suggest that the specific savings in medical training costs to Britain from this medico-economic migration was around US$2.7 billion, and to the United States around US$846.

It's already been noted elsewhere that there is an estimated global shortage of nearly four million health workers, with a particularly serious shortage in

57 countries, 36 of which are in Sub-Saharan Africa. This doesn't just leave these countries under-equipped in terms of a vital human resource: it leaves their health services in a state of low morale as well and at risk of melt-down which means potential catastrophe for their national TB programmes.

An extreme example of this relates to Malawi. Recently there were more Malawian doctors working in the city of Manchester, UK, than in the whole of Malawi.[246, 247] The story from Ghana is similar. According to Dr Ken Sagoe, a senior member of the country's health service, 604 out of 871 medical officers who trained in the country between 1993 and 2002 are now practising overseas. Zimbabwe trained 1,200 doctors in the 1990s with only 360 remaining there today. Zambia has only 50 doctors remaining out of the 600 who trained in the country during the last 40 years.[248]

Some experts actually suggest that the best judge of the strength of a nation's health service is the state of its tuberculosis epidemic. It is also suggested that the biggest driver for growth in drug-resistant TB so far seen has been poverty or deterioration of national health-care infrastructures.

---

[246] Robert L Broadhead and Adamson S Muula - "Creating a medical school for Malawi: problems and achievements", BMJ 17; 325; 7360 (2002) 384–7.

[247] Ruder Finn - blog: "Health systems in Malawi" http://www.ruderfinn.co.uk/blogs/dotorg/2009/01/health-systems-in-malawi/

[248] Laurie Garrett, - "The Challenge of Global Health", Foreign Affairs, 86; 1 (2007) 27.

India versus China

"TUBERCULOSIS IS VIGOROUSLY PUSHING ITS WAY THROUGH THE CROWDED STREETS AND LANES OF THE POPULOUS CITY OF CALCUTTA AND NO STEP HAS YET BEEN TAKEN TO RESIST ITS COURSE. ... WE HAVE HOPELESSLY FAILED TO STAMP OUT TUBERCULOSIS. ... ROUGHLY SPEAKING NEARLY ONE-EIGHTH OF THE TOTAL NUMBER OF DEATHS IN CALCUTTA IS DUE TO THIS CAUSE."

"Progress of Sanitary Measures in India" (1912) [249]

Around 36% of the world's total population and an estimated 50% of the world's MDR-TB population reside in China and India. It may well be more because these two countries between them have an enormous number of prevalent tuberculosis cases and if they are not managing them well there must inevitably be a lot of drug-resistant disease. Both are in the list of 22 high burden TB nations and are also in the list of the 27 high burden MDR-TB nations. Both are middle-income BRICS with rapidly developing economies and are creating massive amounts of wealth, and yet in spite of this a large proportion of both countries' peoples still live in poverty.

Each country can reasonably be described as an economic super-power with their economies depending on their booming populations – in other words their continuing growth is dependent upon their national human resource. Such economic growth can logically only be sustained by nurturing this resource and certainly not by disabusing it. Worrying pictures are merging relating to the TB epidemics in both countries, however, and in both countries they appear to be taking a huge toll on the poor. Reports of insufficient public health initiatives in India are sometimes compared to the more aggressive public health systems of China. They may yet prove to be the Achilles' heels for Indian TB control. Meanwhile other reports from China are worrying for different reasons.

TB is certainly no stranger in either country. Rates of TB generally have been high in both for decades, and the numbers that have been infected have been mind-boggling. It is suggested, for instance, that as many as two TB deaths occur every three minutes in India. In both countries TB is still

[249] His Majesty's Stationery Office, London.

recognised as the number one cause of death from infectious disease. In contrast to Africa, both of their national rates of HIV infection are lower, although there are regional exceptions – in Henan Province in China, for instance, where huge numbers of peasants were infected with HIV as a result of a plasma-donor malpractice scandal in the 1990s.

Both countries have been taking on their respective fights against tuberculosis, but the ways in which they have been doing it include some significant differences. Some of these differences may help tell us more about how global TB might be successfully contained in the next decades, and some may tell us the opposite. Offiocial reports for both countries are frequently presented in positive terms, but there are also alternative disturbing reports of endemically insufficient public health initiatives in India, almost as much as there are consistent reports of aggressive and proactive public health systems in China which may not match the reality.

In this section we will look at whether such assessments are fair, and what the implications might be if they are not.

China

"IF YOU KNOW BOTH YOURSELF AND YOUR ENEMY, YOU CAN WIN A HUNDRED BATTLES WITHOUT JEOPARDY."

Sun Zi – "the Art of War" (c.400 BC)

Tuberculosis control has been a part of China's public health programme since the 1950s. More recently China developed and implemented two five-year national plans in the 1980s, and then another 10-year plan in the 1990s in order to bring the disease under control. According to its national surveys, the prevalence of tuberculosis in the country fell by an average of 3.3% each year during the 1980s, but in spite of this, the country's progress slowed during the 1990s as well as in the first few years of the new millennium. The estimated proportion of new cases of sputum-positive TB that was being diagnosed and treated by the country's public health programme, for instance, had stagnated at around 30%, far below the 70% target that was then being set by the WHO.

This inadequate control of tuberculosis in China can be readily linked retrospectively to its general poorly functioning health systems. From 1978 until 2002 the government's share of total health expenditure reduced from 32% to 16%, a reduction which forced many Chinese health-care facilities and health providers to focus more actively on the generation of revenue with less co-ordinated concern being concentrated on issues of public health – including their TB programmes. Hospitals and clinics in China were essentially functioning at this time as private for-profit independent entities.

By 2000, nearly 90% of TB patients were initiating their diagnostic and treatment process in such hospitals or in such non-public health-care facilities, where they would have to pay for the requisite tests and drugs. Many patients who felt that they had sufficiently improved discontinued their treatment well before completing treatment while others ran out of money. It was being estimated that as few as 20% of patients with tuberculosis who were being treated outside the public health system were taking their tuberculosis medications properly.[250] Such irregular treatment guarantees the growth of drug-resistant TB.

Even for those patients who eventually ended up in the public health system, there was not much in the way of better solutions, and the same patterns were being repeated. By 2002, only about 40% of funding for the country's public health centres were coming from central government and so these public institutions began to concentrate on revenue generation as well – exactly as the non-governmental ones had been doing. There was no effective incentive left for them to engage in the labour-intensive and unprofitable activities involved in tuberculosis control. Worse still, even where government subsidies should have been fully supporting the free diagnosis and treatment of tuberculosis, many clinics were charging for ancillary tests as well as for extra drugs, some of which were of questionable benefit.

In response to this problem, the Chinese government initiated a series of major partnerships with international agencies to try to support its failing efforts, some of which are worth identifying. Early in 2002, the government signed a seven-year US$104 million loan with the World Bank, a loan which included grant funding from the UK's Department for International Development. The Japanese government also began to provide free anti-tuberculosis drugs. In late 2002, China received a US$48 million grant from

[250] Ministry of Health of the People's Republic of China - "Report on nationwide random survey for the epidemiology of tuberculosis in 2000", Beijing: Ministry of Health of the People's Republic of China (2002).

the Global Fund to fight AIDS, Tuberculosis and Malaria specifically to tackle tuberculosis. The Belgian Damien Foundation and the Canadian International Development Agency also supported efforts to control tuberculosis in several provinces. The WHO, meanwhile, continued to serve as the lead technical agency, providing both policy and technical support to the national tuberculosis programme throughout this period.

What prompted the real change for China was the SARS outbreak in 2002-3. Its rapid spread had revealed massive weaknesses in the country's medical infrastructure, something which was being experienced by those in power as an international embarrassment. In the aftermath of SARS the Chinese government set in place a series of measures to strengthen its health systems, and they were measures which included a rigorous assault on its national TB epidemic.

By January 2004, the Chinese Ministry of Health implemented the world's largest internet-based communicable-disease reporting system, one which intended to address the delays and incomplete reporting which had been revealed by the SARS epidemic when governmental authorities had been unable to assess and report on the extent of the epidemic. By the end of 2005 the length of time that was being taken to report any notifiable disease from a county-level health facility to the central level had been reduced from an average 29 days to just a single day. This sort of pro-action was enabling patients with tuberculosis to be dealt with appropriately, ensuring both swift diagnosis and proper treatment.

In March 2004, the central government also revised a law on the control of infectious diseases, a revision which directly addressed the well-recognised under-reporting of tuberculosis by many health facilities. Tuberculosis had now to be reported to local public-health authorities within 24 hours, with failure to report it now defined as being a crime. As a result, hospitals began to take the reporting of tuberculosis very seriously indeed.

By 2006, implementation of the WHO-recommended DOTS programme had increased from 68% to 100% for all counties, and the detection of smear-positive tuberculosis by the public health system had more than doubled – from 30% of new cases to 80%. Together with a reported treatment success rate of more than 90%, China was now achieving the 2005 global targets for tuberculosis control, something that was a rare example of success at the time. What is more, given the huge numbers involved in any report on TB in China, these statistical success stories were, and still are, making a huge difference to the overall assessments of the global pandemic.

It's far from all being good news, however, and the more detailed picture remains much less coherent. The 2000 national tuberculosis survey had already revealed that one in ten TB patients in some provinces were being found to be MDR. This should hardly have been much of a surprise given the known mismanagement of the national programme in the previous decade but it was a shockingly high rate for the time. Without a correspondingly rigorous DOTS-Plus programme in place to deal with it, one that was at least equal to the scope of the DOTS programme, it is unlikely that such a rate could possibly have reduced since. In fact it will far more probably have been doing the opposite. Other studies began confirming this possibility – that there was a really serious epidemic of MDR-TB in several Chinese provinces, with rates of DR disease in previously untreated cases that were five to ten times higher than the global mean.

Such concerns have been more recently underscored by a study that was funded by the Chinese Ministry of Health itself and which was published in the New England Journal of Medicine in 2012. This study retrospectively estimated that one in 10 of ***all*** TB cases in China in 2007 were MDR (which amounts to twice the current estimated global average five years later in 2012), and that 8% of these cases were XDR. This would have been translating to around 100,000 MDR- and 8,000 XDR-TB cases per year in China, far more than anyone was reporting at the time. What was more worrying still was that most cases of both MDR-TB and XDR-TB appeared to have been resulting from primary transmission, and that one ***new*** TB case in every 200 was being exposed as being XDR (i.e. was not a relapsed case), implying that infectious XDR-TB was circulating in the community. China, whilst being officially reported to be the golden child of TB control, was now looking to be in real trouble as regards MDR- and XDR-TB, although there was still little official acknowledgement of this. The conclusions of the study were that:

> "China has a serious epidemic of drug-resistant tuberculosis. MDR tuberculosis is linked to inadequate treatment in both the public health system and the hospital system, especially tuberculosis hospitals."[251]

---

[251] Zhao Y et al. - "National Survey of Drug-Resistant Tuberculosis in China", New England Journal of Medicine, 366 (2012) 2161-2170.

Patients treated in hospitals, according to the study, were now being identified to be 13 times more likely to have MDR-TB than those treated elsewhere. This may not have been that surprising because their diagnosis was probably being made there. But if their hospital treatment was substandard (also a strong possibility) then it might also mean that they were acquiring their MDR-TB from other hospitalized patients in the course of their hospital stays.

So even with an apparent TB success story on our hands (at least as far as reported mortality rates and surveillance is concerned), the drug-resistant genie now appears to be very much on the loose in China, and the previously accepted dogma that almost all drug-resistant disease has been occurring in relapsed cases is also up for a challenge.

Equally worrying has to be the huge contrast between the content of these studies and the current estimates for TB and MDR-TB in China as published by the WHO. The general incidence rates for China continue to be reported as being in decline. In the three-year average for 2008-2010 they were pegged at 80/100,000; the figure for 2012 was just 73/100,000. These sorts of numbers are understandably viewed by the global authorities as good news, particularly since they make such a healthy impression on their elusive global targets because of the size of the population of the PRC. They also may make sense given the known aggressive public health efforts that have been made in the last few years – but can TB really be turned round so fast?

The 2013 WHO report suggested that 89% of all TB cases were being detected in China, but this is also a difficult claim to accept given that China has met only 20% of the global target for provision of sputum smear microscopy centres. Exactly how could 89% of cases have been detected with such a poor diagnostic provision? In fact, according to MSF and PIH "even the best programmes do not detect more than 60-70% of expected new smear-positive cases within a population".[252] And, as we will shortly see, the proportion of smear-positive cases may be less in China even than in Africa.

---

[252] PIH & MSF - "Tuberculosis – Practical Guide for clinicians, nurses, laboratory technicians and medical auxillaries" (2014) page 173. http://refbooks.msf.org/msf_docs/en/tuberculosis/tuberculosis_en.pdf

A national prevalence survey is conducted in China every ten years, and the most recent one (the fifth, completed in 2010) tells an altogether more disconcerting story. It employed standard sampling techniques for surveying a total sample population of 264,000 people aged 15 or over at 176 cluster sites in 31 provinces across the whole of the country. The information gathered related specifically to "active pulmonary TB (all types), smear-positive pulmonary TB, and bacteriologically confirmed pulmonary TB". As such, it did not include EP-TB at all so ignored one part of the epidemic completely.

The figures suggested a national prevalence of "all types of pulmonary TB" of 442/100,000 which extrapolated to more than five million active cases nationwide. These figures dramatically fly in the face of other officially estimated numbers[253] – suggesting that China might be carrying over 40% of the current estimated global burden of prevalent disease which runs globally at around 12 million estimated cases. Regional prevalences were found to be almost double in rural areas when compared to urban ones – and rates of disease were identified as increasing in these rural populations, not reducing. These demographics were also weighted heavily westwards, with far higher rates being found in China's western regions (where rates were also identified as increasing), most particularly amongst the poor. The average family income of those surveyed who had active disease was less than a dollar a day, with the local uninfected averages being three times higher.[254]

According to Chen Yude, a technician who was involved in the study, only 18% of those in rural areas had even consulted a doctor about their symptoms. The study itself reported that 76% respondents said that they would not want to visit a doctor because he/she would "not pay attention" to them – with a further 18% suggesting that it was simply because the doctor would be "too busy". Tellingly, treatment adherence was also recorded as being poor, with only 57% of those surveyed who were already on treatment "regularly" adhering to it.

---

[253] The estimated number of prevalent cases in China in 2012 in the 2013 WHO Global Tuberculosis Report was 1.4 million.

[254] http://www.who.int/tb/advisory_bodies/impact_measurement_taskforce/meetings/lille_oct10_china.pdf

This survey was represented in a quite different way in an article which was published in the Lancet in 2014, however.[255] This presentation of the figures specifically separated out the numbers of cases in the study into three groups: those who were found to have clinical and radiological signs and symptoms of TB ("all pulmonary" 442/100,00); those who were found to be bacteriologically positive by culture (116/100,00); and those found to be smear-positive (59/100,00). There was no explanation provided as to why the numbers of "all pulmonary" cases were so much higher, but what the article did choose to focus on were groups of bacteriologically and smear-positive cases. It thus concluded in its summary that "in 20 years, China more than halved its tuberculosis prevalence". In fact, if the numbers relating to "all pulmonary" were applied in the same analytical fashion as the bacteriologically confirmed cases, then rates would have had to have been reported to have dropped by less than half what the summary chose to claim. This reduction would still have been impressive, it should be added, but China's continuing contribution to global prevalence in the officially published WHO reports would have been proportionately far larger and both the country and the global authorities would have had to accept that it still had a huge epidemic on its hands.

The 'official' story with MDR-TB as published in the Global Reports makes similarly little sense as well. The total estimated MDR-TB cases in China for 2012 was 59,000 (a 6% drop from 2011). And yet the 2012 NEJM study suggested that the numbers of MDR-TB cases five years earlier may have been 120,000 (twice this more recent WHO published estimate). The number of notified cases in the Global Report, however, was just over 3,000, with nearly 2,000 on treatment. A simple question arises out of these figures: with so relatively few MDR patients on treatment, exactly how can the MDR epidemic possibly be reducing as has been being reported?

Several other questions deserve to be asked as well, the most fundamental of which is this: how can such official figures be so readily accepted when they fly so dramatically in the face of other studies? The rates of XDR-TB that have been being quoted in some reports suggest that China may have as much or more of an entrenched problem with extensive strains of resistance as South Africa (which supposedly carries 71% of the disease burden with a far smaller population). And XDR-TB does not just come

---

[255] Wang L et al. - "Tuberculosis prevalence in China, 1990-2010; a longitudinal analysis of national survey data", The Lancet.com, published online: http://dx.doi.org/10.1016/50140-6736(13)62639-2

out of the air – it arises from an established MDR-TB epidemic that has been being inappropriately managed with second line drugs. So if these higher XDR-TB rates are true, the same question returns to haunt: exactly how can the rates of any type of DR-TB possibly be dropping in China? The history of TB control in the country in the 1980s and 1990s right up until 2003 exactly predicted that China should have the sort of entrenched MDR-TB problem that these studies quoted above suggest may now be the case, and there is little evidence of an adequate recognition or response to this probability.

Can the WHO seriously be accepting these rates? It has certainly included them in its report, and, possibly more worrying still, it also appears to be allowing for them in budgets for the Western Pacific Region.

India

"WE HAVE MANAGED BY A COMBINATION OF COMPLACENCY AND INCOMPETENCE TO ALLOW THIS BACILLUS TO MUTATE INTO A VIRTUALLY UNTREATABLE FORM."

Dr Zarir Udwadia (2012)[256]

If you were just to read the WHO's 2010 publication "A Brief History of Tuberculosis Control in India" you could easily be forgiven for concluding that, similarly to China and despite huge challenges, the efforts being made to control the epidemic and to meet global targets have been proceeding pretty swimmingly in the country.

Its National TB Programme (NTP) was launched by the Government of India in 1961. Early TB drugs were implemented and Rifampicin was introduced in 1981. After a joint review by the government in New Delhi, the Swedish International Development Agency and the WHO, the "Revised National TB Control Programme" (RNTCP) was established in 1993 and it promptly identified some serious shortcomings as a result of which a new programme, one which included DOTS, was launched in 1997.

[256] TB specialist in Mumbai and author of "Totally drug-resistant tuberculosis in India: Who let the djinn out?", Respirology, 17;5 (2012) 741-2.

The requisite donor funds to implement the RNTCP were initially provided by the World Bank, helped by the governments of Denmark and the UK. These funds were provided centrally and then were channelled to the respective districts and registered charities, then on to their officers, most of whom were government officials.

The RNTCP included, according to the 2010 WHO report, "flexible funding mechanisms, decentralization, an ensured supply of quality-assured drugs at all times, better supervision, monitoring and evaluation, and technical support via a country-wide network of consultants". By 2006, the whole country was supposedly being covered under the RNTCP, and case detection and treatment success rates were similarly being reported to have improved significantly.

In terms of statistics, the 2010 report was also positive, although it is not at all clear whether it was completely transparent. It quoted encouraging "evidence of a sustained decline in both incidence and prevalence" from a WHO 'Model DOTS Project' carried out in Tiruvallur district, Tamil Nadu in South India. The report then proceeded to discuss the general prevalence of disease, although, given what was available from other sources, it cannot be confidently said that this part of the report related to national figures or to those in the district in Tamil Nadu. If they were national figures, they were certainly widely belied by other evidence, as we will see.

The implementation of DOTS under the management of the RNTCP had, the report suggested, resulted in "improved treatment success rates and probably led to a decline in the duration of disease". WHO estimates prepared in collaboration with the RNTCP suggested that the prevalence of all forms of TB decreased from 506/100,000 in 1995 to 280 in 2007, at a rate of about 6% per year. Incidence rates were similarly decreasing. The nation's mortality rates were similarly claimed to have decreased – from 44/100,000 to 29 in 2007, a rate of decline of 4% per year, still resulting in about 335,000 deaths due to TB in 2007.

The report correctly identified that the prevalence of TB drug-resistance was a good indicator of the effectiveness of TB control. It reported that drug-resistance surveillance surveys had been ongoing since 2005 in Andhra Pradesh, Gujarat, Maharashtra, Orissa and Uttar Pradesh with the prevalence of MDR-TB in new smear-positive pulmonary TB cases was ranging from just 1% to 3% among the different districts. From all the figures presented, it was estimated that 5.4% of all TB patients in India might have MDR-TB, so that there might be about 130,000 incident MDR-

TB cases per year. This figure, however, has been revised downwards in the years since by over 50%. The current official estimate as listed in the WHO Global Tuberculosis Report for 2013 is 64,000 incident cases of drug-resistant disease.

Second line drug sensitivity testing of MDR-TB cases in the Gujarat survey showed 4% XDR-TB among the MDR-TB retreatment cases. An extremely high rate (over 50%) of pre-treatment resistance to quinolones (a group of the second line drugs) was observed, however, among a cohort of 60 MDR-TB cases in Gujarat, and, although this was identified as a matter of concern, the implications of this finding was not further discussed.

Surveys of HIV in TB patients were carried out in four high HIV-prevalence districts in South India between 2005 and 2006, and in 15 districts in eight states from 2006 to 2009. The models used by the report suggested that HIV would not greatly affect the incidence of TB in India.

The challenge in India, the report stated:

> "..was to maintain the present level of programme implementation, whilst incorporating the new components of the Stop TB Strategy, many of which require further policy development, planning and additional financing."

Further specific challenges were also identified:

> "..in regard to engaging the private sector including a common platform to reach the vast network, the years of unregulated practice with ready access to first and second line anti-TB drugs, lack of feasible opportunities for continuing medical education, and the resistance of some academicians."

In 2010 India had four National Reference Laboratories, one Intermediate Reference Laboratory in each large state, and almost 13,000 designated microscopy centres (DMCs). The numbers of DMCs were sufficient for the population but an expansion of both culture and drug-susceptibility testing services was identified as being needed for the management of drug-resistant TB, as well as for the diagnosis of smear-negative pulmonary TB and for extra-pulmonary disease. As of the end of 2009, 12 laboratories had been accredited to perform culture and DST for the RNTCP, and a number of additional laboratories were undergoing further accreditation.

The report was sounding especially encouraging concerning both drug supply and drug quality, however. According to the report:

> "In 2006, the United Kingdom's Department for International Development (DFID) provided a five-year grant to supply first line drugs to about half of the country through the Global Drug Facility (GDF). First line drugs for the rest of the population are acquired through the World Bank loan to the Government of India and Global Fund grants.
>
> "India has developed a unique system of providing drugs in Patient-Wise Boxes (PWBs), which contain the drugs for a complete course of treatment for one patient."

It also optimistically concluded that:

> "Over the last decade, the RNTCP has expanded TB services to over 1.1 billion people,[257] has met the WHO objectives for case detection and treatment success, and is close to fulfilling the TB-related Millennium Development Goal indicators and the Stop TB Partnership targets by 2015. It has also proved that ensuring free TB services via both the public and private sector is a cost-effective and sound investment, providing a significant economic return to the country."

And it concluded that:

> "Most of the work of the RNTCP has been achieved even though the public health infrastructure remains weak, and the success is primarily due to careful planning, thorough implementation, stable funding and the use of an innovative network of technical consultants."

The level of expenditure on activities related to TB control in India was furthermore identified by this report as being "unprecedented":

> "The achievements of the RNTCP, with emphasis on the cost effectiveness of the programme, should help to convince both the Government of India and donors to increase their investment in the country with the world's greatest TB burden, both in terms of drug-susceptible and drug-resistant disease."

Perhaps this is the most revealing sentence of all.

Elsewhere we can find startlingly different assessments of the situation in India. The principal problems which are most regularly identified include a poor primary health-care infrastructure (particularly in the more rural areas), unregulated private health care leading to widespread irrational use

[257] This almost amounted to its entire population.

of both first line and second line anti-TB drugs, a lack of political will to admit to or address the scale of the problem, and, above all, a corrupt administration.

Unfortunately, at least officially, India is essentially in denial of the true scale of risk from this disease in its variety of forms. This culture of denial shows itself to be so deeply rooted that as recently as 2010, in its first ever "Annual Report to the People on Health", the Ministry of Health was reporting that TB was still showing decreasing trends.[258] At the same time, however, several non-governmental sources were already reporting MDR-TB in excess of 25%.[259]

The Indian Public Health system considers TB to be a "facultative" disease for which the required control measures are already in place and functioning. The exact intended meaning of the adjective "facultative" is unclear, but it would seem likely to relate to the capacity of the disease to adapt to and capitalise on its immediate environment. Unfortunately, if this is the case, it just may have been doing so particularly successfully in India in terms of developing drug-resistance. A proper response to such a generally facultative disease in any case should surely also have been to aggressively address reducing poverty whilst implementing effective infrastructures to combat the threat. If such initiatives are indeed "in place and functioning" as was being suggested, its benefits are surely being missed by a substantial proportion of those most at risk from the disease or who are already in the process of dying from it in a country where the gaps between rich and poor is ever widening.

In contrast to China, the Indian Ministry of Health had never even instituted a centralized list of notifiable diseases, so it has been effectively impossible for TB to be appropriately nationally notified as it should have been. Each state in the country has had its own list and priorities have shifted within each state. For Tamil Nadu, for instance, (the state which was quoted in the WHO report as having such encouraging figures) TB was a lowly 11th on its priority list of 24 notifiable diseases.

---

[258] Ministry of Health and Family Welfare - "Annual report to people on health. New Delhi, India, 2010",
http://mohfw.nic.in/WriteReadData/l892s/9457038092AnnualReporthealth.pdf

[259] D'Souza DTB, Mistry NF, Vira TS, et al. - "High levels of multi drug-resistant tuberculosis in new and treatment-failure patients from the revised national tuberculosis control programme in an urban metropolis (Mumbai) in Western India", BMC Public Health, 9 (2009) 9, article no. 211.

The near certainty of under-reporting under such regimes was finally confirmed by the shocking report only a year later than the optimistic "Annual Report" – of cases of totally drug-resistant (TDR) TB in India from a tertiary health care centre in Mumbai.[260] Dr Zarir Udwadia, the author of the report and a well-published expert on TB, was initially vilified for his outspokenness. He maintained nevertheless that the levels of resistance which he was seeing were "relentlessly amplifying".

As late as May 2012 the Indian Journal of Medical Research was still reporting that the country was "on target" to meet the millennium goals and disarmingly added that – "The prevalence of MDR-TB is not increasing in the country."

This turned out to be somewhat at odds to some frightening revelations later that year which suggested that as many as 10% of ***new*** TB cases in populous Mumbai, Bihar and Uttar Pradesh were MDR and also that there were increasing cases that were resistant to all currently available TB drugs. Both of these latter reports didn't just suggest a well-entrenched drug-resistant epidemic in India, they rather indicated its certainty. Dr Udwadia himself described his normal reaction to a confirmation of a case of MDR-TB:

> "Ten years ago, you would have been horrified. Now we say, 'At least she's only MDR…'."

According to Dr Udwadia, the Mumbai findings show that totally drug-resistant TB "was an accident waiting to happen". The evidence suggests that MDR-TB has been smouldering away in considerable proportion to the wider epidemic for years, and that the unregulated private sector has effectively been fanning it into flames. Udwadia explains:

> "To get to this stage, you have to have amplified resistance over years, with loads of misuse of (antibiotic) drugs. And no other country throws around second line drugs as freely as India has been doing."

This flare-up of drug-resistant disease in India has been put down to the unregulated nature of Indian medicine and of its drug provision (in its private sector). These allow patients to 'graze' the TB drugs – including second line ones – without a proper programme in place either to control, reduce or eliminate the risks of increased resistance.

---

[260] Udwadia ZF, "Totally drug-resistant tuberculosis in India", Clinical Infectious Diseases, 10 (2011) 1093.

A discussion paper innocuously entitled "What is the Relevance of Clinical Finding to National Regimen?" investigated at some depth the way the disease has been being managed in India. It revealed that TB drugs were being sold in a "bewildering number of [first line] drug combinations": Rifampicin alone; Rifampicin and Isoniazid; Rifampicin and Isoniazid and Ethambutol; Rifampicin and Isoniazid and Pyrazinamide; and finally Rifampicin, Isoniazid, Ethambutol and Pyrazinamide. All but the last could promote resistance to first line drugs if misused on re-activated infectious disease. Second line drugs are also readily available in the country. Ian Harper, the author of this paper, interviewed a WHO TB Officer who described a "therapeutic anarchy" on the loose in the country, with 50 or more companies "pushing their combinations".

Around 50% of TB patients seek help in the private sector from doctors who are happily doing their own thing in terms of their prescribing practices without consideration of the epidemiological consequences. These patients resort to these doctors because they sadly have even less trust in the country's public sector. Furthermore, 74% of the TB drug market is in private hands, in an industry with an already chequered history and which frequently supplies drugs of inconsistent quality.

As if further evidence were needed, Udwadia's team conducted a study in Mumbai to establish just how well doctors might be dealing with MDR-TB in the city. In one district only five out of 106 doctors in the unregulated private sector could give a correct prescription for a hypothetical patient with MDR-TB.

> "What people say and what is the truth [about TB in India] are two entirely different things."

This statement was made by Dr Shelly Batra, the founder of Operation Asha, and was quoted in the Financial Times on March 22nd 2013. Operation Asha is an Indian NGO operating in both India and Cambodia and it has an impressive reputation. Some of the figures it has published are devastating: it suggests that there were 2.2 million new cases of TB in India in 2011; it further suggests that there are 3.5 million prevalent cases (or 25% of the global TB burden); and it suggests that there are at least 100,000 prevalent cases of MDR-TB (with fewer than 3,000 actually identified).

In the most recent WHO global resistance report, MDR-TB rates for India were reported as being 2-3% in new cases and 12-17% in retreatment cases

– i.e. below the global average. However, these estimates were based on small sample sizes and came from sentinel centres where programme performance almost certainly are exceeding what is being routinely encountered elsewhere. For example, at a private referral hospital in Mumbai, the corresponding MDR-TB rates for new and retreatment cases run at a shocking 30% and 60% respectively.[261]

Similarly, the WHO report reveals that XDR-TB prevalence rates amongst retreatment cases is around 0.5%, yet in the very first report of XDR-TB from Mumbai in 2006, 11% of all MDR samples sent to a private mycobacterial laboratory were XDR-TB.[262]

Summary

It looks to be almost certain that the disease (including rates of drug-resistance) is being consistently under-reported in different ways and for different reasons in both of these TB super-powers. If this is indeed the case, the consequences are likely to be grave.

The table below shows some of the officially published rates and numbers for both countries in relation to MDR-TB. A summary study suggests that the numbers demonstrate almost nothing in the way of consistency - nor much that makes coherent sense. The major anomalies point towards the following:

- India's estimated percentage rates for both new and retreatment cases of MDR-TB is almost certainly massively under measured, and is probably double what was published in the 2013 report.

- China's figures, whilst assuming that 90% of all TB cases are notified in the face of other evidence, is treating less than 3% of its estimated MDR-TB cases and is meanwhile anticipating that this might keep rates of MDR-TB under control.

---

[261] Rodrigues C, Shenai S, Sadani M, Thakkar P, Sodha A, Udwadia ZF, et al. - "Multi drug-resistant tuberculosis in Mumbai: it's only getting worse", International Journal of Tuberculosis and Lung Disease,. 10;12 (2006) 1421-2.

[262] Jain S, Rodrigues C, Mehta A, Uwadia ZF - "High Prevalence of XDR-TB from a tertiary care hospital in India", Proceedings of the American Thoracic Society International Conference (2007) San Francisco, USA.

- Both countries (India meeting only 20% of the global target for drug-susceptibility testing, and China meeting 70%) are barely testing a third of their estimated total retreatment cases for MDR-TB.

	"Official" estimated incident rates and numbers of MDR-TB, (new and retreatment)	Laboratory confirmed MDR-TB cases (2012)	Cases started on MDR treatment	Numbers of new XDR-TB at 9.6% of MDR-TB cases
India	(2.2% & 15%) 48,400 & 42,632[a] **Total – c. 91,000**	16,588	14,143	8,736
China	(5.7% & 26%) 57,000 & 10,873[b] **Total – c. 68,000** (possibly c. 100,000)[c]	3,007	1,906	6,528 (possibly 8,000)[c]

[a] – new MDR cases calculated at 2.2% of 2,200,000 estimated incident TB cases for 2012, and retreatment at 15% of 284, 212 total retreatment cases (WHO - "Global Tuberculosis Report 2013", page 122)
[b] – new MDR cases calculated at 5.7% of 1,000,000 estimated incident TB cases for 2012 (900,678 of whom were notified cases), and retreatment at 26% of 41,817 retreatment cases (WHO - "Global Tuberculosis Report 2013", page 119)
[c] – Zhao Y. et al. - "National Survey of Drug-Resistant Tuberculosis in China", New England Journal of Medicine, 366 (2012) 2161-70.

Mycobacterium bovis (Bovine Tuberculosis) in humans

"TB OR NOT TB?"

Natasha Bolognesi[263]

Whilst *M. bovis* is not a normal "extra-pulmonary" TB disease, neither is it strictly speaking tuberculosis in the sense that it is not caused by the mycobacterium *M. Tuberculosis*. It does, however, behave in an extremely similar way. It does not cause illness in all those it infects, and can also remain latent for years; it replicates slowly; it causes wasting, intermittent fever, and in untreated cases often causes death. It can also, like *M. tuberculosis*, infect a wide range of organs.

In contrast to human tuberculosis, the bovine bacillus has an exceptionally wide host range, one which includes cattle, humans, non-human primates, goats, cats, dogs, pigs, buffalo, badgers, possums, deer and bison and even seals. Many susceptible species, including humans, are described as being 'spill-over' hosts rather than endemically susceptible species – in other words they present themselves as mammalian species in which a primary infection is not generally self-maintaining within the species. It is in the sense of this non-propagating spill-over phenomenon that the risk to humans is most frequently assessed, although there may even be some valid cause for concern in relation to its capacity for self-maintenance in some human populations.

Given that cattle are a major component of family wealth and carry considerable trading value in many traditional economies, there can also be significant secondary financial risks from this strain of mycobacterium for such human populations and communities. During the first half of the 20th century in the UK *M. bovis* was estimated to have been responsible for more losses among farm animals than all other infectious animal diseases combined – in other words it constituted a very substantial loss to the British farming economy.

And *M. bovis* infection is still recognised as a major public health problem particularly when it is transmitted to humankind via milk from infected cows. The widespread introduction of pasteurisation in the 20th century, however, helped eliminate this problem for most of humanity.

[263] Freelance South African health writer.

From the 1920s onwards efforts were made to control bovine infection. First of all, herds that were known to be safe from disease were certified TB-free by tuberculin testing and could then guarantee safe milk. Secondly, a special heat treatment of milk was implemented in order to kill the mycobacteria. Although such pasteurisation had been originally considered as early as 1913, Britain revealingly lagged behind much of Europe and the US (by as much as a quarter of a century) before finally putting it into consistent effect.

The reduction of rates of bovine disease in humans has been remarkable. Whilst *M. bovis* transmission from cattle to people was once common in the US, for instance, *M. bovis* today causes a very small proportion, estimated as being less than 2%, of the total number of cases of TB disease – amounting in fact to fewer than 230 cases per year. This has been achieved simply by decades of disease control in cattle and by routine pasteurisation of cows' milk.

The disease is still found in cattle in much of the world. While most countries have been able to significantly reduce or limit the incidence of the disease by rigorous testing and culling, in some countries the disease has been eradicated completely. In fact the story right across the developed world tells a very similar story. The disease now struggles to maintain any sort of significant pool of infection in cattle, so, in different countries and on different continents, other feral animals are being focused upon having been recognised as the main vector for carrying new disease between herds.

Most of Europe and the Caribbean is now virtually free of *M. bovis*. Australia is officially free of the disease, although small residual infections are still thought to exist in feral water buffalo in some isolated parts of its Northern Territory. In Canada, there remain only small populations of infected wild elk and white-tailed deer in Manitoba.

In the United States *M. bovis* is still endemic in white-tailed deer (*Odocoileus virginianus*) in the states of Michigan and Minnesota. This has prevented what would probably otherwise have been a nationwide eradication of the disease in livestock, but it has also provided an unusual commercial opportunity for the states concerned who sell deer harvest tags to their state-resident hunters to do the culling on their behalf. In 2008, 734,000 licensed deer hunters paid out to harvest approximately 490,000 white-tailed deer between them.

In New Zealand, the common brushtail possum (*Trichosurus vulpecula*) is recognised as the main vector for the spread of the disease which is believed to be still endemic across 40% of the islands. New Zealand's Animal Health Board operates a nationwide programme of cattle testing and possum control with the goal of eradicating *M. bovis* from this wild vector species across 2.5 million hectares – around a quarter of New Zealand's at-risk areas – by 2026 and ultimately of eradicating the disease completely. The programme has been successful so far, reducing cattle and deer herd infection rates from more than 1,700 herds in 1994 to fewer than 100 herds by 2011. This result is mainly attributed to sustained possum control which reduces cross-infection between herds and thus effectively breaks the cycle of disease.

The reason that possums are thought to be such particularly efficient transmitters of bovine TB is because of the way that their behaviours change once they enter the final stages of disease. Possums are normally nocturnal, but when terminally ill with TB they resort to venturing out during the daytime to get enough food to eat, sometimes seeking out buildings in which to keep warm. As a consequence, they stray into farm buildings where they attract the attention of inquisitive cattle and deer and the cycle of infection gets completed once again.

In the 1930s in the UK as many as 40% of cows were estimated to be infected with *M. bovis* and there were as many as 50,000 new cases of human *M. bovis* infection every year. Since mass pasteurisation of milk, however, this incidence has dropped to almost none – with almost all new human cases now being 50 years of age and older and therefore most probably re-activation cases from latent disease. The disease is still found from time to time in cattle and is still dreaded by farmers for good commercial reasons.

In the UK it is the badger (*Meles meles*) that has been identified as being the main vector for infection. The principal method of transmission from badger to cattle is believed to be as a result of cattle grazing over latrine areas frequented by the badgers whose urine and fecal matter are infectious. The anatomical evidence (from the high incidence of cervical, abdominal, glandular and skeletal tuberculosis) indicates that the digestive tract rather than the lungs is the most common channel of entry of the bacilli into cattle.

Badgers were first identified as being potentially the main carriers of *M. bovis* in Britain in the 1970s, but it was only in 1997 that they began to attract specific attention by being proposed to be the main cause for the spread of *M. bovis* between what were otherwise unconnected herds of cattle. In fact a government-sponsored "Randomised Badger Culling Trial" has subsequently established that it is cattle-to-cattle transmission that is the most prevalent route of infection but there is still widespread attachment to the idea of badger culling, both by politicians and farmers alike. Unlike in New Zealand where the culling of possums has become the norm, "to cull or not to cull" the badger has become an issue of some controversy in the UK. There is special sensitivity on the issue because the badger is a legally protected species in the country so slaughtering the animal under the direction of government legislation creates some understandable contradictory concerns. Some scientific findings indicate that the rising incidence of disease in cattle can be efficiently reversed without any culling at all, and that the geographical spread of the disease can be contained simply by more rigid application of cattle-based control measures. It has also been argued that the badger may be not much more than the innocent fall guy, since in some areas the risk of transmission to cattle from fallow deer is suggested to be greater than it is from badgers. It's still far from clear how important the badgers' role in the disease really is – some authorities have even argued that cats create a higher rate of infection of bovine TB than badgers, and that the generally accepted dogma that badgers are such a major vector of disease may be a totally mistaken one.

The culling of badgers has been conducted in Ireland for over a decade, however, and the rates of slaughtering of infected cattle have reduced there during the same period, whilst they have been rising quite fast in the UK. Badgers, however, are not believed to be so densely populated in Ireland as they are in mainland Great Britain, a factor which might have made the Irish targeted culling more effective. The Irish approach, moreover, has been a 'reactive' one – in that culling is only carried out in a limited area around a farm which has had more than three cattle infected with bovine TB. In the UK the proposal has been that it should be 'proactive' over wider areas because it is believed that targeted culling may exacerbate the problem due to population 'perturbation' which, it has been further suggested, will be spontaneously generated as a result of only localised culling.

Currently selective pilot culls are being undertaken in specific regions which aim to kill at least 70% of badgers in each cull zone by free shooting them at night over a period of four years using high velocity rifles and shotguns. At best, it is expected to reduce levels of new cases of TB in cattle by around 16% over the next nine years.

The option of vaccinating badgers is also being explored by some British charities. The UK's National Trust, which manages large areas of British countryside, has been trialling the option at one location in Devon. The cost is reported to be high – at £330,000 for just 20 square kilometres. The badgers are being trapped in cages, injected with vaccine and then released. The idea is to vaccinate the animals annually for four years (badgers live 3-5 years) in order to try and cumulatively create a herd immunity.

The most common test for disease in cattle, as in humans, is the tuberculin skin test (TST) which is normally performed intradermally in the skin of the animal's tail. The injection site is examined for a reaction 72 hours post-inoculation. If there is a reaction (which may be a discoloured raised area) the animal is classified as a reactor and so will be immediately euthanized. Treatment of bovine tuberculosis is not recommended anywhere simply because of its infectious nature.

The BCG vaccine (which was originally derived from *M. bovis* itself) has been widely considered as a way of helping to eradicate bovine TB in cattle, but, despite it having been derived from the bovine bacillus itself, there is still a recognised variable efficacy, exactly as with humans. The vaccine certainly reduces the severity of the disease in animals – and seems to do so more effectively than it does with humans. It usually restricts the bacteria to infecting just a few lymph nodes, but it still doesn't reliably prevent infection *per se*. Much more importantly, however, a vaccinated cow can give a false-positive result after a skin test, which renders testing meaningless should it be deemed necessary because of a newly perceived risk to a herd. It thus would disable what is the greatest tool for disease surveillance – so vaccination is not considered as a realistic strategy to protect herds.

There are current studies researching the efficacy of combining the BCG vaccine with mycobacterium protein and DNA, hoping to develop an enhanced vaccine that might provide guaranteed protection against the disease. If any are successful it would make a big difference, and it could also potentially be given to other wildlife as well. It might even further 'spill-over' and prove to be of use for human disease.

The general greater success in containing and reducing TB in animals stands in painful contrast to the general failure to do the same for the human variety of the disease, and it is worth us taking a few moments to consider why this is so. Two factors basically separate the two campaigns. One is euthanasia: the nearest thing that physicians have at their disposal is the isolation of the patient which today is only very rarely carried out where the disease is endemic. The second is the fact that veterinarians don't use a vaccine on their bovine patients whilst physicians do on their human ones, meaning that the TST in cattle can be assumed to be 100% reliable, whilst in humans it is anything but – at best it offers the possibility of a latent infection.

One other factor exists which makes it easier to specifically diagnose this disease in cows. *M. tuberculosis* (the human disease) can never be seen to be confusing the picture in cattle when they are seen as sickening, whilst *M. bovis* can and does confuse the picture if when it causes humans to sicken with otherwise typical symptoms of tuberculosis.

When humans do have bovine TB they most commonly contract it by eating or drinking contaminated unpasteurised dairy products or by eating inadequately cooked meat. Human infection can also occur from direct contact with a wound, however, such as might occur during slaughter or hunting, or even by inhaling the bacteria in air exhaled by animals infected with *M. bovis.* This is also known to occur during slaughtering, although direct transmission from animals to humans through the air is thought to be, under normal conditions, very rare.

The bovine disease is even known on occasion to be able to be spread directly from person to person when someone already infected with the bovine disease in their lungs coughs or sneezes, although this is certainly rare today in the developed world. There was a tiny unlikely outbreak in the city of Birmingham in England in 2004, however. One man died and five others were infected in an outbreak of bovine tuberculosis that was thought to have been somehow spread in a nightclub. An enquiry eventually concluded that the index source of the outbreak was probably a man who had drunk unpasteurised milk.

One improbable instance again from Britain but this time back in 1944 even exists of an infection spreading from man back to cattle.[264]

The main risk to humans, however, remains from direct infection from animal hosts. In areas of the developing world where pasteurisation is still not routine *M. bovis* is still a not uncommon cause tuberculosis-type disease in human beings. And as unlikely as it might at first seem, with any significant presence of infectious individuals in a community, the risk of

---

[264] Griffith AS and Munro WT -"Human pulmonary tuberculosis of bovine origin in Great Britain", Journal of Hygiene, 43; 4 (1944) 229–40, and also:

Tice FJ - "Man, a source of bovine tuberculosis in cattle", Cornell Vet 34 (1944) 363–5.

person-to-person infection has to be consequentially much higher. Once again this serves to reveal the Great Divide which exists in terms of prevalence and prevention of TB between the developed and the less developed worlds.

HIV, as we have already seen, is widely recognized to have created a massively increased risk of active disease in humans infected with *Mycobacterium tuberculosis*. It is also believed that this same increased risk exists in the case of *M. bovis* infection. In Africa, human TB is known to be caused principally by *M. tuberculosis*, but an unknown proportion of cases are almost certainly also due to *M. bovis*. The consumption of both unpasteurised milk and of poorly cooked meat (as well as from close contact with infected animals) must represent the main source of infection for humans in the region.[265] It remains a complete unknown, however, as to how much the disease might also be carried directly between human hosts in an immune compromised population.

Infection of *M. bovis* in humans is generally under-reported anyway in Africa – in fact it is barely reported at all. None of the national reports submitted to the WHO by African member states, for instance, mentions either the importance or the prevalence of *M. bovis* in human TB cases despite this disease being no less dangerous than common *M. tuberculosis* particularly in the presence of HIV/AIDS. This is hardly surprising: the resource to differentiate the diseases is almost entirely lacking. The bottom line is that little is known about this.

Bovine tuberculosis itself is certainly known to be widespread today throughout Africa and it is also known to infect a variety of animal hosts, both domesticated and wild. Ironically, it may not even be endemic to the continent. European settlers are thought to have originally brought the disease to the continent in the early 1800s. Although its existence has long been acknowledged, the general rates of infection in both cattle and people are simply not known, let alone controlled. It is estimated, though, that approximately 85% of the cattle in Africa and 82% of its human population live in areas where bovine TB is still only partially controlled or is not controlled in any meaningful way at all. In essence, Africa today is still pretty much where both Europe and North America were 80 years ago, but with the telling addition of having HIV at hand as well to make things a lot more complicated.

---

265 Avele WY et al., "Bovine tuberculosis: an old disease but a new threat to Africa", International Journal of Tuberculosis and Lung Disease, 8; 8 (2004) 924-37.

A 1998 article in the Journal of Emerging Infectious Diseases revealed that only seven of all African nations consider bovine TB to be a notifiable disease – still generally perceiving it as an animal and not a human infection. There is probably a good reason for this – and it is because *M. bovis* is clinically so difficult to distinguish from *M. tuberculosis* in the region. The two strains share 99% of their DNA sequences which means that the standard test for TB — microscopic examination of sputum — cannot possibly distinguish which strain might be causing the disease. According to Anita Michel of the Agricultural Research Council's Onderstepoort Veterinary Institute near Pretoria, South Africa, the lack of data on bovine TB relates to this continuing perception as an animal and not a human disease:

> "With the health problems relating to HIV/AIDS and human TB, bovine TB is inevitably assigned an extremely low priority."

Given the treatment resources generally available, it has to be said that discriminating between the strains of disease would hardly make much difference for treatment. The human treatment for *M. bovis* differs from drug-susceptible TB treatment only in that *M. bovis* is known to be inherently resistant to Pyrazinamide, one of the standard first line TB drugs. The three other first line drugs should still be active against *M. bovis* so the disease (as long as it occurs in an otherwise drug-susceptible form in an HIV-negative person and the treatment is adhered to) should still be fully curable.

But controlling *M. bovis* in the animal populations in the region would almost certainly reduce rates of infection (and therefore deaths) in humans as well – but this challenge remains one that has yet to be confronted in Africa. There is good evidence available that *M. bovis* is part of today's human problem. In 2006 in Tanzania, there was a screening programme conducted on both animals and humans. As many as 88% of the villages screened had at least one animal that tested positive for bovine TB, and 10% of people with stomach or lymph gland tuberculosis were identified as being infected by *M. bovis*, not *M. tuberculosis*.

The Tanzanian researchers concluded that:

> "The growing concerns about TB in Africa and the knowledge that *M. bovis* does contribute to the current human epidemic emphasise the importance of integrating veterinary, medical and wildlife sectors in the investigation and control of this disease."

Projects to investigate bovine TB are now underway in Chad, Mozambique, South Africa, Tanzania, Uganda and Zambia. The scientists involved are aware of the importance of quantifying the potential for disease transmission as patterns of animal and human movement change. Efforts so far, however, have been focusing mainly on quantifying the spread of the disease in wildlife before and after the establishment of wildlife parks, and have not yet focused at all on the human bovine epidemic if there is indeed one of any size.

Claire Geoghegan, from the Mammal Research Institute at the Department of Zoology and Entomology in the University of Pretoria believes that *M. bovis* is the cause of an unknown but significant number of human TB cases in Africa:

> "Bovine TB is definitely a developing country problem, but so little work has been done on this disease."

She is leading a South African research programme to quantify the prevalence of bovine TB in poverty-stricken areas, and particularly to establish who is most at risk and why. The study area is KwazaZulu-Natal in South Africa which is already recognised as one of the global hotspots for TB – including drug-resistant TB – and also for HIV/AIDS. Her work is focusing on farming communities there and her results could yet further confound ideas of simpler solutions to TB control in the region.

Geoghegan's research initially aims to discover where bovine TB is occurring in domestic livestock around South African wildlife parks. Earlier research has indicated that there is a high prevalence of bovine TB in buffalo, warthogs, kudu and even in some lions and cheetahs in the Kruger National Park in northern Mpumulanga province and also in the Hluhluwe-Mfolozi park in eastern KwazaZulu-Natal. It is being proposed that this bovine TB was originally passed to wild animals, particularly to buffalo, from domesticated cattle in the 1960s, but that this development only began to be picked up in the 1990s. A TB epidemic is also rife in the buffalo and antelopes of South Africa's Kruger National Park, where cattle are thought to have been the original reservoir. Transmission to wild life weakened by drought is occur at infected water holes or vegetation. It has then spread up the foodchain to lions feeding on infected prey. If all of this is true it may indicate a well-entrenched epidemic in African wild animals, originated from livestock.

Ultimately Geoghegan and her team hope to collate their results with other African data to develop mathematical models that might be used to predict bovine TB incidence throughout Africa. "Once we have the answers to our questions," says Geoghegan, "we can start education programmes to control any spread of the disease."

Geoghegan suspects that her study will show that bovine TB's threat to public health is underestimated, but that it can be effectively controlled and that this might help reduce not only disease but also endemic rural poverty. In Africa, cattle are important for food but they are also important cultural status symbols and signs of wealth: the more cows you have the richer you must be. And it is this close cultural and physical link with cattle, according to Geoghegan, that puts rural communities at such risk of infection.

One other logical possibility exists as well. Drug-resistance is accepted to be a predictable event given any amount of anti-TB drug treatment, the likelihood of which is proportionately higher if treatment is mismanaged. The possibility that the treatment of bovine TB (whilst assumed to be infection of *M. tuberculosis*) is being proportionately mismanaged in similar ways where treatment has been mismanaged in the wider epidemic has to be undeniable. If this has been the reality, it suggests that multi drug-resistant *M. bovis* would have been inevitably created at the same time. Whether this might directly infect another human being must also be considered, and it must be done in the light of this risk being higher in a population with high incidence of HIV/AIDS.

What bovine TB may suggest in relation to human tuberculosis

In 1999 an extraordinarily thought-provoking submission was made by Hellen Fullerton PhD to the UK's Parliamentary Select Committee on Agriculture. It was published as the 29th Appendix in its Fifth Report.[266]

The report itself was considering the problems of bovine tuberculosis in British cattle. Fullerton's submission wondered whether trace element nutrition could have been having an impact on the rising incidence of *M. tuberculosis*, not only in cattle but also in badgers in certain regions in the country. She also shed further fascinating light on the cattle-badger

266
http://www.publications.parliament.uk/pa/cm199899/cmselect/cmagric/233/233app30.htm

connections. Most of her submission was specific to cattle and ruminants, but it also contains food for thought in respect of the development of *M. tuberculosis* in humans.

Fullerton developed several hypotheses, but broadly speaking she advocated that raising the nutrient status of the entire food chain through the soil might result in both cattle and badgers being largely protected from TB.

She focused particularly on the mineral micro-nutrients of selenium, copper, zinc, cobalt and iodine, all of which are known to be essential to a healthy immune response. Subclinical deficiencies in all of these minerals are known to be widespread in UK herds, particularly so in the case of selenium. She considered that the same would probably therefore be the case with most other resident wildlife. An analysis of the fur of 36 badgers supported this idea, showed on average selenium levels of 0.036 mg/kg which was nearly ten times lower than the levels in the fur of domestic mammals fed a more balanced diet.

Certain other factors were identified as being likely to be suppressing these natural mineral-promoted immune resistances in British cattle. The principle cause, according to Fullerton, was simply because of arable and dairy farm intensification since the mid-1970s. Another was because of acid rain, with its sulphate content displacing selenium from its natural binding sites in the soil. A further cause for loss of selenium has been because of fertilisation of soil with ammonium sulphate for the same reasons. Another has been through silage treatments with certain additives that precipitate nutrient loss. A further adjunctive cause has been through the spreading of raw slurry with insufficient time being given for microbial destruction of its pathogens.

Other factors related more directly to the farming of the animals themselves. A failure to feed supplementary minerals in the form of mineral slicks was one contributory factor. A further cause for promotion of immune deficiency was simply from stress from modern more intensive farming methods. Another which related to selenium again) was through bulls being housed with cattle (bulls lose selenium at each ejaculation and so are more vulnerable than cows to TB, and could provide a reservoir of infection). Stress of any sort would also have been having predictable impact, and any pushing by the industry for high productivity would have had to have created stresses on cows' metabolisms. Moreover intensively managed farms pay less heed to cows in need of care or protection. This could manifest in many ways: stress due to short uncomfortable cubicles with inadequate bedding; slippery or uneven yards and walkways; also by competition at the silage face with more timid animals losing out.

Danny Goodwin-Jones of Trace Element Services has been pioneering the restoration of trace elements to depleted soils on livestock farms since 1983, and has reported to be solving problems which arise from depressed immunity. These have included recurring mastitis, failure to thrive and calf mortality, infertility in both male and female animals and also a reduced frequency of difficult births.[267] Appropriate treatment of the soil effectively immediately raises the nutritional status of the whole food chain – of cattle through their pasture, fodder and feed, and of badgers through the worms, insects and small mammals in the badger diet. Once zinc, copper, cobalt and iodine levels have been restored they have been seen to last for years. Selenium losses have to be watched for more carefully and have been found to need to be restored on an annual basis.

If this general hypothesis is correct then, according to Fullerton, by improving the soil the immune systems of UK cattle might be sufficiently enhanced to induce TB resistance, and all of the controversies concerning the routes of transmission would be rendered irrelevant. Interestingly, some anecdotal reports suggest little TB in organically farmed cattle which supports her view.

Fullerton's own suggestion was that TB infection was most likely initially from cattle-to-cattle transmission via exhalation in the crowded conditions of winter housing sequentially followed by the stressors of cold wet springs at turn-out with lower nutrient availability in the grass at this time stoked by all of the other possible stressors. The critical nutrient availability, as far as Fullerton was concerned, remained the key factor. If this were rectified she suggested that there would be no need at all to cull badgers and reactor cattle would quickly be seen to reduce.

She offered some compelling evidence of just how effective such a restoration of soils can be. Goodwin-Jones has had soils analysed from over 2,000 livestock farms throughout the UK. He has taken samples from different soil types and terrain, and even from individual fields on the same farm. Total selenium levels were rarely found to be higher than 0.3 ppm, and in some areas were as low as 0.08 ppm. A New Zealand soil survey rating, meanwhile, has classed anything less than 0.3 ppm as very low and 0.5-0.9 ppm as average. New Zealand is known to have selenium-poor soil,

---

[267] Goodwin-Jones R. Unpublished farm reports. Trace Element Services, Pencnwc, Abergorlech Road, Carmarthen SA32 7BA.

so these British averages should be considered to be very poor as well. Goodwin-Jones then restored the trace elements according to the needs of each individual farm and monitored the results in terms of animal response. For an optimum response in cattle and sheep he found that selenium levels should be boosted up to 0.8-1.2 ppm, a little higher than the New Zealand average. Responses which were specific to selenium levels included the elimination of herd problems of failure to conceive. Farmers reported an increase in cow conception pre-treatment rates of 45 per cent, which is the national average, up to 90 per cent post-treatment.

Fullerton further proposed that badger-susceptibility to TB is similarly exacerbated when their immune systems are depressed by the same selenium deficiency but is also exacerbated if they carry higher than average loads of internal parasites. Whilst acknowledging that the badger has been widely incriminated as the main source of infection, her report also suggested that other forms of wildlife should not be discounted, particularly birds with access to feed stores. Starlings, for example, have been heavily implicated in the transmission of farmyard salmonella.

Badgers turn out to be remarkably resilient to TB infection. In a study of badger carcases in Devon, 118 showed no visible lesions but 15 of them were shown on cultural examination to have been infected with *M bovis*. What was significant was that, of these 15, eight had granulomata which were infested with lungworm parasites, and six contained fungal parasites. This strongly suggested to Fullerton that badgers succumb more readily to TB if their immune systems are already stressed with a parasitic load – in fact that without this they may well be largely resistant. Mammal parasites are controlled by adequate levels of B12, a vitamin which requires cobalt for its structure and zinc for its biosynthesis. Large areas of TB-prone Devon and Cornwall are on granite where cobalt is endemically deficient and these are two of the regions in the UK where the badger link has been most made.

So what has all of this got to do with human tuberculosis? Some connections will almost certainly already have been made in readers' minds.

Whilst it would be wrong to point the finger at selenium deficiencies as being any sort of significant cause for human susceptibility to TB, its phenomenon in animals adds further support to the wider theory that poor nutrition is a major contributory factor. One other nutritional factor that impairs host macrophage function is protein malnutrition, and it is probably this nutritional deficiency, not selenium, which explains why TB is a disease of poverty in humans. Protein malnutrition is frankly unlikely to be ever seen in UK cattle, but if the immune-health of cattle can respond so quickly with a simple micro-nutrient addition in their natural diet, then a similarly rapid response might equally easily be seen in humans with nutritional improvements.

But there still could be an indirect link with selenium levels in the soil because there's some research which indicates a geographical link between regions of selenium-deficient soils and peak incidences of HIV/AIDS infection. Much of the Sub-Sahara is low in selenium; Senegal, however, isn't and has a significantly lower level of HIV than the rest of the continent. If there is any validity in this link, then there is likely also to be an inversely proportional link between incidence rates of TB in Africa and the levels of selenium in the soil.

There is also the matter of the link with parasitic infestations in the badgers. Such infestations could just be another major contributory risk factor in those living in poverty, just as it appears to be in the badgers.

The final link relates to the bulls and their ejaculated selenium. Bulls have a higher natural demand for selenium than cows because they lose a fraction of their selenium reserves with each ejaculation and if they are serving a herd then this loss is significant. If selenium deficiency is a major factor in the depression of immuno-resistance to TB, then this might explain why bulls appear to be more susceptible to TB than cows. It might also help explain why males of the human species might be more vulnerable to tuberculosis as well – exactly as they are in that most sexually active age-range of 15-35 years of age.[268]

---

[268] It should also be noted that low levels of selenium in UK soils are reflected generally in its low levels in food. The average intake in Britain used to be about 60mcg/day until joining the European Economic Community in the 1970s when the country was obliged to cut its imports of high-selenium Canadian wheat by a fifth and then depend on flour for bread on UK wheat which contains a tenth as much. As a result, and in combination with falling soil levels the average Se intake has declined. A 1995 Total Diet Survey showed that the population's intake was as low as 29-39mcg/d. The accepted Reference Nutrient Intake (RNI) given by the Committee on Medical Aspects of Food Policy (COMA) in 1991 was 60mcg/d for women and 75mcg/d for men. There may be other health impacts beyond susceptibility to TB in these findings.

Counterfeit and Substandard Drugs

"THERE'S REALLY NO SUCH THING AS THE 'VOICELESS'. THERE ARE ONLY THE DELIBERATELY SILENCED, OR THE PREFERABLY UNHEARD."

Arundhati Roy (2004)[269]

There were very worrying signs of another contributing factor to the pandemic which emerged early in 2012. A survey of available TB drugs was conducted in the unregulated private pharmaceutical marketplaces of 17 countries with known high burdens of TB (including India and several countries in Africa). The survey identified that 16% of all the tested TB drugs in the African countries failed quality control tests. Overall 9% of the tested drugs in the whole survey failed these tests, and approximately half of these failures were assessed to be sufficiently deficient to actually contribute to drug-resistance if they were used as part of a treatment programme.

It's important to recognise that none of these drugs were part of any national TB control programme in the countries concerned (although there is a risk that drugs like these can percolate into the approved supply chains through fraud). But these drugs were (and still are) readily available to TB patients, sometimes more so than the drugs which are supplied through approved channels.

There are several understandable reasons why patients might choose to resort to the private sector and might therefore expose themselves to these drugs (and also pay for them). One is when there are supply problems with the supply of drugs supplied through the Global Fund (as happened in 2012 for at least three months in Uganda, for instance). It has even been suggested that first line drugs may be cheaper in the private sector than on national programmes for patients in some countries, with Zambia being mentioned in this respect. Another is where there is a lack of confidence in the national provision of TB services – something which is frequently recognised as a common phenomenon in India. And the most probable is when there is existing drug-resistance circulating in the community but no corresponding provision of second line drugs available in the region's public health sector (as is the case in most of Africa and in many other

[269] The 2004 Sydney Peace Prize Lecture.

countries – even in high burden MDR-TB ones). In such cases patients may recognise that their treatment is failing or else they may realise they are relapsing, and then resort to the unregulated private sector because they see it is their only available option.

In June 2013 both epidemiologists and civil society experts publicly appealed to the newly formed government of Pakistan requesting that they crack down on counterfeit drugs in the country. Their appeal was fronted by Tammy Haq, the Executive Director of Pharma Bureau Ayesha. She is anxious to protect what is left of the reputation of her industry. She announced:

> "The Interior Ministry informed the National Assembly sometime back that 50% of all medicines in Pakistan are either counterfeit or substandard … [and] counterfeiting is equivalent to consumer fraud."

The idea that half of all medicines being substandard or counterfeit merely amounts to consumer fraud must reflect more the perspective of a representative of the pharmaceutical industry itself rather than of a physician. Given the estimated death toll that results from counterfeiting drugs, such 'fraud' should surely be more properly considered as a conspiracy for premeditated mass murder. Criminals are apparently widely drawn into the fake drugs business because it's seen as being a low-risk area of activity with a likelihood of a very high return. Whilst a heroin trafficker might receive a death sentence in many of these parts of the world where counterfeiting is rampant, individuals who are caught peddling fake pharmaceuticals may get, at worst, a few years in prison – and might even get away with a fine.

Haq claims that the WHO has assessed that up to 10% of the world's pharmaceutical trade (as much as 30% of it in developing countries) consists of fake medicines, while the global market for spurious/counterfeit drugs has been estimated to have a turn over value of US$431 billion.

Looking more carefully beneath the surface of the fake drug industry reveals a world which is perhaps as shocking as anything previously described on any page of this book. Counterfeiting has been described as 'the crime of the 21st century', but we normally think of counterfeiting as being the far more harmless hawking of fake designer clothes, of counterfeit Rolex watches, or of fake works of art. Even when it comes to fake drugs we tend to think first of all of counterfeit lifestyle medications – for erectile dysfunction or for hair loss. The human consequences of all of these are minimal compared to the consequences of fake medicines being peddled for life-threatening disease.

The production of counterfeit drugs as a criminal activity has been referred to as being a 'perfect crime' because false drugs are so difficult to detect, the criminals behind their manufacture so hard to trace, and the profit for the counterfeiter so high.[270] It can, however, also be perfectly deadly in its consequence.

The principal sources from which such drugs originate have consistently been identified as being Indian and Chinese though self-evidently Pakistan is a substantial source as well. The African continent, in the meantime, has been recognised as being their most frequently intended destination. Counterfeit drugs are now being estimated by some to constitute more than 30% of all medicines sold on the continent. According to the WHO, in fact, as much as 70% of all the drugs that were sold in Nigeria in 2001 were counterfeit.

There is a desperately sad and familiar ring to so much of the authoritative literature on the subject – familiar in that it sounds so similar in both its choice of words and in its tone, reflecting passages written or quoted on previous pages of this book in relation to the more probable prevalence of DR-TB in Africa:

> "Little is known about its true prevalence and impact, supply and demand, existing prevention and intervention strategies and their effectiveness, and other issues critical to understanding its nature and to developing evidence-based strategies to address it…
>
> "Because so little is known about the counterfeit drug trade in Africa it is difficult to provide any solid information regarding regional differences. Much of the published information is 'recycled' in that organizations often cite each others' statistics. Most of the information has been collected by international organizations and local government personnel and there are few empirical studies. Even with limitations, it is certain that the trade of counterfeit drugs is thriving throughout Africa, and most countries have been unable to effectively combat the threat."[271]

---

[270] Kontnik L - "Pharmaceutical counterfeiting: Preventing the perfect crime", Greenwood Village, CO (2004) Lew Kontnik Associates.

[271] Roy S Fenoff, Jeremy M Wilson - "Africa's Counterfeit Pharmaceutical Epidemic: The Road Ahead" (2009). http://a-cappp.msu.edu/sites/default/files/files/AfricaPharmaPaperFINAL.pdf

It all sounds so familiar.

What does seem likely is that anti-malarial and not anti-TB drugs are the principal problem – with the WHO suggesting in 2003 that as many as 20% of the one million African deaths from malaria were totally avoidable because they were the result of counterfeit drugs (the great majority of which would have also been children). The estimated extent of the fake drug trade for TB is still more vague, but there can be little doubt that it is substantial. One study in 2009, in fact, suggested that counterfeit drugs for tuberculosis and malaria together kill 700,000 people every year.[272]

Perhaps the most shocking single piece of evidence of the tragic effects of counterfeit drugs in Africa relates neither to malaria nor to TB, but relates to meningitis. The following is an extract from a WHO report from 2003 entitled "The Nigerian Meningitis Epidemic". It is included here because it typifies the extent of institutional neglect that can occur in matters concerning public health in Africa, neglect that is generally gets ignored by the world's media:

> "In 1995, a meningitis epidemic broke out in Niger. In response to the crisis, Niger authorities organized a country wide vaccination campaign. In an effort to combat the outbreak, Nigeria donated 88,000 vaccines which were given to more than 60,000 people. After the vaccines were administered, more than 25,000 people died. The Niger authorities suspected that the donated vaccines may have caused the deaths and conducted an investigation. The findings confirmed their suspicions that the drugs supplied had been substituted with counterfeit drugs that contained no active ingredients."

---

[272] Harris J, Stevens P, Morris J - "Keeping it real: Combating the spread of fake drugs in poor countries" (2009) - http://www.ncpa.org/sub/dpd/index.php?Article_ID=18062/

"Is Africa lost?"

"WE ARE FACING
ONE OF THE GREATEST PUBLIC HEALTH DISASTERS
SINCE THE BUBONIC PLAGUE."

J L Stanford, J M Grange and A Pozniak (1991)[273]

In 2013, it was being predicted that the 2015 goal of reducing TB mortality rates by 2015 to half of what they were in 1990 was "within reach". Right now, however, death rates in Africa are running at roughly twice the global average.

In fact seven years ago in 2006, 'Part II' of the Global Plan's "Global and Regional Scenarios of TB Control" speculated as to how hard it would really be to halve the death rate in Africa as had just been planned. It identified what it called "serious constraints" that would hamper this goal and then stated that overcoming these constraints would require "massive improvements in general health systems" and an equally optimistic "reduction of 50% in HIV incidence" – all of these in addition to powerful new diagnostic tools and substantially shortened treatment regimes. None of these has appeared as yet.

Unsurprisingly then, given this sober analysis, the authors of the report concluded that:

> "It is unlikely that even massive additional funding or even greater effort would be successful in overcoming the constraints."

Their answer? They chose not to elaborate.

It's difficult not to sound cynical about it, but it looks like there may have been good reasons to have been keeping those TB deaths which were tainted by a co-diagnosis of HIV out of the target numbers, because including them would have revealed such a dismal story. But even with this manipulation, no-one is seriously expecting that the death rate for Africa

---

[273] Stanford JL, Grange JM, Pozniak A - "Is Africa lost?" The Lancet, 338 (1991). 557–558.

could be anywhere near halved by 2015 – although even this isn't true, because a group of politicians (joined by some industry experts) went so far as to suggest in March 2013 that this might still be achievable. Their suggestion was contained in the so-called 'Swaziland Statement'. No-one should be holding their breath on the matter.

In order to better understand the possible prospects for this part of the world, some historical and sociological contexts deserve a little deeper exploration.

The Mining Factor

"TWO HUNDRED THOUSAND SUBTERRANEAN HEROES WHO, BY DAY AND BY NIGHT, FOR A MERE PITTANCE, LAY DOWN THEIR LIVES TO THE FAMILIAR 'FALL OF ROCK' AND WHO, AT DEEP LEVELS RANGING FROM 1,000 TO 3,000 FEET IN THE BOWELS OF THE EARTH, SACRIFICE THEIR LUNGS TO THE ROCK DUST WHICH DEVELOPS MINER'S *PHTHISIS* AND PNEUMONIA."

Solomon Tshekisho Plaatje (1914)[274]

The South African mining industry had its first boom years in the late 1800s. Its workers from the outset were exposed to silica dust, overcrowded hostels, poor nutrition and stress, all of which made them perfect hosts for TB. Not that much has changed, except that many of the mines are now miles deeper.

Silicosis is an occupational lung disease caused by exposure to the dust in mines. Miners affected by it face a consequential risk of developing active TB which is estimated to be almost three times higher than it is for miners free from the latent disease. Add HIV into the equation and things get even worse: HIV-positive miners who are affected by silicosis are estimated to

---

[274] Sol Plaatje (1876-1932) was a South African intellectual, journalist, linguist, politician, translator and writer. He was a founder member and first General Secretary of the South African Native National Congress (SANNC) in 1912, which would become the ANC ten years later.

be 15 times more likely to develop TB than HIV-negative miners free from silicosis.[275]

When miners became too sick to work, they return to their and then spread the disease to their nearest and dearest. The euphemistic term used for this by the industry is that the miners are 'retrenched' but what this really means is that they have been made redundant by the mine because of their failure to work. This action results in a miner's family losing its primary source of income because of a disease which the South African government today recognises is occupational. With no financial compensation provided by most mines because the foreign-owned mining companies continue to refuse to recognise that TB is an occupational hazard of their industry, these men have little means to support their families while they hopefully undergo at least six months of TB treatment.

The South African mining industry was originally pioneered by British immigrant miners from Cornwall and Wales. In "The White Death: Silicosis on the Witwatersrand Gold Mines, 1886-1910", Elaine Katz notes that these immigrants who had been working on the gold mines before the South African War of 1899-1902 failed to return to the Witwatersrand in any large numbers after the war largely because of silicosis. "Almost an entire generation, whose skills pioneered the South African gold mining industry, died from silicosis," she records.

But silicosis was not the only problem. It was soon realised that silicosis rendered miners much more likely to contract active TB and this was seen to particularly affect the black miners who were now taking over from those first miners. Official statistics from the first half of the 20th century show that white miners were suffering from higher recorded rates of silicosis, while black miners had higher rates of TB and pneumonia.

The following is an excerpt from the Milner Report on TB in the mines of South Africa which calculated that the average working life of a machine-driller on the Witwatersrand was seven years, and that their average life-span was 37:

> "The extent to which Miners' Phthisis [TB] prevails at the present time is so great that preventive measures are an urgent necessity, and that such a large number of sufferers in our midst is a matter of keen regret."[276]

---

[275] Reddy, M. et al. - "Deloitte on Mining & Metals: Taking the Gamble Out of Mining Related Risk", Johannesburg: Deloitte Touche Tohmatsu (2006).

This report was written in 1903, and that urgent necessity still exists. Paula Akugizibwe from the Aids and Rights Alliance for Southern Africa (ARASA) describes today's mining industry as being a "TB factory" and reckons that it is over a century behind schedule with regards to its proper response to the problem. Conditions by all accounts remain appalling, and they feed the recent strikes in the country's gold and platinum mines, one of which descended into tragedy and dozens of deaths in August 2012 as police intervened against the strikers in the country's Marikana region – an event which has since been described as a massacre.[277]

Back in 1930, it was already being estimated that over 60% of the black population of South Africa was latently infected with tuberculosis. By 1953 the rate of active disease was being measured to be 780 per 100,000 of the population in the northern and eastern parts of the country. Today, 60 years after TB drugs became available and 110 years after the Milner Report, these regional rates are higher still.

Incidence rates measured from notifications appeared to peak during the 1960s, and then apparently declined, although in reality this was probably only because of changing patterns of data collection, changes which coincided with the creation of the *bantustans*, the areas that were also euphemistically referred to as 'black homelands'. These amounted to little more than marginal territories where as many as 3.5 million black South Africans were forcibly relocated in the early 1970s having been denied their rightful South African citizenship. Because some of these territories were then declared as independent states, those infected with TB who were removed to them also found themselves erased from the reported national figures.

Other apartheid policies were undeniably responsible for much of the tuberculosis during this era, with rural poverty and rapid urbanisation providing further conducive conditions for the bacillus. The South African epidemic largely remained uncontrolled because the health service that was provided for the majority black population was so inadequate. Even today, whilst South Africa as a whole is regarded as a middle-income economy,

---

[276] Cited by Paula Akugizibwe, AIDS and Rights Alliance for Southern Africa (ARASA), SA AIDS Conference, April 1 2008. http://www.ghdonline.org/uploads/Akugizibwe_TB_and_Mines_in_Southern_Africa.pdf

[277] There have even been suggestions that the South African ANC government approved the use of force on the striking Marikana miners.

these *bantustan* areas are largely still recognised as being regions of 'absolute poverty'.

For many years the standard treatment, when it was available, was a 12 or 18 month period in hospital (on PAS, Isoniazid and Streptomycin). Rifampicin was only introduced in 1979 (although this was earlier than most of the rest of Africa). Then the treatment was changed to ambulatory (out-patient) care in order to save hospital costs and (supposedly) to make it easier for patients to access treatment. Such services as existed remained mainly hospital-based, meaning that patients had to travel long distances to access treatment, making it largely inaccessible and unaffordable. Drugs supplies in many areas were also erratic.

Then HIV/AIDS emerged as a problem of its own, and it all got that much worse. By 2007, South Africa's HIV epidemic was being assessed to represent 17% of the global burden of HIV/AIDS.

Today the incidence rate of TB in South Africa nationally is estimated to be a round 1,000 (per 100,000), second only to Swaziland with an even more terrifying rate of 1,350.[278] This makes TB the leading natural cause of death in South Africa.

Whilst underground extracting gold, diamonds, chromite, vanadium or coal, miners are constantly exposed to the silica dust that inflames the lungs and can trigger re-activation of latent TB. Meanwhile they also live in desperately cramped spaces, with the coughed-out mycobacterial content of one infectious miner potentially circulating for hours for others to inhale. These same miners are also at risk of being infected with HIV. Sex work is commonplace around the all-male hostels allowing HIV to finish the job that the working environment has begun, damaging the immune system so that a dormant TB infection can advance much more rapidly into infectious TB disease, now also potentially being composed of multiple or multi drug-resistant strains.

Sick miners return home – not just to homes in South Africa, but in territories ranging from the Southern Cape to Angola, Mozambique and Zimbabwe – and may then spread their disease to their families and communities. More often than not they receive no compensation, nor will they have access to any cross-border health referrals. They will also have no source of income to support themselves and their families while they are out of work receiving any treatment.

---

[278] WHO - "Global Tuberculosis Report 2013".

In this devastating way, mining-associated TB gives rise annually to an estimated 760,000 new cases in wider southern Africa each year.[279]. These new TB cases due to mining are estimated to represent one third of all new cases across sub-Saharan Africa, and 9% of cases worldwide. Inadequate and interrupted treatment can then readily lead to drug-resistant strains of the disease anywhere – and the development of MDR- or XDR-TB is almost guaranteed to be fatal in countries without DST and a regulated and approved supply of SLDs.

In fact, according to the South African Department of Health's "Tuberculosis Strategic Plan for South Africa 2007-2011", the South African gold mining industry may well have the highest incidence of TB anywhere in the world with incidence estimates among the half a million miners running anywhere between 3,000 and 7,000 per 100,000 miners per year. South African Health Minister Dr Aaron Motsoaledi is quoted saying on more than one occasion:

> "If TB/HIV is a snake in southern Africa, we know that its head is in South Africa in the mines."

Since 1956, the National Health Laboratory Service has been performing autopsies on the lungs of dead miners, mandated by law to examine the cardio-respiratory organs of dead miners with their relatives' consent. The institution currently has a data store of 105,000 autopsies carried out over 58 years. Its records tell a frightening story.

Firstly, they record that the data curves for both silicosis and pulmonary TB have been rising continuously since 1973 – from around 50 cases of each disease found per 100,000 autopsies to around 350 cases in 2011. But it is the significant rise since 1993, the year of the dismantling of apartheid, that must give more concern. In 1993 the rate of silicosis being found in the lungs of deceased gold miners was around 125/100,000. For TB it was just over 50/100,000. By 2011 the rate for silicosis had risen to nearly 400/100,000 and for TB to just under 350/100,000.

There ***is*** a compensation system for occupational disease in place in South Africa, but it is widely accepted that, with miners, it doesn't work.

---

[279] Stuckler D et al., - "Mining and risk of tuberculosis in sub-Saharan Africa", American. Journal of. Public Health, 101; 3 (2011) 524–30.

The very first piece of legislation aimed at compensating miners, the "Miners' Phthisis Allowance Act", was passed as long ago as 1911. The original realities, however, were heavily influenced by the politics of race. White miners benefitted from political voices which were legitimately expressed through their labour organisations – black miners, meanwhile, were effectively ignored. By 1973, white miners were eligible for payouts which were estimated to be between 12 and 15 times those being granted to black miners.

In 1993 this explicit racial differentiation within the mineworkers' compensation system was dropped, but more than 20 years later, black former miners and their families are still struggling to access the system's benefits. Currently the South African "Mine Health and Safety Act" requires all mines to maintain a system of medical surveillance as well as to monitor employees who are exposed to health hazards resulting in an annual report covering the health of all employees for every mine. The numbers of occupational diseases recorded are then collated and reported to the "Mine Health and Safety Inspectorate", which has a grandiose mandate to "safeguard the health and safety of mine employees and communities affected by mining operations".

Mineworkers' compensation is handled differently to other forms of worker compensation in the country, something which may account for part of the problem. It is handled under the aegis of the "Occupational Diseases in Mines and Works Act" which is itself facilitated by the Department of Health. Other compensation for occupational disease contracted during the course of work in South Africa is handled by the "Compensation for Occupational Injuries and Diseases Act" which is managed by the Department of Labour. Miners are seen to end up being fundamentally worse off under this system which can be seen to be discriminatory. There is no pension provision for sick former miners, for instance, whereas other sick workers qualify for a monthly pension after a certain threshold of disability. Miners also have to be more severely ill to qualify for even first-degree compensation.

The record of actual paying out of compensation is also appalling. A landmark 1998 study into silicosis prevalence among former Transkei miners in the Eastern Cape found that, of the workers who had been certified as having a compensatable disease, only 2.5% had been paid in full.[280] Other research by consultants from Deloitte from 2003 found that, of 28,161 certified claims, payouts were made in only 400 cases. This amounted to less than 1.5%.

The compensations themselves are supposed to be financed by levies paid by the mining houses which have historically exerted influence to control the amounts. As a result, the compensation fund is reported to be grossly under-resourced. A recent study by Yale University's Global Health Justice Project suggested that:

> "Even under the most conservative assumptions, the fund … is more than R600 million below the level required to cover current liabilities, and may in fact be R10 billion or more below the level required to cover the total annual costs to South African society."

This alone may help explain the rationale behind the bureaucratic failures. The system cannot possibly afford to pay out what it owes.

When miners do succeed in winning compensation, they are generally lump sum payments of between R48,000 and R180,000. It is arguable that these should in fact be pensions, particularly if there is so little alternative work.

Dr Thuthula Balfour-Kaipa, the head of "Health for the South African Chamber of Mines", accepts that there's a problem and agrees that the system itself needs an overhaul. The Chamber (which is part of the industry itself) has apparently been collaborating for five years with the Department of Health and the National Union of Mineworkers to try to improve access to compensation, but there's little evidence as yet of any progress. Balfour-Kaipa has identified that the industry is sitting on a time-bomb if increasing numbers of miners decide to collectively explore a legal route to access the money they feel is owed to them. The government, meanwhile, would appear to be obfuscating around its responsibilities by maintaining a system of unnecessarily impenetrable bureaucracy, whilst allowing most of the blame to fall on the industry. The Chamber's head of Health candidly elaborates:

> "If I were a miner, and I'm out there and I'm sick, I have an occupational lung disease and I know I'm supposed to be compensated – you know, I don't look at who is responsible for ***why*** I can't get access to a service or

[280] Trapido et al. - "Prevalence of Occupational Lung Disease in a Random Sample of Former Mineworkers, Libode District, Eastern Cape Province, South Africa", Americal Journal of Industrial Medicine, 34 (1998) 305–13.

> ***why*** I can't get the compensation. All I know is that I worked at a mine. And so, in a way then, the anger gets directed at the companies. So I would say that it is imperative that the industry … makes sure that the compensation system works."

The major issue for the many former miners who are eligible for compensation is not the mine companies themselves as much as it is the bureaucratic hurdles that have to be jumped through. These appear to be the main reason for the poor success rate of pay-outs. The first hurdle is a medical examination – possibly the most straightforward part of the process. The body responsible for certifying miners' claims is the "Medical Bureau for Occupational Disease" (MBOD), and it requires a medical form, a worker ID (including fingerprints) and labour records. The popular picture of the bureau's operations is far from being an encouraging one. One report has claimed that the MBOD's offices have "towering stacks of claim records requiring evaluation" including ones that were filed as long as 50 years ago.

Once certified, the claims are then referred to the office of the Compensation Commissioner, who sends a form back for the worker to complete. Given the domestic conditions that many sick miners will have returned to, this bureaucratic hurdle alone can be too much. If their resubmission is found to be imperfect (as is often the case) subsequent letters will be sent back to the claimant, but these often go to old addresses and the claim falters through ineptitude.

For migrant miners drawn from areas outside South Africa the challenges of seeking compensation are almost impossible. In a register of cross-border silico-tuberculosis claims for Lesotho from 1998 to 2003, only six claims were successfully filed.

Dr Motsoaledi may say that the mines are the head of the snake of TB in southern Africa, and that if you want to kill a snake you need to stamp on its head – but there has been little evidence of any serious stamping getting underway. There are some signs, however. In August 2012 the 15 Southern African Development Community (SADC) heads of state signed the "SADC Declaration on TB and the Mining Industry". This declaration committed the countries to "moving towards a vision of zero new infections, zero stigma and discrimination, and zero deaths resulting from TB, HIV, silicosis and other occupational respiratory lung diseases".

Over a year later and a "Code of Conduct" was still being developed to accompany this ambitious declaration. This document is intended to provide a legal framework which might hold mining companies accountable for improving working conditions and also specifically for addressing TB. The delay in developing this code has been explained as being because direct representation from the mineworker and ex-mineworker community was bafflingly left out of the initial consultation process.

The 'Swaziland Statement' came next, signed in March 2013. It saw regional governments being joined by members of the donor community as well as by multilateral organisations like the World Bank, Global Fund, International Organization for Migration, UNAIDS and international NGOs. The document is a pledge to renew efforts in the last 1,000 days of the Millennium Development Goals to halt and reverse the spread of TB, especially in relation to TB in mining.

The mining companies themselves are still showing a lack of commitment to working with government to form any sort of harmonised response to the issue, evidenced by their notable absence from the signing of the Swaziland Statement. But the government of South Africa has hardly hurried on the matter either given that it's been 20 years since the dismantling of apartheid when this job should have properly been begun.

With US$2.5 trillion in mineral reserves, South Africa still has the largest mining sector in the world. Half a million miners are employed in the industry, and migrant workers are actively welcomed because they contribute to the nation's wealth. The industry itself, meanwhile, is still owned by multi-national companies that are largely head-quartered in the capital cities of Europe and North America.

This disease takes a heavy economic toll as well as a human one. It's been shown for a long time that tuberculosis is a source of financial loss to a community in terms of the wage-earning power of its individual members. This is something which 70 years ago was recognised as "too frequently bringing its victims individually and collectively to localised poverty and destitution".[281] What is only becoming properly clear today, though, is the truly devastating effect that this can have on a country and its whole economy.

[281] Sir Arthur S. MacNalty, UK Chief Medical Officer, Ministry of Health (1939).

According to a study commissioned by the Southern African Development Community, TB costs South Africa alone US$886 million each year. This figure includes not just health-care costs, but allows for the impoverishment that is promoted when family providers are either too sick to work or die. But this is only part of the picture regionally because it is having massive economic effects on neighbouring countries too.

The TB incidence rate for Swaziland, one of the countries which feeds the South African mining industry with workers, is currently estimated to be the highest in the world, over 30% higher than its nearest rival at the top of this list, although the country still fails to claim a place in either official list of high burden countries.

Its HIV infection rate is also unprecedented and is possibly the highest in the world at 26.1% of all adults, and at over 50% of adults in their 20s. This combined epidemic (sometimes described as a 'syndemic') has effectively stopped its national economic and social progress, and is at a point where it endangers the existence of Swazi society as a whole. The United Nations Development Program has suggested that, if the expansion of disease continues unabated, the "longer term existence of Swaziland as a country will be seriously threatened".[282]

This syndemic has reduced life expectancy so that the country also has the highest age- standardised death rate in the world, and one of the lowest life expectancies at birth. With an unmatched crude death rate of 30 per 1,000 people per year, about 2% of Swaziland's total population dies of TB/HIV every year.

February 2014 saw three major events that have the potential to finally catalyse genuine change towards reducing the burden of TB and other occupational lung diseases among miners. A Mining and TB Summit was organised by the Stop TB Partnership, intended to bring together the SADC Ministers for Health, Labour, Mining and Finance to meet with the CEOs of the major mining companies and also the miners' representatives to attempt to decide on a programme of action along with practical steps and targets for industry and governments to take.

[282] United Nations Development Programme - "Draft country programme document for Swaziland (2006-2010)".

This summit was directly followed by the Mining Indaba, which is the largest annual conference on mining and mine investment in the region. In addition, the World Bank was scheduled to release an economic analysis of the regional impact of the TB epidemic in the mines. This was expected to highlight the potential financial incentives for mining companies if they invest more in TB prevention, diagnosis and treatment.

To date there is no evidence of this report nor of any other progress beyond an ongoing mining strike at platinum mines owned by the British company Lonmin which is the longest in South African history .

Looking ahead

"..AN EYESORE SPOILING AN OTHERWISE BEAUTIFUL VIEW.."

Steve Biko (1978)[283]

The world during Cold War years was divided into three, the bottom tranche of which was commonly referred to as the 'third world'. More recently it has become customary to divide the world for similar purposes into two – with the lower tranche termed the so-called 'developing world'. The experience of Swaziland suggests that a third (lower) descriptor may yet again be needed – one that marks countries out as being in an almost hopeless plight – what might be termed the 'currently undevelopable'. And by implication, despite other more encouraging indicators suggesting reductions in rates of absolute poverty, more countries than tiny Swaziland may yet join this club.

So which other countries are most at risk? First and foremost they are the countries which lie to the north of South Africa: Namibia (655), Zimbabwe (552), Lesotho (630), Botswana (408), Mozambique (552), and Zambia (427) and Malawi (354).[284] The clues as to why this possibility exists are there in the figures identified in brackets beside each country – figures which relate to the incidence rate of TB per 100,000 population, almost all of which are amongst the highest in the world. More worrying still is the fact that all of them have a known rate of co-infection of over 50% and so

[283] Steve Biko - "I write what I like", London, Heinemann (1978).
[284] These figures all relate to the 2013 WHO Global Tuberculosis Report.

are also particularly vulnerable not just to TB, but to developing MDR-TB (or worse).

And how many of these countries (along with South Africa and Swaziland) are listed in those 22 high burden TB countries? Just three – South Africa, Mozambique and Zimbabwe, although all eight do fall in a list of the 12 countries in the world with the highest estimated incidence rates of TB.

And how many find a place in the 27 high burden MDR-TB countries (HBMDR-TBCs)? Just one – South Africa itself.

Is it reasonable to suggest that all nine might already have problems with MDR-TB which may reflect and might even approach South Africa's? Of course it is, and there is even evidence of this possibility. Swaziland was reported in 2009 to have had the highest level of ***primary*** MDR-TB ever reported in Africa at 7.7%.[285] If this isn't evidence of drug-resistance imported by migrant workers, it's difficult to decide what might be.

Meanwhile the world has largely been choosing to ignore this possibility. In 2009 the WHO's annual global report on drug-resistant TB barely raised its eyebrows as it recorded reported incidence of drug-resistance from around the world, including data from only four countries in Africa only one of which was in the south. Since Africa was already recognised as having the highest regional TB mortality rates along with 13 of the 15 countries in the world with highest incidence rates of disease, the fact that so little attention was being paid to the continent in the report was concerning to anyone who cared to notice.

Few apparently did, although the general regional situation with TB was recognised by some, summed up in the following critique that was published by a panel of experts in 2012 in the Journal of Infectious Diseases:

> "It is worrisome to note that…only half of the estimated total tuberculosis caseload is detected in the WHO Africa region, implying that more than

---

[285] Seddon JA, Hesseling AC, Marais BJ et al. - "Paediatric use of second line anti-tuberculosis agents: a review", Tuberculosis (Edinburgh), 92 (2012) 9–17.

> half of active tuberculosis cases remain undetected and remain a source for continued transmission of *Mycobacterium tuberculosis*."[286]

The WHO Global Task Force on TB Impact Measurement had been established in mid-2006. Its mandate was to ensure the best possible assessment of whether the 2015 global targets for reductions in the burden of disease caused by TB were going to be achieved. It reported on the progress in the years leading up to 2015 and the strengthening of the capacity for monitoring and evaluation at country levels. Since 2011 (which was arguably a little late in the day) one of the Global Task Force's three priorities has been focused on developing and applying standards and benchmarks for TB surveillance. Its long-term goal is to directly measure the burden of disease caused by TB from routine surveillance data using notification data to measure TB incidence and using VR data to measure TB mortality. The Task Force's subgroup on TB surveillance set to work on a TB surveillance checklist of standards and benchmarks, to assess a national surveillance system's ability to accurately measure TB cases and deaths, and to identify any gaps in national surveillance systems that need to be addressed.

This was completed for the African region and reported upon in the 2012 WHO Global Report. It revealed that (with the single exception of one carried out in Eritrea in 2005) the most recent national surveys in the African Region were undertaken between 1957 and 1961.

At long last we may now be seeing better progress. The 2013 Global Tuberculosis Report announced that a total of six had been planned for Africa, and that one (in Nigeria whose frightening findings have already been discussed) had already been completed.

Five years earlier in 2008, a paper which was published in the Journal of Emerging Infectious Diseases had already very politely and cautiously suggested that everyone might be missing something that could well prove to be very serious indeed. The paper began by pointing out the anomalous

286 Alimuddin Zumla et al. - "Eliminating tuberculosis and tuberculosis–HIV co-disease in the 21st century: key perspectives, controversies, unresolved issues, and needs", Journal of Infectious Disease, 205, supplement 2 (2012).

fact that, despite a "dramatic" increase in TB rates in Africa, the region was reporting the lowest median levels of drug-resistance in the world.[287]

The authors then went on to explore the possible explanations for this, positing first what they described as the "most commonly put forward" explanation. This suggested that there were "well-functioning control programs in Africa," and that "89% of the population in the WHO-defined region of Africa" was covered by DOTS. They then pointed out that this purported DOTS coverage failed to accord at all with the fact that the countries with lowest rates of both detection and cure were also clustered in Africa. They didn't go so far as to suggest that such a theory was ridiculous, although, given the facts it surely was. They did, however, suggest that things weren't adding up to a more probable reality, and concluded that this first explanation just didn't really hold water at all.

The second explanation they reviewed was that, since Rifampicin had been introduced later in Africa than in other regions, there had simply been too little time for any meaningful MDR-TB epidemic to develop in the region. Their report was written in 2008, and Rifampicin was first developed in 1966. So just how "recent" had this delayed introduction of the TB wonder drug been? The earliest known introduction of Rifampicin in Africa was in 1979 in South Africa and the latest was 1989 in Zambia, 23 years after the drug's discovery. This itself should have constituted a public health concern at the time, but be that as it may, the study's authors also discounted this second theory by explaining that TB is known to develop resistance to Rifampicin "rapidly" in the presence of HIV/AIDS. They also believed that there would have been time enough for this to happen despite this original delay in the introduction of the strongest drug in the pharmaceutical cabinet.

They then went on to develop a far more probable explanation, one which is also the most obvious – that the field results for the African region concerning drug-resistance were simply "still incomplete, despite the recent publication of the WHO Fourth Global Report". They added:

---

[287] Yanis Ben Amor, Bennett Nemser, Angad Singh, Alyssa Sankin and Neil Schluger - "Underreported threat of multidrug-resistant tuberculosis in Africa", Journal of Emerging Infectious Diseases, 14; 9 (2008).

> "Furthermore, one might speculate that those countries capable of providing DRS data may have been the ones most likely to have a well-functioning NTP, laboratory structures, and transport networks, which would bias overall reporting."

And they further wrote that:

> "Even if this is not the case, overall low levels of reporting make the findings of the [Fourth Global Report] report questionable."

They even went so far as to suggest that the accepted report and its associated explanations might not be "an accurate reflection of reality", and stressed that:

> "In light of the added threat of XDR-TB within the African context of high HIV prevalence, a thorough assessment of TB drug-resistance and evaluation of data-specific deficiencies is urgently needed."

The report was concluded with the cautious suggestion that:

> "MDR-TB is likely to be more prevalent in Africa than previous reports indicated."

There really should have been no surprise here at all because a survey from 1999 (a full nine years before the paper quoted above) had attempted to review available global trends in drug-resistance at the time, and one of the fingers which it pointed was in the direction of southern Africa.

Mozambique was one of only eight countries in Africa that had responded to the report – and, significantly, was the only one with a survey purporting to be of the whole country, so was also perhaps the only one that could have been really treated seriously. The numbers it submitted reflected not only the largest national cohort surveyed but also cast Mozambique as the country with the highest percentage prevalence as well (at 3.5% which was high at the time).[288] So the writing was already on the wall back in 1999 for anyone who cared to read it.

---

[288] Marcos A. Espinal et al. for the World Health Organization–International Union against Tuberculosis and Lung Disease Working Group on Anti-Tuberculosis Drug-resistance Surveillance - "Global Trends in Resistance to Antituberculosis Drugs", New England Journal of Medicine, 344 (2001) 1294-1303.

The 2008 paper on under-reporting in Africa had also discussed the possible ramifications of Category II retreatment failure rates and its association with MDR-TB. Such retreatments, the authors suggested, could fail in many instances simply because a given patient may already have MDR-TB – and high rates of failure should thus be seen as being a possible marker for pre-existing MDR-TB. In fact, in environments where DST is absent, it may be the ***only*** real marker. But the paper also went further. It suggested that this WHO-recommended retreatment regime might itself be a major cause of both MDR-TB and XDR-TB because the suggested retreatment regimens amounted to adding just one drug to an already failing regimen, potentially intensifying or amplifying the levels of drug-resistance.

There was nothing new in their theory, and solid evidence of it had already revealed itself on African soil more than two years earlier. It happened in 2005, at the Church of Scotland Hospital in the village of Tugela Ferry in KwazaZulu-Natal, South Africa. Doctors at the hospital, already used to deaths from both TB and HIV, became worried when patients who had been responding well to HIV drugs began dying very quickly from TB.

Of the 542 people with TB at the hospital in 2005 and early 2006, 221 (41%) had MDR-TB - but 53 of them were found not to respond to ***any*** of the available second line drugs. Of these 53 patients 52 died, half of them within 16 days of diagnosis, a full four weeks before any drug-susceptibility test available anywhere could have been completed to properly inform their treatment. And six of them were health workers.

This particularly deadly strain of tuberculosis was subsequently found to be resistant to seven of the nine drugs that were tested, and the remaining two drugs that would have been active against it were not available in South Africa at the time. According to Salim Karim, an epidemiologist who was working on the outbreak at the Nelson R. Mandela School of Medicine in Durban, the patients were "dying like flies".

This event comprised the first major outbreak not just of XDR-TB, but of what is now referred to by many as extremely drug-resistant (XXDR-TB). In fact this single outbreak accounted for 16% of the known XDR-TB cases worldwide at that time. What was even more worrying was its having been so spectacularly and rapidly lethal. The entire episode was fully reported by the WHO in 2006, and offered a chilling wake-up call to the world that the resurgence of TB might be taking a terrible turn for the worse. People simply didn't die from TB in a matter of days – they should have been taking months or even years to do so. The one factor which the world decided to largely ignore was the fact that this event took place on African soil where continental rates of DR-TB at the time were supposedly so low and where supplies of second line drugs were also poor – because mismanagement of second line drugs ***had*** to have been part of the cause of the outbreak. The local epidemiologists may not have ignored this, but the official response to the outbreak suggested that the global authorities were still glossing over this in any of their calculations which were intended to model where rates of DR-TB might be being most underestimated.

It certainly wasn't being ignored by everyone. Dr Mario Raviglione, WHO's Stop TB Department Director, reported on it in 2006:

> "Tugela Ferry was a wake-up call that there were problems in the management of TB in southern Africa."

By November 2007 a further 205 cases of the strain had been discovered, but bad news had already been breaking in South Africa for years before this. Some scientists had begun sounding the alarm as early as 2003, having identified new XDR-TB superbugs which they said were circulating in communities over on the Western Cape. One particular variant, simply termed DRF150, was found to be resistant to almost all of the antibiotics used to treat drug-resistant TB.

This newly emerging mutant strain had not been identified before anywhere else in the world. This outbreak had had its focal point in George, where 60 patients had been affected, but another 20 cases had also been found in other areas north of Cape Town. The team which had identified the strain was led by Professor Tommie Victor of Stellenbosch University's Faculty of Health Sciences, one of South Africa's major TB research facilities. They also reported that more than 60% of the drug-resistant TB which they had identified was being transmitted from person to person. Up until then, expert opinion conformed to the idea that almost all drug-resistant TB occurred in people who did not take their TB medication regularly. The team's findings turned this idea on its head.

It is not unreasonable to suspect that such strains were simultaneously circulating not just in both the Western and Eastern Capes, but also in the neighbouring countries in southern Africa, having been carried there by migrant workers. At least as far as public health strategies are concerned, it would have been wiser to assume this to be the case until proven otherwise rather than await scientific confirmation, since such confirmation invariably (and inevitably) lags so far behind the development of the disease.

Some level of confirmation of this probability has been published quite recently. A new paper published in the Centres for Disease Control and Prevention's 'Emerging Infectious Diseases' journal warned that the first cases of "totally drug-resistant" tuberculosis had been found in South Africa and that the disease was "virtually untreatable".[289] It also repeated the suggestion that the absence of routine second line drug-susceptibility testing was concealing the problem and suggested that the treatment of MDR-TB with an inadequate standardised regimen in accordance with 2004 guidelines may have led to inappropriate treatment of undiagnosed pre-XDR-TB cases.[290] If so, this regimen would have prolonged the period of infectiousness and would have led to transmission to close contacts as well as having increased the risk of amplification of resistance.

Further confirmation of the critical state of affairs in South Africa has been provided by Professor Nulda Beyers, the Director of the Desmond Tutu TB Centre at Stellenbosch University. He cited a list of challenging factors that have been contributing to the South African epidemic, including poverty, the prevalence of HIV/AIDS, the legacy of apartheid, and individual health-seeking behaviour.

What concerned him most was that, in contrast to an apparent decrease in TB levels in some other countries in the region, and despite South Africa's status as a middle-income developing country with a substantial spending on health, TB incidence rates continued to rise and rise. In fact he described them as being at levels that he considered now to be out of control:

> "When something is out of control it's exactly that – one can't get away from it. Here in the Western Cape, one in every three minibus taxis has a person with infectious TB in that taxi. Once it has reached those proportions it's very difficult to unravel what was the reason the figures got so very high."

The possibility that one person in every three passing minibus might be actively infectious suggests that one person in 45 in the Cape Town townships may be actively infectious.

---

[289] Klopper M. et al. - "Emergence and Spread of Extensively and Totally Drug-Resistant Tuberculosis", South Africa Journal of Emerging Infectious Diseases. 19; 3 (2013).

[290] www.sahealthinfo.org/tb/mdrtbguidelines.pdf.

Another earlier report, one of the few that has ever specifically reviewed the situation in Africa, had offered an uncomfortable question in its final sentence:

> "If the continent is finding difficulty addressing TB, a well-defined disease caused by a well-defined agent, which is fully treatable with effective and affordable drugs through internationally recommended guidelines, then how will the continent fare against MDR-TB and XDR-TB?"[291]

One of the many paradoxes in the fight against TB is that, as a basic rule, no TB control programme at all is better in the longer run than a poorly managed one, because a poor programme allows the disease to smoulder and then re-ignite into a drug-resistant epidemic. With an existing MDR-TB epidemic, however, there should no doubt at all that this basic rule is even more relevant, and ignoring it is also far more dangerous.

[291] Amor Y. et al. - "Underreported Threat of Multidrug-Resistant Tuberculosis in Africa", Emerging Infectious Diseases, 14; 9 (2008) 1345–52.

Migrant workers

"ON THE EDGE OF THE CITY YOU'LL SEE US AND THEN
WE COME WITH THE DUST AND WE GO WITH THE WIND."

Woody Guthrie (1960)[292]

One group which remains of special concern in relation to the spread of the pandemic are migrant workers. They are a phenomenon all of their own within the epidemic, and they have been that way before.

In the early and mid-20th century, the wider TB epidemic in Japan was fuelled by migrant workers who had come to the cities, working and staying in conditions that were conducive to tuberculosis, and who then went home sick, subsequently spreading the disease to the countryside. In that instance, the phenomenon affected young women working in the country's newly industrialised textile industry. Today it primarily affects men, whether in China, India or the mines of South Africa – or indeed in any low-income country anywhere in the world.

Most often they are poor but in spite of this they often travel far looking for work, crossing borders both legally and illegally. Many leave villages and join one of the ever growing shanty towns and slums in the burgeoning megacities in Africa, Asia or South America. In every instance, these floating migrant populations carry higher rates of TB than the national averages. More often than not they both work and live in conditions that promote transmission of tuberculosis and make its diagnosis and treatment more challenging if not impossible. They are also usually so poor that the cost of adequate diagnosis and treatment is prohibitive if they have to pay for it – and they are often legally excluded from any local health service. If they do start treatment they are also more likely to relapse than patients with better residential stability, and they are almost impossible to track if they disappear.

If migrant workers sicken to the extent that they are unable to work they frequently find themselves dismissed and unable to earn further income. If they cannot access treatment locally they may well return to their homes because subsidized management of tuberculosis may be only available to them there.

[292] From the Guthrie song "Pastures of Plenty".

Additionally, such migrant workers also sometimes recourse to unprotected sexual intercourse with sex workers, and thus run the compound risk of infection or co-infection with HIV or other sexually transmitted disease.

In China migrant workers number over 260 million men and women and the country's recent rapid economic growth has largely been dependent upon them. At least 160 million of them (mostly men) live in cities far away from their home regions. They might earn an average of US$3 per day (a lot more than they can earn in their home regions) but they are notoriously exploited and marginalized in the process. Furthermore, their general welfare rights are severely restricted by the *Hukou* system of residency permits which ties individuals to their originally registered residence for any subsequent social welfare benefits. The system dictates that citizens born in rural zones can't switch registration to become urban residents. Originally the policy was intended to restrict movement that was considered undesirable, but since 1992 citizens have been allowed to leave their area (albeit only temporarily) for more remunerative work. As such, millions of Chinese live outside their officially registered areas with minimal eligibility for access to local government services. They then find themselves living in conditions which have been described as being much the same as those of illegal immigrants. If they then contract tuberculosis the only way that they can access treatment is by returning home, something they are understandably reluctant to do. As a result they often remain infectious while doing their best to tough out the disease.

India not only has a similarly massive migrant workforce of over 80 million within its borders, but it has a massive number engaged in migratory employment outside the country as well, both in South East Asia and throughout the Middle East. At any time, there are estimated to be around 7.5 million Indians in the Gulf States alone.

The tradition of the Indian migrant worker is a longstanding one, but the background to its current episode had its beginnings in social tragedy. In the 1990s Indian agricultural economy collapsed having become increasingly non-remunerative and leaving much of its workforce destitute. Between 1996 and 2003 an estimated 100,000 peasants took their own lives (amounting to a suicide of an Indian farm worker roughly every 45 minutes for a period of seven years) whilst millions more deserted the countryside looking for work.

Of the 80 million migrant workers within India itself around 40 million are said to work in the construction industry, 20 million are domestic workers, two million are active sex workers, five million are call girls, and between one and two million work in illegal mines – the most conducive working environments of all for tuberculosis to thrive as we know from the longstanding South African experience.

In South Africa the relationship between migrant workers and TB is particularly well-recognised. In March 2013, Dr Aaron Motsoaledi, the Minister of Health for South Africa, described those migrant workers who come to his country from neighbouring countries Africa specifically to work in its highly profitable mining sector:

> "Mineworkers come from the whole sub-region; they come here to our mines to catch TB and HIV and take it back home."

Somehow he managed to make it sound almost as if they do so on purpose. It's clear from his observation that he is well aware that this particular phenomenon of economic migration is far from being solely a South African problem, since Motsoaledi is also fond of calling the mining industry the "head of the snake" of the HIV and TB epidemic in the wider region of southern Africa which includes eight other countries.

All such groups, whether they work in mines, brothels or sweatshops, are vulnerable to tuberculosis, and collectively they form a significant single component part of the overall global TB burden. Tackling this group presents an enormous challenge, but failing to do so means that a large residual epidemic is bound to remain whatever new developments occur in terms of drugs or vaccines.

Infection Control, the 'Q' Word and the "Swamp of Ideology"[293]

"AT THE TIME, I WAS PRACTISING IN A FAR DISTANT LAND WHERE TUBERCULOSIS WAS BY FAR THE MOST COMMON DISEASE; SO COMMON THAT EVERYTHING WAS CONSIDERED TUBERCULOSIS UNTIL PROVEN OTHERWISE."

Theodore Dalrymple (2008)[294]

The general tendency for media reports on DR-TB has been to feed (or, worse still, feast) on the instinctive human fear of foreign disease because doing so sells papers. Such fear can certainly help raise awareness, something which still remains in far too short supply, but the awareness which it raises can just as easily become misplaced or even misdirected, almost always on account of the issues being over-simplified in the telling by the media.

The first fear that is peddled is that we are all facing a new type of Black Death – one that might sweep around the world killing half of the population in its path. With TB today, even with the more virulent drug-resistant strains, this is extremely unlikely – not just because it spreads so slowly, but because it is not super-infectious like bubonic or pneumonic plague must have been, and because the disease is dependent on contributory social factors for it to flourish. With such a degree of inefficient transmission the global pandemic of DR-TB should be relatively efficiently stalled and controlled in all better resourced countries. It should certainly not be allowed the opportunity to maintain any sizeable infectious base by developing a critically sized pool of latent disease with which to feed an ongoing epidemic.

Even this may be an oversimplification, however, because recent developments in the understanding of infectivity suggest that some individuals can be dramatically more infectious than others. This was the case with SARS, for instance. It was finally realised from contact tracing that most people who had contracted the virus either didn't infect anyone else at all or only passed it on to a single person. During this short-lived

[293] The "swamp of ideology" was a phrase used by Paul Farmer to describe the complexities of quarantining HIV patients.

[294] Theodore Dalrymple, - "Too posh to infect?" the BMJ; 337: a1354 (2008).

micro-pandemic, however, a few individual people inexplicably did infect many others, and it was these few who had turned a disease that might otherwise never have even been spotted on the infectious disease radar into a four-month global panic. In fact SARS is now believed to have only gone global at all thanks to one individual – a so-called 'disease super-spreader', a Chinese doctor who infected more than a dozen people at a Hong Kong hotel, with one of the people he infected subsequently bringing the virus to Canada.

It is now being realised that something similar could be happening with DR-TB at a much slower speed. It is recognised, for example, that most of the current primary DR disease in South Africa is being transmitted by only a small fraction of the country's drug-resistant infectious patients: today 80% of new DR-TB in South Africa is believed to be being caused by person-to-person transmission, but nevertheless it is thought that only a relatively few individuals are doing most of this transmission.

Such ideas raise huge ethical and moral issues. Should such people be sought out and isolated for the good of the community? This has happened once already – in 2007, a supposed XDR-TB case (who turned out to be actually misdiagnosed) was put into forced isolation in the US simply out of a reactive fear of his transmitting deadly disease. Perhaps after all there is some justifiable cause for the fear that media reports tend to promote, although such fear can too easily be twisted towards other agendas, ones which may be as much intended to deliberately marginalise vulnerable minority communities or restrict immigration as much as they might be intended to prevent spread of drug-resistant disease.

It certainly would seem sensible for a country that is largely clean of DR-TB to monitor access to it by peoples from other countries that are known to have high rates of the disease. If this merely results in public fear, however, the result will do no more than stoke an obsession directed towards keeping disease out rather than promoting efforts to holistically confront what is a global problem. In fact it may be that such an obsession will ultimately be seen as one of the humanitarian obscenities of our age – even as a crime against humanity. It will be difficult to see it otherwise if today's developed countries remain focused on keeping disease out while at the same time continuing to recruit qualified doctors from those affected countries for the benefit of their own relatively wealthier, healthier and more fortunate citizens.

It cannot be denied that something of this sort is already happening in Britain, for instance. Potential immigrants from high incidence countries are now being screened by X-ray back at their source countries rather than on arrival in the UK itself. Such a policy is agreed to be a sensible one from the perspective of the UK, but if Britain is simultaneously recruiting the very resource which can best be put to use to fight the disease in the source country for its own benefit (i.e. its trained doctors and health workers) this hardly amounts to an ethical immigration policy.

Everyone agrees that the two most important factors for infection control are early diagnosis and prompt implementation of effective treatment. The first, as challenging as it is, offers a compellingly simple solution: get the resources in place and then track down the disease. It is the second of these which poses the real problem though, because the idea simultaneously assumes that effective treatment is available. The WHO itself, for instance, "strongly recommends" that all governments should ensure, as their top priority, that every patient has access to high quality TB diagnosis and treatment for TB which includes drug-resistant forms of the disease. But, as we well know, this is exactly what ***isn't*** being provided on the ground where the problems are the greatest.

So what about the idea of quarantining (or more technically, of legally enforced isolation) as a way of protecting the majority when so many national systems are in varying degrees of melt-down?

Unfortunately, things are far from simple in this respect. The WHO gets as close as it can to a fighting stance by strongly recommending a right to the provision of decent TB treatment for all. In doing so it sets out a number of "rights" and "responsibilities" for TB patients anywhere in its "Patients' Charter for TB Care".[295] These rights include a right to free and equitable access to tuberculosis care, a right to receive both proper medical advice and treatment (including for those with multi drug-resistant tuberculosis), and a right to benefit from proactive community outreach, education, and prevention campaigns as part of comprehensive local care programmes.

Under the terms of this charter, the patients themselves have responsibilities of their own, however, and these include providing health care providers with as much information as possible about themselves as well as about their immediate family, friends, and others who might be vulnerable to tuberculosis or who might have been infected by contact. They are also expected to follow any prescribed treatment, and accept a

[295] http://www.who.int/tb/publications/2006/patients_charter.pdf?ua=1

moral responsibility to share information and knowledge gained during the treatment itself. This last idea is a laudable one – including passing their experiential expertise on to others in the community, helping to making patient empowerment as contagious as the disease itself, whilst at the same time engendering a collective moral responsibility to make the community tuberculosis free.

What can be seen here is a contract which might work rather well in a more perfect world. In the real one in which tuberculosis reigns, however, things are a little different and policies are dictated much more by what is actually available rather than by what may be seen to be most desirable by panels of experts.

In the early days of MDR-TB in South Africa patients were being virtually imprisoned, treated in isolation units for months at a time until they were no longer infectious to prevent a wider spread of infection. Today, with only 2,500 available beds and a prevalence burden of infectious drug-resistant TB that is probably well over 25 times that number (in 2012 the number of laboratory-diagnosed cases alone was nearly 16,000) the idea of hospitalisation, enforced or otherwise, has been dumped. This has happened out of pragmatic necessity but the likes of MSF and PIH have embraced the challenge by embracing the idea of patient-centred community care as the only real way to fill the gap in provision. What this has meant is that infectious cases are now being dealt with in community settings, which makes it a far riskier business as far as infection control is concerned. Where they are well-managed, it is one thing; but when they are barely managed at all, it is entirely another.

In all circumstances simple measures for infection control for TB should be being undertaken for patients with active risk of transmitting disease, drug-resistant or otherwise. These should ideally include:

- Gathering information about how many people share accommodation
- Screening all contacts
- Ensuring that children under five spend as little time as possible in the same room as any infectious person
- Ensuring that mothers always wear masks while caring for a child while sputum-positive
- Educating patients in cough etiquette and providing masks
- Keeping patients in a separate room at night

- Ensuring common areas are well ventilated
- Encouraging the patient to spend time outside if weather permits.

It should be noted that this last recommendation, while harking back to the days of the sanatorium, makes a lot of sense – because droplet nuclei are known to be able to hang around for several hours depending on levels of ventilation and UV light.

Is this happening in the way that is being expected? MSF suggests that any professional attending to the infectious patient should wear a personal respirator - these are fundamental items which remain in desperately short supply where they are needed.[296]

But we should to take another look at that Patients' Charter. Under its terms, if an XDR-TB patient were to refuse treatment he might be seen to be wilfully presenting himself as an active danger to the public. The threat thus posed might make it seem preferable to limit that individual's human rights by instituting quarantine or isolation so as to protect the rights of the wider public. Such an action could be seen as necessary for the public good, and even be considered legitimate under international human rights law. A set of international legal guidelines have been developed exactly for such occasions – the so-called 'Siracusa Principles'. In such a case, each of the following five criteria would have to be met in order for an isolation order to comply with international law, and in any case any restrictions that might be imposed could only ever be of a limited duration and would have to remain subject to both review and appeal.

These Siracusa Principles dictate that:

---

[296] "Personal respirators are fundamentally different from, and more expensive than, the more familiar surgical masks which they resemble. Surgical masks are designed to protect the operating field from relatively large respiratory droplets generated by surgeons and surgical nurses. They are relatively loosefitting and made of paper or cloth but are inadequate for prevention of TB infection. Masks that prevent TB transmission are known as 'particulate respirators' or simply 'respirators'. They are designed to protect the wearer from tiny (1–5 μm) airborne infectious droplets. The filtration media through which air passes must capture these minute particles; most importantly, the respirator must fit tightly on the face, especially around the bridge of the nose." WHO – "Guidelines for the programmatic management of drug-resistant tuberculosis. Emergency update 2008".

- The restriction is provided for and carried out in accordance with the law;
- The restriction is in the interest of a legitimate objective of general interest;
- The restriction is strictly necessary in a democratic society to achieve the objective;
- There are no less intrusive and restrictive means available to reach the same objective; and
- The restriction is based on scientific evidence and not drafted or imposed arbitrarily i.e. in an unreasonable or otherwise discriminatory manner.

A general principle prevails that isolation should be exercised only as a last resort, may only be temporary, and can only be legally justified after all voluntary measures to isolate such a patient have already failed.

So far so good, because in our hypothetical case the reason for the enforced isolation was on account of the individual failing to meet his or her own responsibilities by refusing to take his drugs. But what if the state itself has failed to meet its own obligations that are written into the charter? Does this make a difference? The WHO's charter assumes that the state (or at least its National TB Programme) will actually be able to provide effective treatment. But what if it can't do this, either because of lack of resource or because the patient has functionally untreatable drug-resistant disease? In fact, what if it is the WHO itself which is falling short of its own responsibilities and principles?[297] What rights do patients then have? More importantly still, what rights do communities have for their better protection when other parties, for any reason at all, are unable to fill their own obligations in either the citizen/state contract or the Patients' Charter?

The global emergence of MDR- and XDR-TB offer good circumstantial evidence of a general failure of public health systems to control TB as both hoped and intended. TB is a disease which is still, despite being both

[297] There is good reason for the WHO to share responsibilities here: the "WHO Guidance on Human Rights and Involuntary Detention for XDR-TB Control" of 2007 specified exactly in this respect that national programmes should ensure, "that the capacity to identify and treat drug-resistant TB is in place" but then added that this should be accompanied by "a secure supply of second line anti-TB drugs required for treating multidrug-resistant TB obtained through the Green Light Committee (in resource-limited settings)". Seven years later this can hardly be claimed to have been achieved.

infectious and lethal, generally recognised to be normally treatable. If this was the case, however, all communities would have been secure in expecting their public health systems to have been able to protect them from the disease by properly implementing treatment programmes. The prevention of the development of drug-resistant disease could only ever have been reasonably guaranteed if health systems had ensured, as their first priority, that individuals suspected of having all types of TB had had universal access to rapid diagnosis, appropriate treatment, and adequate support systems to ensure treatment completion. This self-evidently has never happened, so, in the very different scenarios that are now increasingly being seen to occur with DR-TB, it is difficult to see exactly how these charters and principles should now apply.

From a public health perspective, any general approach which advocates that government policies should be directed towards providing for the greatest good to the largest component of its population must make most sense. With smouldering tuberculosis (as opposed to quick-fire infectious epidemics) this idea creates real dilemmas, however, particularly because the development of both MDR- and XDR-TB can be so readily blamed on an inadequate implementation of government policies in the first place.

XDR-TB, once it occurs, has to be the real bugbear, however, because it often turns out to be functionally untreatable. For such unfortunate cases, infection control that involves restrictions of movement which was initially imposed for a limited duration could really mean confinement until death, or, if the patient were to survive for any length of time, it could even be redefined as being indefinite. Both scenarios run contrary to any policy enshrined in the Siracusa Principles.

South Africa, as much as any country, is currently wrestling with this problem. Its current health legislation empowers its authorities to detain patients with an infectious disease if it sees it as being necessary – at least until the disease no longer poses a public health threat. It thus allows quarantine or isolation to be enforced for a limited period exactly as described above. But functionally untreatable XDR-TB was never considered within this legislation. From a human rights perspective any sort of prolonged isolation would violate the country's hard won constitutional rights as well as contravene international human rights law as well. This is a very delicate affair.

In 2012, 1,646 South Africans were diagnosed by DST to have XDR-TB. No-one has any clear idea how many others may be out there, but unquestionably these 1,646 individuals were posing the biggest identifiable active threat to public health in the country. Less than half ended up being put on treatment. Of the ones that were, a large proportion would have been expected to end up failing to respond, and therefore inevitably remain infectious as long as they survived. Yet, despite this, the policy now is to return them to their communities so that their hospital beds can be better used by others with more recent infections who still have hope of cure. Of course, it's also safe to assume that, when they get home they rejoin those undetected others who never had any treatment in the first place.

No-one yet has any real idea of the longer term consequences of this change of policy, but it doesn't require a Masters degree in epidemiology to figure out a few probabilities. The University of Cape Town has been reported to be tracking some of these individuals using 'smart mast' technology – analysing their movements to see how they behave and assess what risk they might present to their community – to see whether they use public transport, shopping malls or supermarkets.

The WHO's "Guidelines for the programmatic management of drug-resistant tuberculosis Emergency update" of 2008 was initially explicit on its recommendations:

> "XDR-TB patients should be placed in isolation until no longer infectious."

It also accepted the probability that, in many cases, treatment of XDR-TB would have to be withdrawn. Under such circumstances, the document was equally clear:

> "It is very important that medical visits continue and that the patient is not abandoned."

So should these patients not be being quarantined? Should they not at least be forced to wear masks if they are mixing with members of the community? Even the doughty MSF becomes coy on this subject. One of itsr experts says that they prefer to approach the problem by using the term 'infection control' rather than 'quarantining', seemingly resorting to euphemism rather than addressing this thorny subject head-on – including those sensitive issues around human rights. These issues were well summarized by three experts of bioethics in 2009:

> "Autonomy has become a prominent first principle in modern bioethics and is enshrined in human rights doctrine. However, there is an equal need for communities to be protected from harm. Infectious diseases underscore

> our universal vulnerability – how individuals can be both victims and vectors of disease and how we are related in a common cause in controlling diseases. Relationality and solidarity may serve as important principles in our response to TB. We also need to embrace reciprocity and put it into action – articulate what we can do for each other in order to build healthy communities. This is only possible if we create communities in which individuals with infections are facilitated and supported in discharging their obligations to others."[298]

The story of AIDS control in Cuba can offer food for thought on this. When cases of HIV began to be seen amongst the *internationalistas* returning from Angola, Mozambique and the Congo in the late 1980s, efforts were swiftly made to contain and treat them in a segregated unit. Initially it was run by the military but, as its initial residential population began to include a growing number of gay and bisexual men, management problems began to develop and the project was handed over to the Ministry of Public Health. From one perspective the strategy looked like straightforward quarantining, and in some quarters was described as such (including in the American media). But from another it appeared that it had developed into something that was altogether more sophisticated, particularly with similar units appearing in every province. Essentially they were not just 'sanatoria of consent' (which they definitely were), but they were also both person-centred and educative, in terms of promoting responsibility for those within the institutions and also for raising appropriate awareness outside well. And because the conditions inside the sanatoria were so good, most patients chose to stay there of their own free will. The results have to be seen in hindsight to have been impressive because rates of HIV remained lower in Cuba than in the rest of the Caribbean.

The political systems which exist today in a country like South Africa are certainly different to those which existed in Cuba in the 1990s. In Cuba there was certainly a more serious general commitment towards social equality, as well as a political will to address a serious medical problem.

If back-up provision and support in the community were ready and widely available in South Africa it would be one thing, but unfortunately even this doesn't yet appear to be the case with the situation deteriorating. In New Crossroads (a township in Cape Town) in the Western Cape, for instance, the author knows of XDR-TB patients who are being cared for by health

---

[298] Upshur R et al. "Apocalypse or redemption: responding to extensively drug-resistant tuberculosis" the Bulletin of the World Health Organization, 87 (2009) 481-83.

workers who have been neither properly equipped nor trained to administer to them, nor appropriately advised concerning their infectious status. If this is the case across the rest of the country in its many drug-resistant hotspots, both residents and health workers must be being unnecessarily put at risk of infection with untreatable disease. In these sorts of contexts, the idea of any sort of enforced isolation becomes an extremely compelling one.

This ethical and humanitarian conundrum is not unique to South Africa. It's not even unique to the HBCs or to developing countries because it even presented a problem to a country with one of the lowest rates of TB and DR-TB anywhere in the world – the USA. For a few weeks in 2007 the actions of Atlanta attorney Andrew Speaker focused global attention on the role of compulsory isolation and quarantine in drug-resistant tuberculosis control. In May that year, after being diagnosed with a drug-resistant form of TB, Speaker had chosen to fly to Europe for his wedding and honeymoon – he had been told that he was not actually infectious, but he did travel against medical advice although not against any specific instruction or restriction order. While abroad, laboratory tests back home mistakenly indicated that Speaker's infection was extensively drug-resistant and therefore much more dangerous. Accounts of what followed vary a little. Because he feared isolation in an Italian hospital, Speaker appears to have hatched a plan to get back into the US under the radar of homeland surveillance in order to be able to access what he saw to be the best possible treatment. He knew that he would be prevented from boarding any plane flying directly to America, so he flew to Prague and from there on to Montreal. Then he rented a car and drove south into the United States, presenting himself at a New York hospital where he was immediately met with a CDC isolation order restricting his movements and requiring him to cooperate with health officials – supposedly the first such federal order issued since 1963.[299]

---

[299] The US federal statute granting quarantine authority allows isolation or quarantine but only for individuals coming into the country from a foreign country or territory – as such it seems that it would have been impossible for the order to have been issued if Speaker had not just entered the country from Canada. Actually, while Speaker's detention is frequently quoted as having been unique, it wasn't. In 1993, in response several outbreaks of multidrug-resistant strains of TB, New York had amended its health code to allow officials in the city to detain persons who were no longer infectious but were merely completing their course of therapy. As of 1999, the city had detained more than 200 such people in a special facility, Goldwater Memorial Hospital, for periods of as long as two years.

Ironically, some weeks later, laboratory tests revealed that he wasn't infected with XDR-TB at all but was MDR exactly as the earlier tests had shown – a difference that might well have made the media attention his case received a degree less high pitched than it became. In a Senate hearing, for instance, the chair of the House Homeland Security Committee said: "We've dodged a bullet. When are we going to stop dodging bullets and start protecting Americans?"

It seems that potential tuberculosis carriers today are seen by some to threaten a nation as much as terrorists and so should be thwarted by similarly enhanced security measures which necessarily include the vigorous application of isolation and quarantine. In our post-9/11 and post-SARS era it feels like governments have become ever more ready to award themselves such powers. But perhaps even this isn't true – it should be remembered that, prior to 9/11 and the invasion of Afghanistan, Guantánamo Bay was being used as a detention centre for Haitian immigrants suspected of being infected with HIV/AIDS.[300]

A postscript to the Speaker story illustrates the chasm of realities that exist between an affluent country with low incidence rates of DR-TB like the United States and countries like South Africa or India. Nine people subsequently collectively filed a US$1.3 million lawsuit against Speaker for "possibly exposing" them to the disease on the flight from Prague to Montreal and for their consequential "loss of opportunities". Seven were Canadians and two were Czech. Eight had been passengers on the flight but the ninth was merely brother and roommate of one of the other plaintiffs.

Montreal lawyer Anlac Nguyen presented the case in words which both sum up and mock the situation for perhaps half of humanity since they so aptly sum up the true reality that exists for them:

> "They do not have tuberculosis, but nobody can say that they won't have tuberculosis either, and that will not be known, not now, not next year, but for many years in the future, so the pain and suffering that the people have gone through are real. They continue to suffer now because of the uncertainty."

---

[300] See Paul Farmer - "Pathologies of Power", University of California Press (2005). 51-69.

Speaker later chose to sue the CDC himself, alleging that details of his medical history had been unlawfully released as well as of his alleged condition, wedding and identity – "none of which needed to be released to the general public in order to accomplish any legitimate public health purpose". The case was dismissed twice, once in 2009 and again when he tried again in 2012.

Are such legal sensitivities ever being explored in the courts of South Africa or India because of exposures in the shopping malls of Cape Town or in the cinemas in Mumbai where the disease is out of control? A more fundamental legal question also deserves to be asked in such places – whether less restrictive tuberculosis-control programmes (i.e. DOTS and DOT-Plus) should be in place and be effective before even short-term isolation can even begin to be considered to be legal in the first place since only then could the WHO charter be seen to apply. And if they are not in place, then who exactly should be responsible for those who are innocently infected? Whether asking such questions might be as appreciated by members of communities under active siege of an infectious disease which had been spawned by the failure of their own public health programmes as much as it might be by a human rights lawyer is a moot point.

As yet no-one is offering any answers to these sorts of question, but failing to have much on the table for debate to help resolve these dilemmas looks likely to give the XDR genie another extra edge.

To some degree XDR patients can be likened to TB patients in the era before the discovery of drugs. At that time 50-70% of cases would have been expected to die, 20-25% would have 'spontaneously cured' (although exactly what that really meant remains debatable) and 20-25% would have been expected to develop chronic smear-positive infectious TB. With HIV co-infection, these percentages can be expected to be vastly different, with a far higher proportion of deaths and few chronic infectious cases, but any long-term cases of chronic infectious untreatable disease at all circulating freely in a vulnerable community still present a huge predictable public health threat.

In that same earlier era, the answer to the problem was seen to be the sanatoria. Whilst they may never have been as effective at curing the disease in the way that had been hoped, they certainly helped contribute to the reduction of epidemics by separating infectious individuals from their communities. Should something similar be attempted today, modelled on what might help the current problem – a humane combination of two different movements in health care – one the sanatorium and the other the hospice? They could offer a refuge where patients could be looked after even if they fail treatment and could be offered proper palliative care. It could amount to something not unlike what was being done in Cuba with HIV patients actually wanting to stay because of the conditions created rather than feeling like prisoners on death row.

One further question does deserve to be asked as well. If there really is such a phenomenon as a 'super-spreader' in XDR-TB (as is increasingly being believed), then should at least these individuals be proactively sought out, identified and then lodged (or even forcibly confined) under a revised set of principles in some sort of isolated community? They should hardly be that difficult to identify once identified by a failing treatment regimen, being that all that should be required would be a single decent sputum sample with a heavy bacillary load identified by smear microscopy. These cases, at least, should surely never be being discharged at the end of a course of unsuccessful treatment.

Reducing disease

"EVERY TIME WE LOOK THE PROBLEM IS WORSE THAN WE THOUGHT. NOW IT IS COMING TOGETHER WITH HIV IN SUB-SAHARAN AFRICA, AND IT COULD BE THE MOST FRIGHTENING THING WE ARE EVER GOING TO SEE."

Dr Jim Yong Kim[301]

Reductions in diseases can normally be predicted by three factors:

- A decline in the virulence of the pathogenic micro-organism
- Changes in the environment which may reduce exposure to the pathogen
    - perhaps as a result of an immunisation programme
    - perhaps as a result of a public health programme
- Improvements in the hosts' defensive resources after initial exposure
    - perhaps by improved scientific treatment methods
    - perhaps as a result of improved nutritional intake or living conditions

Unfortunately, it seems that the general virulence of *M. tuberculosis* has not been in any way weakened by 50-plus years of pharmacological assault on it, and once extensive resistance has developed, its relative virulence increases as it becomes less and less treatable with any existing drugs. The bacillus is also, without any doubt, far more virulent when it is active in the company of its viral buddy HIV. It may even be that in certain populations some strains of the disease are more virulent than others. While this idea is promoted it is still not proved conclusively – but then nor was the idea that drug-resistant strains are inherently 'less fit' than normal susceptible strains of disease as was previously being assumed to be the case. So the first

[301] Co-founder of Partners in Health, former Director of the WHO HIV/AIDS Department, and currently President of the World Bank.

option as suggested above that declining virulence might reduce the pandemic does not currently seem to be a likely possibility.

The second option includes both better immunisation and more committed public health programmes. The existing vaccine, as we have comprehensively discussed, is known to be inadequate. We have already considered the possibilities and problems of developing a new vaccine and concluded that, wherever latent infection is common, the possibility of a new vaccine making any serious short term impression on the pandemic is very limited. We have also identified the unfortunate fact that, with a global shortage of nearly four million health workers, the idea of mobilising a concerted and uncompromised public health assault similar to the ones in the industrialised countries in the 1950s and 60s is also unlikely in the short- to medium-term unless strategic public health policies experience a major shift of emphasis.

So we are only left with the third option, which, in the case of TB, means both new drugs and a reduction in poverty (and needs to be both) if the analysis developed in the previous pages is in any way accurate. Africa may be being promoted as the world's second fastest growing region, but its rates of reduction of extreme poverty are still not on track to be halved by 2015 as was planned. There is a lot still to be done in this respect if serious progress is to be made. Meanwhile, globally, the gaps between the rich and the poor can be seen to be widening almost everywhere.

It has to be recognised that more impoverished nations, whether in Africa or elsewhere, will simply not be given meaningful access to new drugs if they lack the medical infrastructure with which to administer them in a way that will deprive the disease of fresh opportunities to mutate. If any resistance to a new drug occurs then all the precious progress that has been made will have been lost at a stroke and a further cycle of drug-resistant disease may have been begun.

In the meantime we encounter three units of measurement with which to monitor how this struggle is being progressed, each of which gives us a slightly different window into how the disease is faring.

The first is the rate of prevalence. This standard epidemiological measure is the number of people 'per 100,000' that are infected with active disease during a period of measurement (which is normally a year). The WHO, very understandably, is particularly alert to this measurement with TB since, with such a slow burn disease, it gives a very useful indicator of the amount of active infectious disease there might be in a community. The rates of prevalence would always be expected to be higher than the rates of incidence (which we will come to shortly). Curiously, on the odd occasion this does not seem to be the case in the official per-country figures.

As with almost everything with TB, this prevalence measure is not as simple as it might first appear. If the disease were to run its normal course, it would certainly be a useful measure (with the important further proviso that the numbers were being accurately measured). But with any positive active pharmaceutical intervention, the picture is almost immediately rendered less useful. A patient may self-refer, may then be diagnosed AFB positive, and then may be put on immediate DOTS treatment. As a consequence, this same patient might be rendered non-infectious in as little as a month, and so should be no longer the lingering epidemiological threat that he would have been. Meanwhile he or she must remain on the prevalence books for either a further five or seven months.

If the patient is MDR, these periods would all correspondingly extend. She may be infectious for four months as the slower second line drugs take control, but will then remain on the prevalence books for a further 20 months beyond this, although hopefully would have no further effect on the epidemic beyond adding to the prevalence statistics during this period.

But in any case, how long might a patient have been prevalently infectious before self-presenting, and yet never contributed to the numbers? We have no way of knowing, but this is another key factor in the estimation of real prevalence of an infectious disease like TB.

Nevertheless, as an available measure for deciding how much potentially active infectious disease there may be in any community, prevalence must in some sense still be the best indicator we currently have despite these limitations.

The second measure is that of incidence. This, again, is measured per 100,000 population, but gives us a slightly different feel for the disease. It is intended to count the number of new cases (or retreatment cases) which present in a given period (again normally a year). As such, it tells us how things are going on several levels.

One window which it opens for us reflects the state of the pool of latent infection that might be feeding the epidemic in any locality. In other words, if the incidence rate is high, it strongly suggests that the pool of latency is high as well since new cases must be spitting out of it so efficiently. If the incidence rate drops, it would suggest that the efficiency of the feeder mechanism that is part of the latent epidemic must be sputtering too. This might indicate positive effects from Isoniazid preventative treatment if it were being employed locally, which would certainly be an encouraging sign.

Incidence rates can reflect something else important as well – the effects of any measures which may be being implemented to more directly combat the disease, measures such as vaccination campaigns, or improvements in social policies. The former might be expected only to show slowly as it might cumulatively eat into the percentage of latent disease, the latter potentially more swiftly as improved living conditions or nutrition might provide an effective buffer against progression to active disease. Either factor should be easily corroborated from other available data if they were indeed impacting on the measured incidence rates.

The third measure is the rate for mortality. Again, these have been being measured as a number 'per 100,000 population. This measure gives us an idea of how effective a given intervention might be (and/or possibly how immune-compromised the host population might be). If the figure drops, it suggests that the treatment might be desirably effective, particularly so if it drops faster than the other rates. If it rises, then it suggests that treatment might be ineffective or that population demographics are shifting.

In fact, even this is questionable, and in any case the measurement may well be in the process of being slightly recalibrated. Instead of numbers of death per 100,000, it is being suggested that the ratio of 'deaths to notified patients' (M:N) would offer a much clearer picture of treatment efficacy. Significant variations in this M:N ratio have recently been observed in the European region, with high levels in the Russian Federation (M:N ratio of 20%), lower levels in Estonia, Latvia and Lithuania (11%) and even lower levels in the high-income western European countries. Such variations are highly informative and probably shed better light on the situation. They also are suggested as being reflective of the differences in the burden of drug-resistant TB and also as possibly showing key indicators of the effectiveness of efforts to treat MDR-TB. Simple mortality rates as they have been being used up unti now aren't able to show these differences nearly so clearly.

We can see from this that each of these measures presents its own individual problem. The universal and most important one must relate to their accuracy in the first place. We have already learnt that rates of TB are seen as a good measurement of the effectiveness of a nation's health infrastructure. Of course, this need not always be the case: low rates of any of the methods of measurement we have just just discussed might equally indicate under-reporting or misreporting, both of which also indicate a potentially weak infrastructure although they may not be so readily recognisable as such.

Another problem for all of them is that they present risks of oversimplification. This can already be seen in the way that mortality rates have been being used in the Partnership's targets, currently excluding those who die from TB who are also HIV-positive. This is a policy which renders the window on the disease less than desirably clear. The same could easily be said of both prevalence rates and incidence rates. Neither measure offers us that useful a tool without further complex elucidation.

How many incidence cases are retreatment cases, for instance? Retreatment cases clearly aren't being fed by the pool of latent disease, but their number may be fed by poorly managed treatment. How long was the gap between first treatment and relapse? Was the first treatment completed or not? How many retreatment cases in a national epidemic are MDR? How many are XDR? Each of these further measures offers us the only really useful window into how any localised epidemic might be really developing, and most may be immeasurable given the local diagnostic resources.

When it comes to measurements of prevalence, the drug-resistant component becomes an even more significant factor, since patients will remain in the system for three or four times longer than with straightforward DOTS patients and will therefore substantially skew the numbers.

And, of course, how many of each of these different types of patients are co-infected with HIV?

All of these measures are already being collected, but, at best, this is still being done inadequately. Why? Because the self-same deficient health infrastructures which dictate that TB might be rife in any particular country will almost inevitably also dictate that the data will be poor too.

The most recent total figure of 38,000 MDR-TB cases for the African region aptly illustrates this problem. As we have earlier identified, the most recent total TB incidence estimates for this region is quoted as being 2,300,000, which in turn suggests the rate of MDR-TB is as little as 1.7%.

It's impossible to believe that this can possibly be the case, being as it is about a third of the current global average rate for incident MDR disease.

In fact there is every reason to suspect that it might be ***higher*** than the global average since it is a given that drug-resistance occurs wherever there is a dilapidated health infrastructure. Unless we choose to disagree with this generally accepted idea, then it seems logical to assume that rates of MDR disease that are above the global average will be occurring almost everywhere where medical resources are poor. In other words, in the absence of surveillance data, ***every country with a known limited medical resource and regular access to first line drugs should be considered a probable high-burden MDR-TB country*** (at least until it can be proven otherwise).

Today this is the only precautionary position that it is sensible for the global authorities to take.

The potential impact of XDR-TB is also still being relatively ignored in both the Global Plan and the most recent WHO reports, despite this emerging as the next problematic wave of the pandemic. No publication attempts to properly monitor the absolute numbers in the XDR-TB epidemic – they limit the data to the numbers of countries reporting a single case of the disease, and to the overall estimated global percentages of MDR-TB cases which are XDR.

More worryingly still given the negative experiences with MDR-TB in the last 20 years, no publication yet elucidates any sort of specific plan to get ahead of this secondary wave of more extensive drug-resistant disease. In fact almost every reference to XDR-TB in the Global Plan simplistically links it to MDR-TB, when the challenge of both diagnosing and treating this frightening type of TB is infinitely more challenging.

Addressing latent TB

Finding and reducing actual active disease is a vital part of a meaningful global strategy. Any drug treatment that works, whether it takes six months or two years to potentially affect a cure, can stifle the spread of disease if it can swiftly render the patient no longer infectious. As succinctly identified by PIH affiliate Edward Nardell at the 2012 World TB Conference of the International Union against TB and Lung Disease:

> "Once appropriate treatment is initiated, the risk of transmission to others declines precipitously."

As rapidly as this may occur, if the infectious condition didn't happen in the first place it would be better still, of course. It's the huge pool of latent infection which feeds the active epidemic, so addressing the size of this pool should, in the longer term, serve to starve the epidemic at its source and reduce the opportunities for further infectious cases.

At the APRC conference in 2013 Dr Christian Lienhardt gave a thought-provoking presentation on this subject. He pointed out that current strategies not just for patients' treatment of TB, but also for its control, have been primarily focused on those populations with active TB disease. With nearly nine million people estimated to contract active TB disease each year such a strategy appears to be entirely logical, but the size of the global population with TB bacteria walled off in their lungs remains even more mammoth – at between two and three billion if WHO estimates are correct.

The ultimate aim, Dr Leinhardt reminded the conference, was still to eradicate the disease "in our lifetimes" (the words of the Stop TB Partnership). He wondered how this could possibly be achieved unless people with latent TB in their systems are not somehow rid of their bacteria.

Ramping up Isoniazid preventative treatment (IPT) might therefore be seen as a vital as well as a still underutilised component of the wider campaign. It is a viewpoint which at first seems hard to argue with – particularly as it is estimated that it is both cost effective and underused (with fewer than 1% of latent TB infections in 2006 estimated to be under treatment).[302]

---

[302] Szakacs TA, Wilson D, Cameron DW, et al. - "Adherence with isoniazid for prevention of tuberculosis among HIV-infected adults in South Africa", BMC Infect Dis 6 (2006) 97.

But even this isn't that simple. There is still, as is explicitly stated in the 2013 report, only a "limited understanding of the fundamental biology of latency" and still "no diagnosis and treatment for people who are latently infected with drug-resistant strains of tuberculosis". This is a massive shortcoming considering what may be in store for us, so developing better tools for its diagnosis and safe and effective treatment must still be a major part of any serious new strategy.

According to studies presented at the 43rd Union World Conference on Lung Health in 2012, IPT on its own is unable to provide lifetime or long-term protection against TB – its protective effect fades soon after stopping the treatment. In high incidence environments, therefore, both diagnosis and treatment almost certainly may require frequent repeating.

One stumbling block to more widely accepting this necessity to get to grips with the plague of latent infection also relates to the same risks from non-adherence to the DOTS treatment regimen, which with IPT ranges from between six and 12 months, as well as to the inadequate existing resources available to properly manage such a huge endeavour. Another relates to the risk of using IPT on TST positive cases whose disease has already progressed to a more active state - a significant risk which we already considered in some detail when we first discussed the treatment used for latent infection.

Wherever there are minimal rates of drug-resistance, and medium to low incidence rates of susceptible disease, a good infrastructural resource and any rate at all of HIV co-infection, IPT should unquestionably be considered as a vital component of any plan to combat the disease. It must be as important a component as any other currently – but wherever there is any known or suspected level of drug-resistant disease IPT amounts to playing Russian roulette with the risks of stoking a potentially untreatable epidemic.

IPT uses a single drug over a period of six-12 months with the intention of eradicating the latent infection. The logic behind the treatment is thus different from that used to treat the active disease. With multiple drug treatment of active disease the basic idea is to consistently keep at least three active agents at work, employing the principle that failing to do so promotes the possibility of fresh resistance to one or more of the otherwise active members of the combination. Such an approach is completely different from a single drug regimen such as IPT. IPT cannot be predicted to amplify multi drug-resistance in the way that inadequately managed polydrug combinations might do, but where there are already high rates of MDR-TB there remain worrying uncertainties.

MDR-TB (and XDR-TB) are both defined by being resistant to Isoniazid along with one or more other drugs, so patients latent infected with such strains can be predicted to remain nonresponsive to Isoniazid treatment. We can therefore reasonably predict that any widespread application of IPT will not be as effective as might be hoped in any communities with high rates of drug-resistant disease – proportionately so in relation to the amount of DR-TB in the community. Sputum-positive Isoniazid resistance has been found in as many as 20% of patients in some parts of South Africa, so IPT for this region must certainly be seen to be fundamentally as questionable.[303]

Two further effects might also be expected to occur, however.

One is that the proportion of DR-TB might increase in relation to the overall epidemic, as the DR-TB component will numerically maintain itself (or organically increase) while the drug-susceptible pool of disease would hopefully reduce. This in some ways may be seen to be a good result (as the overall size of the epidemic may thus simultaneously be measured to be reducing), but in any population which has no longer-term protection against re-infection or access to second line treatment this may not be a good thing at all.

The second potential effect is from the long-term antibiotic treatment which is likely to cumulatively further weaken the host immune systems of those being treated by it. If this were to occur even those who successfully respond to the treatment might not benefit from if they are already immune-compromised. In fact they may find themselves more open to re-infection (and this might be with a more dangerous resistant strain) or more susceptible to other opportunistic infectious diseases.

It is also worth considering the effect of blanket TST-triggered implementation of IPT in any population with bovine TB within it. Bovine TB is naturally resistant to Pyrazinamide, in other words in its 'natural' susceptible state it is already only vulnerable to three of the four first line drugs. The possibility of promoting Isoniazid resistance by mismanaged IPT treatment in such a population presents a further serious risk, since this would leave only two of the four FLDs still active against the disease.

[303] Dheda K, Gumbo T, Gandhi NR, et al. - "Global control of tuberculosis: from extensively drug-resistant to untreatable tuberculosis", Lancet Respiratory Medicine (2014). http://dx.doi.org/10.1016/S2213-2600(14)70031-1

Technically this would not be MDR since it would remain vulnerable to the more potent Rifampicin, but it would still be far less likely to be successfully treated by standard short course treatment, and also far more likely to morph into a more drug-resistant strain.

Such a blanket treatment of a higher incidence population using IPT regardless of whether or not individuals are actually LTBI has, in fact, been the subject of one recently completed study. The only criteria for exclusion was a diagnosis of active disease, formally entitled "A Trial of Mass Isoniazid Preventive Therapy for Tuberculosis Control" but less formally referred to as the "Thibela Study", its results are believed to be imminently publishable in the New England Journal of Medicine.

The study was designed as a cluster-randomized trial in order to explore whether such a blanket strategy might see a reduction of incidence of active TB among South African miners. The study was founded on two assumptions. One was that the overwhelming majority of workers within South African gold mines have existing latent tuberculosis (the assumed rate was over 80%). The other was that the re-activation of the latent disease (often triggered because of the working conditions) is the main factor that contributes to the remarkably high prevalence of active TB in these mining communities. Being as this was estimated by the study authors as 3,000 cases per 100,000 miners, this is over 10 times the threshold for an official national emergency.

The investigators first identified 15 suitable South African gold mines and then randomised them into two groups – eight mines in the intervention arm, and seven as the control. The study began with a total of 78,744 miners in the 15 mines, all of whom were offered screening and treatment for active (but not latent) TB if it was found. In the eight mines randomized to the intervention arm, the workers without active TB were then offered a nine-month course of Isoniazid. In the seven mines which were randomized to the control arm, those without active TB received "standard diagnostic and treatment services" but were not offered Isoniazid.

As might be expected, the incidence of active TB was lower in workers in the mines which had been randomized to the intervention arm during the period in which the miners were receiving Isoniazid. Unexpectedly, however, this difference vanished entirely during the year following the completion of IPT. In other words, the blanket treatment had no further effect on the control of TB in these eight high incidence environments beyond having had a modest and short-lived effect. This may have been disabled either by a re-activation of inadequately treated latent TB or by re-infections because of the high incidence rates in the localities.[304]

As a result, it certainly looks like alternative strategies to IPT may be needed, and thankfully new drugs are now being tested for treatment of latent infection. Rifapentine (a rifamycin-type drug with a longer half-life than Rifampicin) is being tested in combination with Isoniazid. The course of treatment consists of 12 doses of both drugs, administered on a weekly basis. It costs four times as much as a nine-month course of Isoniazid alone, however. Given that there may well be cross-resistance of Rifapentine with Rifampicin, it seems less likely that this would prove a solution anyway in higher MDR-TB burden countries. An Isoniazid-

---

[304] There are several factors which are of some concern in relation to this study. First of all there was no HIV testing of those taking part – at the request of the mining unions. Since IPT is considered to be a standard treatment for PLWH this has to be considered as a questionable policy given the normal stringency of ethical approvals for such studies. By agreeing to this stipulation, the researchers were potentially denying those taking part in the control arm a standard treatment. Secondly, the fact that there was not any testing for LTBI either by TST or IGRA (merely the assumption of high rates of LTBI) is also of concern. As a result an anticipatable proportion of miners who would not have been expected to be LTBI must therefore have received a nine-month course of treatment for a disease which they didn't have with probable side effects. Of more concern, however, was the possible secondary issue created by this decision not to test for latency, because the standard treatment for latent infection is IPT. By not establishing whether the study's participants were LTBI, its designers effectively avoided the thorny ethical issue of whether this standard treatment should have been provided to those in the control arm who would reasonably be anticipated to be LTBI. Since the standard treatment was what was being tested, having had to provide it would have derailed the study's fundamental intention but, given that the ethical gold standard of medical research requires that standard treatment should be provided in clinical trials, this begs the question as to whether the study would have been allowed to have been carried out at all in a different environment. This must have presented a tricky dilemma for those who approved the study as well as for the editors of the NEJM. Finally, the fact that there are high rates of Isozianid resistance in South Africa (as much as 20% of sputum-positive cases) strongly suggests that there must be equally high and probably higher rates in the latent epidemic, meaning that IPT is a questionable treatment for the country in which the study was carried out. The study was, in fact approved by the ethics committees of the University of KwaZulu-Natal and the London School of Hygiene and Tropical Medicine as well as by the South African Medicines Control Council and the South African Safety in Mines Research Advisory Committee.

Pyrazinamide combination is also under test, but the same issues of risk with drug-resistant strains seems to be a probability, and in cases of bovine TB it would in any case add up to standard IPT treatment.

The possibility of the discovery of readily detectable biomarkers indicating the likelihood for progression of LTBI to re-activated disease must be the ultimate aim, particularly if the triggers which promote the actual re-activation of the bacillus from its latent state can be identified and then disabled. Focusing resources on this thus far invisible brief moment in the longer progression of the disease process might be the best research strategy of all, since it just could prove to be the mycobacterium's final undoing.

"Apocalypse or Redemption?"

"DRUG-RESISTANT TB ... IS EVIDENCE OF A NEW FORM OF REGRESSION:
WE HAVE TAKEN THE CURABLE AND MADE IT NEARLY INCURABLE.
THE TENDENCY HAS BEEN TO BLAME THE MOST VULNERABLE AND POWERLESS.
IT IS TIME TO RECOGNIZE THAT WE COLLECTIVELY BEAR RESPONSIBILITY FOR THIS."

Ross Upshur , Jerome Singh & Nathan Ford (2009) [305]

Given any reasonably comprehensive analysis, the scale of the problem confronting us, specifically with growing drug-resistant tuberculosis in much of the world, is enormous. It may yet prove to be both the humanitarian and public health problem of our age, especially given that it is so tied up with issues of inequality and social neglect.

Any sorts of strategies are inevitably complicated at first base by practicalities. Creative ideas are cheap – but implementing them with TB can be extremely expensive, and are also risky because their consequences (whether good or bad) take such a long time to show. Implementation also requires proper recognition of the problem in the first place along with an appropriate political commitment to confront it.

There is a pervasive modern idea that solutions can be found to almost any proble. It's also one which is reflective of the developed world in which not much TB exists. But is there ***any*** real solution – or is the best that we can hope for just an economically feasible one? In other words, is there truly any real 'solution' out there for the two billion people most at risk from this disease?

A host of TB patients have been effectively treated with DOTS in the belief that it was the only answer to the epidemic. The fact that the epidemic is now almost certainly slowly morphing into a plague of drug-resistant disease caused largely by treatment mismanagement suggests that this belief may have been at least partly misplaced. Plainly DOTS hasn't been the comprehensive answer it was believed to be by many experts. This was

---

305 "Apocalypse or redemption: responding to extensively drug-resistant tuberculosis", the Bulletin of the World Health Organization, 87 (2009) 481-83.

exactly what was demonstrated in the MDR-TB outbreak in Lima, Peru in 1995, with the authorities politically wedded to DOTS, whilst it was being shown as clearly as could have been wished that DOTS wasn't working and that something more sophisticated and more complex needed putting in its place. But DOTS-Plus seems not to be so practically implementable alongside it if the evidence of the last 13 years is anything to go by. There simply doesn't appear to be an available resource to properly support any roll-out, nor a political commitment to do something about this. Meanwhile the complexities and risks involved are seen to be getting greater and greater.

Dr Ernesto Jaramillo has lamented that the implementation of treatment for DR-TB has too often been:

> "… hampered by poor health systems, which might mistakenly be using old TB thinking to treat a new drug-resistance threat."

If only it were that simple. It's very reasonable to suggest that the entire global strategy and response to the disease has been hampered by exactly such "old TB thinking" given that it is so wedded to DOTS and has been so reluctant, for many reasons, to accept that other approaches might be vital to confront the emerging threat. This thinking is dependent upon providing a one-size-fits-all treatment, but such an approach falters if it works effectively on easier patients but leaves the tougher cases still free to infect others. These are the very cases who are epidemiologically the most dangerous.

Professor Robin Wood of the University of Cape Town has pointed out that a large part of the problem has been that, at least with regards to DR-TB, the world has been stuck on debating what he has called the "ineffective" (i.e. DOTS) versus the "unobtainable" which (amongst other things) involves not just complex treatment but also wider social development.

Meanwhile two of the world's experts (Paul Farmer and Salmaan Keshavjee) have suggested that barely 0.5% of those with newly diagnosed MDR-TB have been receiving treatment that would be considered the standard of care in the United States. If this is true, it looks like we have a long way to go if we hope to find any sort of real 'solution' to the emerging problems. Both Mario Raviglione and Margaret Chan have unequivocally warned that the momentum to break the disease is now in real danger. The 2012 Global Tuberculosis Report in fact explicitly identified what was still required – "Achieving universal access to treatment requires a bold and concerted drive on many fronts of TB care, and increased financing" – but the same report offered no real idea how these might be achieved.

Whilst the 2013 report was relatively mute concerning the significance and true prevalence of drug-resistant TB, the 2012 report had explicitly discussed why keeping tabs on prevalence rates is still so important for properly understanding this part of the pandemic.

> "The reasons are that MDR-TB is a chronic disease and without appropriate diagnosis and treatment for most of these cases many more prevalent cases than incident cases are expected ... and the number of prevalent cases of MDR-TB directly influences the active transmission of strains of MDR-TB."

"Many more prevalent cases than incident cases are expected," the report suggested. Well, leaving aside the earlier discussions on the accuracy of its focus, the WHO certainly does recognise the risks not just from the rising trends, but also of inadequate treatment.

Its focus, however, has still been homing in on those Millennium Goals for 2015 (and the ultimate goal of eradication by 2050). That left a hiatus period of 35 years between 2015 and 2050 for which a strategy has only just been developed.[306] It will certainly be a period which will be more and more dominated by drug-resistant disease, so if strategies for this period don't properly anticipate and allow for this there will be some serious problems ahead. A major if not a radical shift of focus and resource between what was expected to work and what will be required is going to be needed.

Those tensions which Robin Wood described (between the "ineffective" and the "unobtainable") seem likely to have to be dramatically dissolved by the new strategies, with the focus of effort having to change alongside them. The proportional split in funding is already visibly shifting: the proportion of resource was 4:1 in favour of DOTS in 2011, and is being budgeted to shift to something nearer 5:2 by 2015. It looks like it will have to shift very much further still. While only 2.5% of all enrolled cases on treatment were diagnosed as drug-resistant, the cost of treating them with second line drugs that year took 68% of the national Tuberculosis Budget. This was not a 5:2 ratio in favour of DOTS as is planned by the WHO, but it is potentially 1:17 against it. What is perhaps more disconcerting still is that, despite this focus of funding and effort for MDR-TB already being in

[306] We will be reviewing this post-2015 strategy in a later section.

place in South Africa, the general incidence rates in the country are still rising year on year and the battle against DR-TB continues to be lost.

In 2008, The EXPAND-TB project was launched as a global initiative of multiple partners aiming to strengthen laboratory capacity for detecting drug-resistant TB and establish rapid diagnostics in 27 countries. There is still far too much work to do in this respect, and it will need to be on top of the rolling out of the GeneXpert device with the sort of national coverages we have seen to date. Laboratories which can effectively carry out comprehensive drug-susceptibility system ***must*** still be developed wherever they are needed if effective drug treatment is seriously intended to be properly implemented. The existing supranational reference laboratory network remains desperately imbalanced. While Europe has 12, Africa has just four and two of these are in unlikely locations (in Algeria and Egypt with the others in Uganda and South Africa) and with one further candidate laboratory in development (in Benin).

Meanwhile increases in the number of cases of MDR-TB being reported by selected countries participating in the EXPAND-TB project between 2008 and 2011 have been telling the same story. If you go looking for drug-resistant disease, you will find it in dramatic proportions, particularly if you take a better look for it where you should have been looking already (i.e. in India). But you may also find it in larger numbers than expected even where you ***have*** been looking (i.e. Uzbekistan), and also in larger numbers where you hadn't thought it previously worth looking at all (i.e. Haiti).

The following is a table of selective countries which serves to illustrate exactly these sorts of increases.

	2008	2011	Factor of increase
India	308 cases	4237 cases	13.8
Uzbekistan	342 cases	1385 cases	4
Cameroon	26 cases	63 cases	2.4
Haiti	43 cases	86 cases	2

This situation wasn't helped by the fact that, despite official endorsement by the most important organisations, some other key global health agencies still weren't keen on promoting universal access to treatment. Neither PEPFAR nor UNICEF included universal access to MDR-TB treatment as part of their global strategies despite the substantial risk of death for patients co-infected with HIV and MDR-TB and the possibility that more than 10% of patients with DR-TB may be children.

At this point, it may be helpful to review exactly what DOTS and DOTS-Plus entail.

Since the 1990s, DOTS has been the modern internationally recognized composite strategy for delivering the basics of TB case-finding and cure. It is not just a clinical approach to patients, but comprises a wider strategy for the management of a major public health issue. The strategy is dependent upon a raft of complementary components: on political commitment, case-detection through quality-assured bacteriology, directly observed short-course chemotherapy, patient adherence, adequate drug supplies, passive case-finding, and sound reporting and recording.

The WHO has gone so far as to define DOTS as being a "multi-dimensional approach", and in some sense this is true in that it never solely comprised just that single component of directly observed treatment. But, at least in respect of the directly observed short-course treatment itself, it has elsewhere been described as an attempt at a "one-size-fits-all" strategy which has essentially failed to fit anywhere near as much of the disease as it was originally intended to do.

The original DOTS strategy had been built on "five pillars":

1. political commitment and continued funding for TB control programmes,
2. bacteriological diagnosis by sputum smear examinations,
3. uninterrupted supply of high-quality anti-TB drugs,
4. drug intake under direct observation and
5. accurate reporting and recording of all registered cases.

None has been seen to be quite as sturdy as first intended.

Regarding (1), there is strong evidence that TB has been very seriously neglected in many countries in favour of HIV/AIDS and malaria.

Regarding (2), given that sputum smear microscopy was always an inadequate and unreliable diagnostic it only ever promised to partially address the pandemic. Even today around half of all notified cases are sputum-negative. The microscopy resource has also remained inadequately distributed even where the disease burden was the worst.

Regarding (3), stock-outs have been frequently recorded even in high-burden countries, and the quality of a proportion of a large proportion of TB drugs on the open market in these and other countries is known to be suspect.

Regarding (4), whilst valiant efforts have been made to implement directly observed treatment, it would be naïve to believe that it has been anywhere near as comprehensively implemented as intended in some countries with low incomes and insufficient human resource in their medical sector. There may be very good reasons for the authorities in such countries to want both the WHO and donor countries to believe otherwise if the realities might have negative impact on their funding.

Regarding (5), whilst accurate reporting and recording may also have been valiantly attempted, it remains totally inadequate to the pandemic in comparison, say, to the H5N1 epidemic of 2009 that killed an infinitely more closely monitored, but relatively speaking diminutive, 285,000, and even more so in comparison to the SARS outbreak of 2003 that killed less than 1,000.

The first and last of these factors demonstrate the same fundamental flaw, in fact: as far as TB is concerned, political will seems still to be in too short supply.

DOTS-Plus

DOTS-Plus had been originally officially launched back in 1999, specifically to manage multi drug-resistant TB with second line drugs – including in resource-poor settings. The "Stop TB Partnership's Working Group on DOTS-Plus for MDR-TB" was then established in 2000 in order to help develop the policy.

The Stop TB Partnership itself had been established as a global movement hosted by the WHO in 1998. It was set up to accelerate social and political action to stop the spread of TB. The Partnership's goal was (and still is) to eliminate TB as a public health problem and, ultimately, to secure a world free of TB. Not much appeared to really happen to help this in the next few years, at least as far as drug-resistant TB was concerned.

Then, in May 2005, the World Health Assembly passed a resolution concerning the Sustainable Financing for TB Prevention and Control. Within this resolution the Assembly encouraged all its member states:

> "... to ensure that all tuberculosis patients have access to the universal standard of care."

In other words, the decision-making body of the WHO was unequivocally intending that ***all*** patients should have access to second line drugs via DOTS-Plus as a matter of principle if they were seen to be needed. And that year the Assembly also specifically requested that the Director General of the WHO should:

> "... implement and strengthen strategies for the effective control of, and management of persons with, drug-resistant TB."

The World Health Assembly determines the policies of the World Health Organization. It meets annually in Geneva and is attended by delegations from all the WHO member states. Generally it focuses on a specific health agenda on each occasion, one which will have been previously worked on by its Executive Board. Those responsible for ensuring that TB was set as the topic of the Assembly that year should be credited for having possibly set the highest water-mark of advocacy for TB in the last 20 years.

It was in response to this Assembly request that the WHO launched its Global Plan for TB 2006-2015 in Davos, Switzerland, at the World Economic Forum. It was a plan which purported to contain within it what were described as "ambitious but realistic goals". According to the plan all regions were still expected to see rates of incidence, prevalence and death drop "rapidly over the next 10 years as a result of the various planned TB control activities".

It is something of an irony that this optimistic plan for the poorest of the world's poor was being initially launched not just in one of the favoured playgrounds of the super-rich, but also in the very town that the phthisic elite of Europe had retreated to in the 19th century. This cannot have been missed by everyone involved. Some of those attending the forum were even staying in the Berghotel Sanatorium Schatzalp, a huge art nouveau building situated 300m above the town itself. It is now a luxury hotel but was originally purpose built as a sanatorium.[307]

The plan anticipated generating "potentially enormous progress in all regions".

The global authorities were at least now both recognising and accepting the epidemiological risks arising from drug-resistance, and the plan also set down an immediate principle, one which followed directly from the World Health Assembly's directive of the previous year. It stated that:

> "DOTS-Plus is an effective, feasible and cost-effective intervention."

It also recognised that:

> "The main challenges today are to expand drug-resistance surveillance (DRS) and monitor drug-resistance trends worldwide, and to scale-up implementation of DOTS-Plus beyond the pilot phase as an integrated component of DOTS."

It made a further vitally important link: it specifically defined all countries with a high MDR-TB prevalence as also having a history of poor TB control.

There is one question, however, that few were caring to ask.

Do DOTS Programmes do what they set out to do?

"WITH TB, NOTHING IS STRAIGHT LINE STUFF."

Dr Ibanda Hood (2012)

DOTS has remained the cornerstone of the global strategy to combat TB for over two decades, with its initials well engraved into all of the existing strategies for addressing DR-TB as well. One question does deserve asking, however: does it actually do what it is believed to be already doing?

---

[307] In his novel "The Magic Mountain" Thomas Mann described how, in the winter, the bodies of the dead would have to ferried from the hotel down to the town on toboggans.

Between 1995 and 2011, the WHO reckons that 56 million people were successfully treated for TB in countries that had adopted the DOTS/Stop TB Strategy. This, it is claimed, has saved as many as 22 million lives.

This is a huge achievement, but it also serves to identify the scale of the death toll in the last 25 years if we choose to add in the contribution to the TB death toll from HIV/AIDS and take another look. This estimated gross death toll from TB was running at just over 1.4 million in 1990, and is only a little under 1.4 million today. In 2001 it was actually peaking at nearly two million a year. Its average has been around 1.7 million deaths each year since DOTS was implemented – in other words, the total estimated death toll between 1995 and 2012 has been around 27 million. Add in the lives estimated to have been saved by DOTS, and it makes the total lives that would have been lost without the WHO intervention a massive 49 million. DOTS can therefore be construed to have at the very least staved off a catastrophe – and 45% of those potential deaths may have been saved by it.

One study from 2007, however, suggests that this contribution may not have been so significant.[308] It comprised a systematic review which took a look at the evidence for classic DOTS, and then compared it with either a self-administered regime (i.e. by the patient) or an alternative DOT method, reviewing the evidence from 11 trials comprising a total of 5,609 participants. The results were rather startling and turned out to be not exactly what was being expected. Whether the treatment was applied in low-, middle- or high-income countries, the researchers found:

> "No statistically significant difference was detected between DOT and self-administration in terms of cure ... with similar results for cure plus completion of treatment."

In other words directly observing treatment seemed to be offering no specific advantage over the practice of simply giving the patient the drugs and then encouraging him or her to take them as directed – although things may well not be quite as simple as this summary suggests. It does, however, suggest that the belief that DOTS alone saved those 22 million lives may be slightly mistaken.

---

[308] Volmink J, Garner P - "Directly observed therapy for treating tuberculosis", Cochrane Database Systematic Reviews (2007) 4:CD003343.

Another study by the same authors (this time with two additional researchers) discussed this suggestion in more detail.[309] First of all they reviewed the premise that "tuberculosis (TB) is a good test of a health system". Their research enabled them to recognise that DOTS had unquestionably made a difference if only in that it had both focused approaches and set targets globally. The bottom line, however, was that patients still needed to consciously choose to take their drugs themselves for any system to be as effective as intended.

The problem is that patients everywhere have a habit not just of not taking their drugs as prescribed, but also of becoming demotivated in the course of their treatment if they don't see good results – especially if they simultaneously suffer from debilitating side effects. With TB regimens this unhelpful habit can end up having fatal consequences for the patient, but it can also have wider consequences for both immediate family and community.

Two distinct and divergent fundamental perspectives on patient compliance began to materialize from the review, ones which the researchers saw as acting as brackets at each end of a spectrum of opinion that existed within the community of TB expertise and policy governance.

At one end of the spectrum the dominant viewpoint suggested that it was the right of global public health authorities to ***demand*** adherence to treatment – in other words an overriding public health imperative demands that all patients with positive sputum tests simply ***must*** take their treatment. This imperative, in the opinion of these experts, needs to be legislated for and should be accompanied by some capacity for its strict implementation and enforcement. This was a necessity because these patients posed such a profound risk to others.

The view at the other end of the spectrum suggested that it was much more the responsibility of the policy-makers and health-care providers to devise and deliver interventions that would be more acceptable and still effective. For this approach to succeed health-care practitioners would have to be working within effective health systems so that the most appropriate care

---

309 Paul Garner, Helen Smith, Salla Munro and Jimmy Volmink - "Promoting adherence to tuberculosis treatment", the Bulletin of the World Health Organization (2007).

could be delivered to meet people's differing needs and be more readily accepted by them.

With the first idea the fundamental principle is coercive. In essence, poor adherence (which has been widely seen as being the main reason for drug-resistance) is seen as being caused by recalcitrant patients – ones who don't know, care or understand the importance of completing their full course of treatment. The natural response to this should be to devise a menu of policies to better educate, motivate, watch and even punish patients if they do not do as instructed.

This second idea assumes that, if a large proportion of people are not completing treatment, then it is probably not the patients who have failed the system, but the system that has failed its patients. The proof of this is, as far as proponents of this idea are concerned, is exemplified by the fact that the system can be seen to be failing to deliver what it was supposed to do.

The authors of the review then explored the more uncertain ground which lay between these two points of view. They concluded that any strategies that seriously intended to improve adherence where it is known to be poor had to fundamentally improve the available health services ***and also*** ensure that such services are appropriate to patients' needs. Sometimes (but not always as far as the researchers were concerned) direct observation might help this process.

They also concluded that a model of direct observation which is actively executed by a health worker rather than by a family member or friend addressed the problem of treatment delivery more from the health service's point of view than from the patient's. Modifications to this model, including ones that might more involve family or community members, could provide better opportunities to tackle the barriers which relate to both society and family. Such a policy might then address the problem from what would be a perceptibly different direction, potentially helping to reduce stigma at the same time as encouraging completion of treatment.

Community health staff with good communication skills whilst also being charismatic advocates of good TB control might positively influence these barriers. Unfortunately the community health workers' records from the 1980s which the researchers had reviewed suggested that most community health staff didn't have such skills and were far more likely to be seen as just 'another pair of hands' operating on behalf of an anonymous and megalithic health service.

The experience in India following the so-called Madras study of 1956 strongly supports these conclusions. It may be recalled that this study first revealed the unexpected finding that the hospitalization of patients (which was standard at the time) offered no advantage in terms of successful treatment outcomes. As such, it effectively turned both the received and perceived wisdom of the time on its head. Following the Madras study's completion, however, the research staff who had been actively involved in the study itself had been replaced by health workers who were not so well trained, were less motivated and must also have been experienced by the patients as being that much less 'charismatic' as well. The positive responses which had been seen in the Madras study itself while it was still in action were swiftly seen to deteriorate with relapses becoming commonplace. A subsequent sociological study in Bangalore concluded that this had been caused because of a "slippery slope of sloppy treatment organisation".

There are issues of simple pragmatism at play here as well. In an environment in which there are not enough health workers to implement DOTS, then there is no choice but that a default model should be used. In Uganda, for instance, this has been carried out with a 'buddy' system, whereby a family member or friend comes with the patient and promises to monitor their treatment. Unfortunately there are no studies to help us judge how well the model works. But in cases where the patient's life is dysfunctional because of domestic or alcohol problems such a policy may well not be effective at all. Certainly, the so-called default rate amongst such patients is anecdotally reported to be much higher than the perceived average.

The second 2007 study concluded that the current dominant paradigm is too weighted on the side of trying to control patients rather than trying to find the best way to enable them to co-operate in taking their drugs. Such an approach was not always of benefit to the patients – and therefore neither was it of benefit to others because of the consequential risks of poor adherence, transmission and drug-resistance. They suggested that the basic DOTS approach could be modified towards one that is more focused on developing stronger health systems which could respond to patients' health-care requirements in order to help them to choose to complete their treatments themselves.

This might well have seemed to be a useful and more flexible approach, but just how easily can it be implemented? Actually, there are some signs that it is already in process. The 2013 Global Tuberculosis Report included a set of new definitions of disease, some of which included fresh categorisation of TB patients. Retreatment cases will no longer be sub-categorised as 'defaulted' – they will now less judgmentally be re-categorised either as 'treatment after failure' or 'treatment after loss to follow up'.

When it comes to this issue of control and coercion, however, there is also the equally vital matter of appropriately controlling the other players in the supply chain. This includes drug manufacturers who are known to offer sub-standard drugs on the global market place, manufacturers of diagnostics who supply them in full knowledge that they are unapproved, and criminals who are selling fake drugs on the open market. It should also include officials who might be taking backhanders in any part of these processes.

It should also cover those entrusted with both the immediate accurate notification of infectious cases and of reporting outcome data. In China today, for instance, it is a crime if notification is not promptly made. This policy involves a degree of enforcement that is not matched in any other country – indeed it might not even be possible to consider it in many. But (at least according to figures that are accepted by the WHO) the story of TB control in China in recent years has been a more successful one to the extent that it has largely swayed the global trends in favour of general reductions, with the country also reporting an extremely high treatment success rate.

Then there are the unregulated practitioners operating all over in both low- and middle-income countries who are neither properly trained nor equipped to treat TB to standards which are requisite for the containment of drug-resistance. These players need to be much better controlled as well.

Paul Garner, who played his part in both of these review papers on DOTS, had already taken an earlier stab at the subject in 2006 asking a similar question as to whether DOTS-Plus is cost-effective or (more importantly perhaps) even feasible.[310]

His team started out by accepting the premise that a basic requirement of DOTS-Plus is the existence of advanced medical care, of good infection control measures and of a good capacity for following up patients. They then asked whether such specialist medical services could ever be provided at appropriate scale in any but high-income countries. What concerned them was whether the efforts required to provide such treatment might divert political attention, resource allocation, specialist medical attention, and public health management capacity away from vital first line treatment – and even from other functions of primary care. In other words, it might threaten to imbalance the wider project of providing public health care.

The Stop TB Partnership recommends that DOTS-Plus programmes should only be instituted where there are already effective DOTS programmes in place. DOTS-Plus programmes are distinguished from DOTS by the provision of expensive second line TB drugs, ideally given as individualised treatment according to case-by-case susceptibility. Whenever diagnostic facilities are fewer, however, DOTS-Plus may be given as empirical treatment in people that have presumed MDR-TB rather than other more extensively resistant strains of disease.

There is a terrible catch which reveals itself within this recommendation because the existence of an MDR-TB epidemic is broadly indicative that the local DOTS programme has already failed. If an effective DOTS programme were in place and there is any MDR-TB present, such outbreaks of drug-resistant disease should be both limited and limitable if an appropriate response is swiftly mobilised. So whilst it is entirely logical that DOTS-Plus programmes should only ever be instituted where there are effective DOTS programmes already in place, they should never be that widely needed in such places and will only ever need to be small in scale in comparison to the DOTS provision. Where DOTS-Plus programmes can be predicted to be most needed, however, are exactly where basic DOTS programmes are failing or have already failed. As such they remain

---

[310] Paul Garner, Marissa Alejandria and Mary Ann Lansang - "Is DOTS-Plus a feasible and cost-effective strategy?", PLoS Med 3;9 (2006) e350. doi:10.1371/journal.pmed.0030350.

effectively unimplementable at any sort of scale under the terms of Partnership's TB recommendation. Again we encounter the same sorts of confounding conclusions.

It should also not be forgotten that, whenever rates of XDR-TB are being quantified behind or within an MDR-TB epidemic, they are invariably found to be increasing. In fact, they are not only found to be increasing, but they are almost always found to be higher than expected and rising proportionately faster than the MDR epidemic. This in turn is most probably occurring because of high rates of failed treatment of MDR-TB. As a result it can be surmised that empirical treatment of MDR-TB without DST of second line agents is far from being without significant risk of further promoting more lethal extensive resistance from its very outset.

As such we can recognise that we now have three separate waves of disease to anticipate. The first one is of drug-susceptible disease (which looks to have peaked). The second is MDR disease (which is rising). The third is XDR disease (which is probably rising faster than the second wave since measured rates of XDR-TB rose by 52% just between 2011 and 2012).

Towards the end of their paper the authors struck right at the very heart of the matter:

> "At the end of the day, it is the responsibility of national policy makers to maintain control of their own health-care system, whatever external experts are pushing and whatever funding is on offer. These responsibilities mean having to balance primary care with the need for difficult and expensive treatment for a few but increasing number of patients."

These papers are now six and seven years old with the territory changing rapidly since their publications.

'Mentalities of Scarcity' and 'Droughts of imagination'[311]

"THE RESPONSE TO THE DRUG-RESISTANT TUBERCULOSIS EPIDEMIC SEEMS TO BE INEFFECTUAL, WITH [A] PROJECTED RAPID INCREASE IN THE GLOBAL INCIDENCE OF MDR-TB."

Professor Alimuddin Zumla (2012)[312]

The Millennium Development Goals

The United Nations Millennium Development Goals (MDGs) consisted of eight goals that all 191 UN Member States agreed to try to achieve by 2015. The United Nations Millennium Declaration was signed in September 2000, and committed world leaders to combat poverty, hunger, disease, illiteracy, environmental degradation, and discrimination against women. The MDGs themselves were derived directly from this declaration, and all had specific targets and indicators.

Those eight Millennium Development Goals still exist:

- to eradicate extreme poverty and hunger;
- to achieve universal primary education;
- to promote gender equality and empower women;
- to reduce child mortality;
- to improve maternal health;
- to combat HIV/AIDS, malaria, and other diseases;
- to ensure environmental sustainability; and
- to develop a global partnership for development.

With a year to go the prospects for adequately meeting any of these goals remains poor, although the loose wording of some of them mean that it

[311] These are two phrases used by Carole Mitnick of Partners in Health to describe the existing response to DR-TB.

[312] Professor of Infectious Diseases and International Health at University College London Medical School.

will be easy to make some claims of success. It will be noted that, while HIV and malaria received special mention, TB didn't get any specific attention at all in this 'first edition'. This was surprising given the prevalant scale of the pandemic at the time the goals were set and the fact that the disease had been proclaimed in an unprecedented fashion as a global emergency seven years earlier with all rates rising during the following years. Tuberculosis was specifically identified in "Target 8 of sub-clause 6' (as one of the "other diseases that were being intended to be combatted) and the goal that was set for its control was as bland as some of the other targets – nothing more than "to halt the spread of TB by 2015 and begin to reverse the worldwide incidence". It certainly sounds unambitious, and if this doesn't stand as testimony to the lack of advocacy and activism in relation to tuberculosis control in the 1990s nothing does.

Despite the goal having been so bland and unambitious, and in spite its having been overwritten by other targets eight years ago, it is still being brought out and quoted – perhaps because it is one of the only success stories that can be.

Global Plans and the Partnership's Targets

In March 2000 the Stop TB Initiative produced the Amsterdam Declaration, calling for action from ministerial delegations of 20 countries that were assessed at the time to have the highest burdens of TB. That same year the World Health Assembly endorsed two goals for 2005, effectively superimposing its own targets overt the MDGs: to diagnose 70% of all those estimated to be infected and to cure 85% of the diagnosed cohort. The WHO then set its Global Plan for 2001-2005.

This plan set two specific targets – one for 5 years (as above) and the other one for ten: "By 2010: to reduce the global burden of TB disease (that is, death and prevalence rates caused by disease) by 50% from year 2000 levels".[313]

The rates of disease, meanwhile, continued to rise.

---

313 WHO – "Global Plan to stop TB 2001-2005"

In January 2006 the Stop TB Partnership launched its second Global Plan to Stop TB, this time for 2006-2015. It included some specific slightly more modest targets:

1. by 2015, to reduce the global burden (in terms of both prevalence and death rates) of tuberculosis by 50% relative to what had been the global burden in 1990 to:

    i. prevalence to less than 150/100,000 population; and -
    ii. deaths to less than 15/100,000 per year

2. by 2050, to eliminate tuberculosis as a health threat (defined as a global tuberculosis incidence of less than one case/1 million population/year).

The combined focus on these two factors was clearly correct. The idea was to see less active prevalent disease in the global community, and to see fewer deaths as a result.

At the same time the Partnership launched a six-part general strategy which extended the WHO's previous goals of a 70% global detection rate and an 85% cure rate to 2015 (both supposed to have already been met by 2005). The ultimate aim of this revised global strategy, though, was to achieve the elimination of TB as a public health concern by 2050.

In order to do this, the new six-point strategy was built on what was being described as "existing success" while recognising the key challenges of TB/HIV and MDR-TB. It stated its intention to adopt "evidence-based innovations in engaging with private health-care providers, empowering affected people and communities, to help strengthen health systems and promote research". The authors claimed that their plan "also responds to access, equity and quality constraints".[314]

These were the six components to the plan:

---

314 Mandeep S Jassal and William R Bishai - "Epidemiology and Challenges to the Elimination of Global Tuberculosis", Journal of Clinical Infectious Diseases, 12;50 (2010) 156-64.

1. **To pursue high-quality DOTS expansion and enhancement** including to the poorest and most vulnerable, and enabling DOTS expansion to even the remotest areas.

2. **To address TB/HIV, MDR-TB and the needs of poor and vulnerable populations.**

3. **To contribute to health system strengthening based on primary health care** focusing on facilitating national TB control programmes including innovative service delivery scale-up.

4. **To engage all care providers** recognising that TB patients seek care from a wide array of public, private, corporate and voluntary health-care providers.

5. **To empower people with TB, and communities through partnership** recognising that community care projects can help mobilize civil societies and also ensuring political support and long-term sustainability for TB control programmes.

6. **To enable and promote research** recognising that elimination of TB would depend on new diagnostics, drugs and vaccines.

This general strategy was still being maintained when the plan was revised once again four years later, this time to become the "Global Plan to Stop TB 2011-2015". The targets were still being set for 2015. The key difference was an increasing recognition of the need to roll out proper treatment to combat drug-resistance, with targets for this component of the pandemic being added.

Some of the figures that are being reported today do look encouraging. Currently prevalence rates are said to have reduced by around 36%, running at a little below 170/100,000.[315] Curiously, however, incidence rates haven't correspondingly dropped as might have been expected alongside them, dropping by less than half this rate, by 16%. It's possible that this difference is partly because of higher rates of HIV co-infection, with TB essentially speeding up where and when the two diseases occur together whilst it may have been slowing down elsewhere.

[315] WHO - "Global Tuberculosis Report 2013".

All of these goals and targets continue to be used in a confusing fashion, however, with both authorities and media frequently quoting the fact that the MDG target of "halting and reversing the TB epidemic by 2015" has already been met as if this were still the main goal, and sometimes choosing to ignore the Partnership's own later goals completely.

But other parts of the story are now very far from encouraging at all. A recent prevalence rate made available for the African region was 450/100,000 (which is a 150% rise rather than a 50% reduction), and the mortality rate was 50/100,000 (which is a 166% rise instead of a 50% reduction). The general failure for the African region to address its epidemic is appalling.

The second Partnership Goal (of eliminating the disease as a health threat by 2050) was laudable but was always going to be a huge challenge. The current rate of decline (which started after a period between 2000 and 2008 when disease had been rising sharply) is stable and running at about 2% per year. This year-on-year percentage rate of decline requires that, in order to consider the possibility of elimination by 2050, it should be nearer 20% (and this calculation ignores the drug-resistant component completely). So the goal of elimination by 2050 was never really much more than a pipe dream without massive developments in resource being applied along with huge changes of fortune. Raviglione himself has suggested that, if current rates of decline are maintained, TB cannot seriously be expected to be eliminated before the end of the 21st century.

In fact, because of an increased global population since 1990 the total ***number*** of people who are now being newly infected each year with TB is actually as high today as it has been in any other time in history.

But even in 2006 it was already being recognised that specific challenges were restricting the programme's progress. These were separately being identified as:

- funding shortfalls,
- HIV co-infection, and
- drug-resistance.

There had certainly been clear shortfalls in funding. Even at its launch in 2006 there was an estimated funding gap of over US$30 billion in the programme. (The 2006 total budget for the plan was US$56 billion – US$47 billion for currently available treatment and US$9 billion for R&D).

Regarding both HIV and DR-TB there was already an emerging consensus that the impacts, both separate and combined, of these two components of the pandemic had not been adequately allowed for either separately or together. Nor, in fact, had they even been seriously anticipated in the original development of the DOTS strategy. HIV had been having lethal influence on the African epidemic so it could still, even in 2006, be viewed as being largely regionally specific. But the scale of its effect has nevertheless been colossal. Drug-resistance, meanwhile, has been occurring everywhere, and has remained the major blind-spot in the WHO's policy with nowhere near enough co-ordinated effort being put into its containment in either the first or the second decade of the global emergency.

The Global Plan was now intending to introduce both preventive and restorative strategies to combat these deficiencies – essentially by combining and enhancing DOTS and DOTS-Plus. The plan anticipated that, during the nine years of its existence, a total of 778,000 MDR-TB cases would be treated according to the approved WHO guidelines. At the same time, the intention was that the estimated global percentage of re-treatment TB cases would decrease from 20% of incident cases in 2005 to 11% by 2015, simply as a result of better-managed treatment.

With regards to MDR-TB itself, the implementation of the 2006 strategy was expecting that the prevalent number of MDR-TB cases would reduce from an estimated 533,000 in 2005 to a more manageable 193,000 by 2015 – in other words by a hugely ambitious 74%.

The plan itself included a set of five specific objectives, each accompanied by identifiable or measurable milestones that could be used to monitor progress. They've pretty much been missed, and this was first being identified soon after the Plan's implementation.

The first major update to the MDR-TB component of the plan was made in mid-2007, with more ambitious specific targets being set for the 27 high MDR-TB burden countries. A new general target was established in the 2007 'Global MDR/XDR Response', which was to reach 85% of MDR-TB cases with accurate diagnosis and effective treatment by 2015.

Then a ministerial conference held in Beijing in April 2009 brought together high-level representatives from the 27 high MDR-TB burden countries – those countries that collectively are supposed to account for around 85% of the world's cases of MDR-TB. The conference led to a formal "Call to Action" to both governments and international agencies. Less than two months afterwards, the 62nd World Health Assembly passed a further resolution on MDR-TB, this time calling on all countries to implement the measures needed to achieve "universal access to diagnosis and treatment of MDR-TB" by 2015.

As a result, the Global Plan was redrafted again. Instead of the '2006-2015 Plan', it now became the '2011-2015 Plan', and was published as such in 2010. Essentially it reviewed the progress to date and re-wrote the strategy based on the lessons learnt, particularly recognising the budgetary necessities if the targets were to be met as it was still hoped they could be.

The general final targets for TB for 2015 (of reducing rates of prevalence and mortality by 50%) remained the same. Instead of the five objectives regarding DR-TB contained in the 2006 Plan, however, there were now six, and there were significant differences among them, not least of which was that the intention to reduce rates of MDR-TB by 74% was modified to more realistically just to "reduce the global burden of drug-resistant TB". The target now was a requirement that the incidence of MDR-TB should be "declining by 2015", and no more. In other words, in contrast to the six-year evolution of the Millennium Goals into the Partnership Goals (developing from being unambitious to challenging), with MDR-TB it had taken just four years to devolve and dilute in the opposite direction. And even this goal won't be achieved by 2015.

Some of those troublesome milestones were also now being dropped, but in other respects the objectives were actually hardening up.

A list of the objectives follows. Those of the earlier 2006-2015 plan are shown in italics milestones, and the correspondingly numbered objectives of the more recent 2011-2015 plan follows for the comparison:

> ***2006 Objective 1**: by 2015, representative and reliable data should be available on the global magnitude of MDR-TB, as well as trends in high MDR-TB prevalence countries, and the relationship between MDR-TB and HIV/AIDS.*
>
> **2011 Objective 1**: By 2015, 100% of people who have been previously treated for TB should be tested for MDR-TB. New cases should also be tested for MDR-TB if they have a specific risk, such as contact with a person with confirmed MDR-TB.

2006 Objective 2: *By 2015, all regions should carry out DST for all previously treated TB patients.*

2011 Objective 2: All people who are found to have MDR-TB should receive testing for susceptibility to second line drugs, so as to diagnose or rule out XDR-TB.

2006 Objective 3: *By 2015, all 'detected' MDR-TB patients should be treated with quality-assured second line drugs in line with WHO guidelines, and 56% of the global estimated MDR-TB cases should be being treated.*

2011 Objective 3: All patients with confirmed MDR-TB should be treated according to international standards. The number of patients being treated for MDR-TB should reach around 270,000 per year in 2015. The total number of people to be treated in the five years 2011–2015 should reach approximately one million. Around seven million people would have been tested for MDR-TB by 2015. The treatment success rate among patients with confirmed MDR-TB should increase from the 2009 baseline of 60% to ≥75% by 2015.

2006 Objective 4: *By 2015, the price of second line drugs will have been further reduced, and quality-assured second line drug will be produced by manufacturers based in countries with a high burden of MDR-TB.*

2011 Objective 4: Scale up TB infection control in MDR-TB hospital wards and outpatient clinics. Countries with a high burden of MDR-TB should have instituted a recommended package of infection control measures in hospital wards and outpatient clinics.

2006 Objective 5: *Provide technical direction and strategic planning for the management and co-ordination of global MDR-TB surveillance and control. By 2015, all regions and countries will include DRS and MDR-TB management in regular TB courses and workshops.*

2011 Objective 5: High-quality drug-resistance surveillance data should be available for 110 non high-income countries instead of the 78 for which data were available in 2009.

2011 objective 6: Expand country capacity to scale up the management of drug-resistant TB through global advocacy and policy guidance.

There were some curious changes, omissions and additions, but there was one massive difference which revealed itself in the later plan. One of the specific targets in the original 2006 plan regarding MDR-TB had been to be diagnosing and treating 110,000 patients with MDR-TB per year by 2015, with 100% of confirmed cases treated in programmes following international guidelines. The plan now was to be diagnosing and treating around 270,000 MDR-TB patients per year. In other words, the size and the scale of the problem had been reviewed and judged to be at least two and a half times larger than originally estimated. In 2006 the number that had been identified as being treated that year was just a "few thousand"; in 2009 (at the halfway mark of the plan) it was identified as being 11,000 a year – so at halfway, it was still just a tenth of the 2015 target set five years earlier.

Similarly, at the halfway stage:

- the estimated percentage of previously treated TB patients tested for MDR-TB was running at just 7% – with a target of 100%;
- the estimated percentage of new TB patients tested for MDR-TB was also running at just 7% – with a target of 20%;
- the number of countries among the 36 combined HBCs and high MDR-TB burden countries with one or more culture laboratories per five million population was just over 50% (the actual number, which must have been the easiest number to count in the whole Plan, wasn't defined) – with a target of 100%;
- the estimated percentage of confirmed cases of MDR-TB enrolled on treatment was 36% – with a target of 100%;
- the estimated percentage of people living with HIV attending HIV care services who were enrolled on IPT, among those eligible was less than 1% – with a target of 100%; and
- the percentage of national reference laboratories implementing a quality management system according to international standards was less than 5% – with a minimum target of 50%.

Despite the first item identified in the new plan describing the reasoning for revising the plan as being because of "a need to take into account actual progress made since 2006", as far as MDR-TB was concerned, the progress that had been made was worryingly difficult to identify.

The original Working Group had identified four major areas of risk to its original 2006-2015 Plan, all of which it now sought to address. These had been:

- a deterioration in the global MDR-TB situation and a continued misuse of second line drugs,
- a lack of well-functioning laboratory networks providing culture and drug-susceptibility testing,
- a lack of political will,
- a lack of global coordination.

It is difficult not to conclude that the objectives are almost all at risk, with major milestones having been missed already. Not only that, but it is almost certain that it has been ***exactly*** these four areas of risk that have largely accounted for this happening so they have self-evidently failed to have been addressed.

In an interview in 2011, Mario Raviglione, the WHO's Head of TB, directly addressed part of this problem discussing the consequences of serially misdiagnosing TB, particularly MDR- and XDR-TB. He identified that there were four separate fronts on which the WHO considered that the war against TB needed to be fought: effective TB programmes; free and accessible health provision; comprehensive laboratory systems; and alleviation of the social and economic factors which contribute to the epidemic.[316] They were far from all under the possible control of the WHO, because the last front would have to involve "interventions for poverty, bad housing, nutrition, education, etc., that are beyond the reach of the health community alone".

He also identified how even the existing drugs remained a challenge because they remained both too expensive and insufficient in quantity. He stated unambiguously that the ***only*** alternative to not successfully managing the campaign on all of these fronts was simple straightforward "failure", at

[316] Rebecca Kennedy and Karuna Luthra - "Diagnosing Inaccuracy: New WHO Policy Shift to end ineffective TB Practices", the National Bureau of Asian Research – Center for Health and Aging. http://www.nbr.org/downloads/pdfs/CHA/NBR_Raviglione_interview.pdf.

the same time as acknowledging that those targets that had been enshrined in the MDGs had, indeed, been "unambitious".

He went on to observe that the basic understanding of the pathogenesis and immunology of TB was still insufficient for him to believe that we might really have an effective vaccine within the next ten years. He stated:

> "I find it hard to believe that we will have an effective new vaccine that truly allows elimination within a decade."

It looks like he may be proved right with best dates for any new vaccine being pushed back despite more candidate vaccines appearing.

In strong contrast to the resigned tone set by Raviglione, Martha Benezet, a TB expert who works for Abt Associates,[317] offered a more upbeat analysis in 2013. Abt Associates is an organisation involved in research and programme implementation in global health as well as in social and environmental policies relating to international development. The organisation has been particularly recognised for "its rigorous approach to solving complex challenges" which sounds exactly what is needed.

Benezet felt that local country partners should be "more courageous" and "creative" in finding innovative solutions to the problem, observing that the world had so far only been scratching the surface in terms of the potential of public-private partnerships for fighting TB. Her views are resonant with those that have more recently been emerging from the WHO as it grapples with the rising incidence of cases of multi drug-resistant TB and the higher incidences of HIV and TB co-infection. For Benezet, the most effective solution is for the affected countries to work better with their partners, and, in her opinion, these partners are principally within their private sectors. She elucidated further:

> "TB has been an area that has long been pointed out as underfunded. In many ways it has. But in many ways, there's a lot of progress in securing funding and a lot has been done by countries themselves.
>
> "I think now is the time for us to be creative and courageous and work with our country partners to figure out other ways to implement their TB programmes, because research says that TB programmes, once funded, are

[317] "How to fill the TB funding gap: Creativity and Courage" (2013) https://www.devex.com/en/news/how-to-fill-the-tb-funding-gap-creativity-and-courage/80547.

very cost-efficient and the outcomes are very good. I think we must work with countries to help them find ways to fund these solutions themselves.

"..Governments [must] have a clear view of how much they would have to set aside to deal with their own issues. I think that [some] sort of rigorous analysis is essential.

"I would also say that I think we have just scratched the surface of the potential in public-private partnerships. I think there's a huge potential there to be latched onto. There have been several successful public-private partnerships. We have some work in high-burden countries such as Ethiopia and India that have really brought the private sectors into the health system as effective TB caregivers.

"I think there are solutions that are there already. We just have to look at it in a different way and find them together within the context of each country.

"Even in high-burden countries, sometimes TB is not the top priority. I think there needs to be a lot of advocacy work. There are many, many HIV-related organizations, for example. There are fewer TB-related organizations, but there are many people suffering from TB.

"MDR-TB is no doubt a global threat right now. The issue is [that] even in high-burden countries, case finding is low for MDR-TB. This is well-documented within WHO. I think the first concern is that, before countries can figure out how much they need to have in their coffers to pay for MDR-TB, they have to really understand what is their prevalence, what is the incidence rate, so that they can actually understand the figure that they're coping with.

"In general, case finding of MDR-TB is a tougher nut to crack. It can be frighteningly expensive to manage. But there are resources through the WHO and the Stop TB partnership to access second line drugs at a more affordable price. I think a lot of countries have taken advantage of that to their benefit."

On the basis of recent experience, her ideas certainly sound both considered and exciting but they also come fraught with risk. The idea that the private sector in India has offered effective care for TB patients (as she appears to intimate) is contradicted by evidence which suggests the opposite. Nevertheless we can see signs that such initiatives are now being seriously adopted by policymakers but it may be only because they appear to be the only thing available.

The idea that resources within the WHO have made second line drugs that much cheaper at any sort of scale is also disingenuous: it ignores a decade of lack of progress by the GLC initiative and the GDF. Suggesting that TB programmes are cost-efficient and have good outcomes is also misleading given that the same statement is linked to programmes for MDR- and XDR-TB. Furthermore, the idea that the scales of prevalence and incidence rates of MDR-TB can so easily be measured smacks more of an accountant than of someone who accepts the scale and complexities of the problems being confronted by middle- and low-income countries today. It also suggests a 'can-do' mentality towards solving a very complex problem that just may simple solutions.

Perhaps this may seem a negative response, but the WHO's own global report of 2012 candidly states that:

> "The suboptimal levels of coverage of DST [drug-susceptibility testing] in many countries are one of the main reasons why the number of people who are diagnosed with MDR-TB remains low."

The implicit (and very logical) suggestion contained within this statement is that, if the DST resource were more, the DR-TB epidemic that needs addressing would be measurably larger too, and yet existing resources can't treat anywhere near enough patients. Given that this has to be accepted, Raviglione's resigned tone is surely understandable. Since there is such a dearth both of continuous surveillance and drug-susceptibility testing in low-income countries, there has to be an awful lot of work done before even the faintest outline of realistic budgets and effective strategies can be properly developed.

In the 2013 report, however, this picture of dearth of data went one step further:

> "One of the main reasons for low case detection rates [of TB] in many parts of the world is the existence of a significant private sector in which providers frequently diagnose people with TB but fail to notify these cases to the national authorities."

In other words it recognised that a part of the problem has been created by one of the key players in the innovative solution that is being envisaged.

Benezet does, however, recognise the success of the many HIV advocacy groups who have made such progress in the fight against HIV. There's good evidence of this in the proportionately huge (nine-fold) increase in the numbers of TB patients who have known HIV status in comparison to the slow rise in the number of known MDR-TB case detections.

Her ideas also seem to bend towards the idea of awarding individual countries the right to find their own solutions to their problem rather than having ones foisted upon them. This sounds a laudable idea, and in some situations such a policy must be the right one, but with TB (particularly the global problem of drug-resistant TB) such ideas should be approached with caution. Awarding individual countries too much control over a global problem could be dangerous when given over to local politicians with their own agendas. The culture of denial that was foisted on the HIV epidemic in South Africa by Thabo Mbeki has been estimated to have cost at least 330,000 lives.[318] A similar culture of denial has already been discussed in relation to the management of TB in India. It should always be born in mind that no TB programme at all, in certain situations, can be better than one that is being misapplied particularly if this were to occur because of political and prejudices.

The predictable problem is that, when existing strategies are seen to be failing, measures which may be seen by some as being desperate may be seen by others as offering the only possible solutions – forcing authorities, as Richard Coker described, into doing "all sorts of stupid things".[319]

The problems that perpetuate have been summed up by Carole Mitnick, a TB researcher at Harvard Medical School:

> "The prevailing attitude among those responsible for global TB policy has been that what we had – a six-month, four-drug regimen good for most patients – was the best we could hope for. The battle in TB control, its

[318] Pride Chigwedere et al. – "Estimating the lost benefits of antiretroviral drug use in South Africa", Journal of Acquired Immune Deficiency Syndrome, 9; 4, (2008):

"More than 330,000 lives or approximately 2.2 million person years were lost because a feasible and timely ARV treatment program was not implemented in South Africa. Thirty-five thousand babies were born with HIV, resulting in 1.6 million person-years lost by not implementing a mother-to-child transmission prophylaxis program using nevirapine. The total lost benefits of ARVs are at least 3.8 million person-years for the period 2000–2005."

[319] Richard Coker - "From Chaos to Coercion: Detention and the Control of Tuberculosis", Palgrave MacMillan (2000).

> architects maintained, was simply about rigorous, widespread delivery of the existing tools: drugs that are more than 50 years old; a diagnostic that is now more than 125 years old; and a vaccine that is more than 100 years old. There was a mentality of scarcity among those most concerned about TB, which seemed to preclude demands for innovations in treatment, diagnosis, and prevention. Since drug and medical device research and development is a lengthy process, this drought of imagination has delayed harvest of new technologies for decades."

She describes the general policy as reflecting a "drought of imagination" – strong words to describe a policy which has been elsewhere described by the Director General of the WHO as "in some ways a glowing success story".

The 2012 & 2013 Global Reports

HOW MANY TIMES MUST A MAN LOOK UP
BEFORE HE CAN SEE THE SKY?
YES, 'N' HOW MANY EARS MUST ONE MAN HAVE
BEFORE HE CAN HEAR PEOPLE CRY?
YES, 'N' HOW MANY DEATHS WILL IT TAKE TILL HE KNOWS
THAT TOO MANY PEOPLE HAVE DIED?
THE ANSWER, MY FRIEND, IS BLOWIN' IN THE WIND
THE ANSWER IS BLOWIN' IN THE WIND

Bob Dylan (1962)

Two years after the revised Global Plan for 2011-2015 was published and the Global Tuberculosis Report of 2012 offered up further food for thought. Epidemiological indicators were now indicating (not that surprisingly) that the Goal of TB elimination by 2050 would not be achieved. This was now being accompanied, however, by a further recognition that:

> "… the persistence of TB in the setting of poor existing health infrastructure has led to an increase in drug-resistant cases, exacerbated by the strong association with human immunodeficiency virus co-infection. Spreading drug-resistance threatens to undo decades of progress in controlling the disease."

Yet again this direct link between poor existing health infrastructure and drug-resistant TB was being made, and in this instance a link with HIV was being made as well.

The report further suggested that "several significant gaps can be identified in various aspects of national- and international-directed TB-control efforts" although it remained unclear as to exactly what these were. What it was clear about, however, was that "existing economic and social obstacles must be overcome if TB elimination is to be a reachable goal".

Particular strategies were reported to be already being worked on to help all of this happen.

One was to bring private practitioners more into the DOTS team. We have already looked at this, accepting that it may be seen as a realistic way of attempting to utilise a visible available resource, but that it is arguably a high-risk strategy. It was evidently becoming clear to the WHO that incorporating more private health care providers remain one of the only options for ramping up any sort of potentially effective resource at all.

In much of the developing world, private practitioners are already the major primary care providers anyway, often because of inadequate governmental health care provision. In Pakistan, for example, it is suggested that as much as 79% of first-line health care is in private hands. Unfortunately, it is also recognised that these private health care providers are also often neither well trained nor properly monitored, particularly in regards to proper adherence to national TB programmes or international treatment guidelines. It cannot be seen by anyone as being an easy task to bring them effectively into the fold. TB epidemiologists elsewhere, however, could be seen to be advocating the same thing:

> "If any effective diagnostic and therapeutic modality to enhance DOTS coverage in the world is to occur, private health care providers must be in line with any current and newly adopted standards of care."[320].

(The key here is that they must be kept "in line with any current and newly adopted standards of care" and not allowed to be operating outside of them at all in respect of both treatment and diagnosis.)

So while we may wonder whether this strategy can seriously be ramped up to do what it hopes to do and do it safely, key epidemiologists say that it simply ***must*** do. But if government health care services are so deficient that their populations don't trust them, whilst the private sector is recognised to have been prescribing what has been termed a "therapeutic anarchy", who exactly will be left on the ground to properly co-ordinate this ramping up of resource?

There is a secondary consequence as well to bringing private practitioners into the mix because it will almost certainly have an effect on the figures. The 2013 report suggested that one of the main reasons for the stubborn 34% gap between national notification surveillance systems and the estimated number of incident cases 'still out there' is "because private sector providers fail to notify cases". This isn't the only reason, because poor access to health care or failure to actually detect cases when they get to a health centre contribute to this problem as well.[321] So bringing private practitioners properly into the fold should go some way to enable that first (still-elusive) 2005 goal of 70% case detection or the current one of 87% for 2015, but it may also adjust some of the rates themselves in the process.

---

[320] Mandeep S Jassal and William R Bishai, - "Epidemiology and Challenges to the Elimination of Global Tuberculosis", Journal of Clinical Infectious Diseases 12;50 (2010) 156-64.

[321] WHO- "Global Tuberculosis Report 2013".

The current estimates of incidence cases are arrived at based on notification data (which is essentially accurate) combined with "country consultations in which in-depth analyses of the available surveillance, survey and programmatic data are undertaken". To achieve this "***expert opinion about the fraction of cases diagnosed but not reported, or not diagnosed at all, is elicited*** and documented". (My italics). These estimated rates vary dramatically between countries. In Africa, for instance the percentage estimates of notified cases as opposed to total incident cases vary between 32% in Sierra Leone and 81% in Ghana. In Pakistan, with 79% of front line care in the hands of private practitioners, it is suggested to be as much as 65% (or just one point below the global average). In India it's estimated to be 59% (with as much as 50% of patients resorting to the private sector). In China the percentage is reckoned to be 89%, in a country which has met only 20% of the global target for provision of sputum smear microscopy centres and with rural patients reported to distrust doctors so much that 76% of them said in a study that they wouldn't want to visit one. It's not difficult to begin to question the reliability of these opinions, and to wonder what the real global percentage might be given that these latter two countries have the highest national numerical burdens of disease.

A far better picture of the true state of the pandemic might therefore emerge if these private care providers can be effectively co-ordinated as intended. The deal for them is to be this: work to our guidelines and you receive free drugs, supervision, quality assurance and "financial or non-financial incentives". It sounds quite reasonable, but how will these deals really work out where things are working so poorly already, especially in countries where corruption is a commonplace?

Be that as it may, the general tone of any WHO report on TB follows a standard pattern – it starts positively and then develops a more cautionary tone. Initially such reports invariably identify the successes that have been made, particularly in halting and beginning to reverse the trends in global prevalence of the disease before the 2015 target date, although such exhortations must be beginning to sound hollow to anyone who knows much about the complex nature of the pandemic. Margaret Chan's statement for World TB Day 2013 was typical of this. She started on a positive note:

> "On many levels TB control is a glowing success story ... The epidemic which, in 1993, looked set to spiral out of control, peaked ten years ago and began a slow but steady decline. The [UN's] Millennium Development target of halting and reversing the TB epidemic by 2015 has already been achieved. Overall, the world is on track to meet the [Stop TB Partnership's]

> target of a 50% reduction in deaths compared with 1990.[322] An unprecedented number of vaccines are now at various stages of development. The end of last year saw regulatory approval of the first new TB drug in 50 years."

Given that the state of emergency was declared 20 years before and it took over 12 years to even begin to reverse the upward trend of disease, this may not be quite as accurate a summary of achievement as it sounds. Certainly, given what we know, it can hardly be cast as any sort of "glowing success story". But a far more cautionary note normally follows any such optimistic WHO pronouncement on TB, and this one was no different. Dr Chan continued:

> "The negative side has three dimensions.
>
> "The first dimension is scale. Despite recent success in shrinking the epidemic, the global TB burden remains enormous.
>
> "The second dimension is the rise of TB strains that are resistant to multiple first line drugs or extensively resistant to second line drugs as well ... In some countries, as many as 35% of new cases have MDR-TB at the start. This gives you an idea of the powder keg we are sitting on.
>
> "The final dimension is financial. The funding gap for TB care and control is substantial."

This acknowledgement of the scale and nature of the drug-resistant problem has become increasingly emotive. But this doesn't just relate to bog-standard MDR-TB (as if that weren't challenging enough). It also means XDR-TB which we know is also out there, but which failed to get mentioned (even though it may be the most explosive component in Dr Chan's powder keg).

Global targets are the main tools to keep track of controlling any pandemic. What is repeatedly identified is that certain targets which were set for 2015 are going to be hit (albeit that one of them will ignore deaths amongst the co-infected) and some will only be near missed. What rarely gets mentioned

---

[322] Invoking this as a "reduction in deaths" was an unfortunate choice of words. The goal was in fact a reduction in the ***rate*** of deaths. In terms of absolute numbers of TB deaths, the total has actually risen since 1990, and according to the WHO's own figures from its 2012 report has only recently even begun to fall at all. Quoting the earlier Millennium Goal of "halting and reversing TB" was also an interesting choice, given the more recent Partnership goals which included intending to halve the prevalence rate - a target that is not being met..

is the number of targets that are almost certain to be catastrophically missed, most of which relate to drug-resistant disease.

Here are some specific targets for TB that were set for 2015:

- DOTS: a case detection rate (CDR) of 84% and a treatment success rate of 87% by 2015. The CDR is the number of notified cases of TB divided by the estimated number of new (incident) cases of TB that occurred in the same year. The treatment success rate is the percentage of patients cured plus the percentage that completed treatment but for whom cure was not confirmed. Both are heavily dependent on data input and expert opinion. The latter is also a matter of debate given the ongoing issues of definition of treatment success that we previously addressed.

- New diagnostics: a point-of-care test for TB by 2010 and a test allowing detection of latent TB infection and to predict which people will develop active TB by 2015. Neither are on the horizon.

- New drugs: a novel TB drug introduced by 2010 and the duration of treatment for drug-susceptible TB reduced to 1–2 months by 2015, with regimens also active against MDR-TB and compatible with ART. Two new drugs are now approved but they are far from being widely implemented.

- New vaccines: two vaccines in 'proof-of-concept' trials by 2010 and one new safe and effective vaccine available by 2015. No new vaccine is yet visible in an immediate pipeline.

The tools that were needed to enable control of the disease have still not come on stream as hoped.

Page ix of the 2013 report did summarise the current position with the MDR-TB targets:

> "Progress towards targets for diagnosis and treatment of multi drug-resistant TB (MDR-TB) is far off-track."

This sentence was qualified by a further statement that "less than 25% of the people estimated to have MDR-TB were detected in 2012". History may yet reveal this to have also been an understatement.

Immediately below is a table of some of those targets for MDR-TB for 2015, along with their baselines from 2009, and their current situation as far as it is available from within the pages of the 2013 report. It doesn't make for cheerful reading. Some targets show little or no progress, only one seems remotely close to being met, and one (the rate of successful treatment for MDR-TB) even shows a significant reversal from the baseline.

	2009	**2012 (2013 report)**	**2015 (target)**
% of previously treated TB patients tested for MDR-TB	**7%**	**9%**	**100%**
% of new TB patients tested for MDR-TB	**7%**	**5%**	**20%**
Number of countries among the 22 HBCs and 27 high MDR-TB burden countries with ≥1 culture laboratory per 5 million population	**18-21**	**19**	**36**
Number of confirmed cases of MDR-TB enrolled on treatment according to international guidelines	**11,000**	**77,321**	**270,000**
% treatment success rate among confirmed cases of MDR-TB	**60%**	**48%**	**75%**
% of national reference laboratories implementing a quality management system	**<5%**	**No data**	**>50%**
% of confirmed cases of MDR-TB enrolled on treatment according to international guidelines	**36%**	**92% of notifications**	**100%**

There is no time for any more of the inertia that seems to have bedevilled policy making for the past two decades. A post-2015 strategy is now materialising, however, as we will shortly see. In the 2012 report it was already uncertain whether the goal of eliminating the disease by 2050 was going to be retained. It looked like too much political credibility might be lost if it were dropped, despite its being, even at 37 years' distance, already only a very remote possibility without "dramatic" changes. Meanwhile the 50% mortality target was looking to be almost certainly extended to 2025

In June 2013 a high level panel established by the Secretary General of the UN submitted its own report to the WHO containing recommendations for the new plan and the principle of universal health coverage was definitely being included within it. Exactly what this health coverage target was going to be pegged at must have been being fiercely debated. The new draft strategy then showed its face in October 2013 and, instead of aiming to eliminate TB by 2050 it included the goal of "ending the global TB epidemic by 2035", with milestones and targets being set for 2020, 2025, and 2030. Things were starting to look even more impossible, but it was being intended for the plan to be reviewed by the WHO executive board in January 2014 and then be discussed and ratified by the World Health Assembly in May.

The future that was being envisaged included "a thorough review of the current epidemiological and modelling methods", as well as a set of revised definitions for TB cases – which are far from as semantic as they might first appear. They reflect a rethink which intends to incorporate the new data which must be expected to be coming on stream from the new generation of diagnostics, specifically including the GeneXpert. Does this all add up to a thorough or innovative shift? Not with the current available evidence.

The unifying theme that runs on seems to be much the same as ever – a desperate need to strengthen national TB programmes, and to improve surveillance, diagnostics, treatment and prevention. And the fact remains that these still need to happen both at national and regional levels.

The post-2015 Strategy

"IT ALWAYS SEEMS IMPOSSIBLE UNTIL IT'S DONE."

Nelson Mandela

On the 19th May 2014 the World Health Assembly approved a resolution to accept and adopt the new post-2015 strategy to fight this ancient disease. It was unanimously endorsed by all of the WHO's member governments who made up the Assembly. By endorsing the resolution the governments of the world have committed to a new and ambitious strategy to end TB as a global pandemic by 2035 (reducing it to a global average of less than 10 new tuberculosis cases per 100,000 population each year). This still means over three-quarters of a million new cases in 2035 but, given the story so far, it is still an astonishing ambition. As things stand it would almost certainly seem to be an impossible one.

The World Health Assembly (WHA) determines the policies of the World Health Organization (WHO focusing on a specific health agenda which has been previously worked on by its Executive Board. In this particular instance the proposed resolution has been painstakingly developed by experts within the WHO itself over several years, as well as by a high level panel established by the Secretary-General of the UN which submitted its own report to the WHO with recommendations for the new plan.

The Assembly has passed resolutions in relation to TB before. In 2000, for instance, it endorsed two targets fort 2005 (neither of which have yet been achieved). Then in May 2005, the World Health Assembly passed a resolution concerning the Sustainable Financing for TB Prevention and Control. Within this resolution it encouraged all its member states "to ensure that all tuberculosis patients have access to the universal standard of care". In other words, the decision-making body of the WHO was unequivocally intending nearly ten years ago that ***all*** patients should be having access to diagnosis and treatment by second line drugs if they were drug-resistant. This aspiration is repeated in the current edition as if it were the first time it had been made. In 2005 the Assembly also specifically requested that the Director General of the WHO should "implement and strengthen strategies for the effective control of, and management of persons with, drug-resistant TB". This can hardly be claimed to have been achieved since the drug-resistant component of the pandemic remains comprehensively uncontrolled and is still rising.

At face value it may sound like the WHA has effective powers of direction over the implementation of strategies by the WHO, but practicalities mean that it is more the reverse. The WHO, by submitting the resolution to the WHA, asks the assembly to ratify its own strategy. Meanwhile there remains a chasm of reality between a resolution made in the comfort of a convention centre in Geneva and what happens on the ground. This alone might help explain why, nearly ten years down the line, such little progress has been made in implementing those earlier directions or meeting those targets.

This new plan has set a further set of new targets. The strategy to achieve them this time is intended to be built on three main pillars. We will look at these in more detail shortly, but first we can take a look at the plan itself.

The principal targets (for 2035 now) are as follows:

1. A 95% reduction in tuberculosis deaths (compared with a 2015 baseline)
2. A 90% reduction in tuberculosis incidence rate (to less than 10 tuberculosis cases per 100,000 population)
3. No affected families facing catastrophic costs due to tuberculosis.

There are also milestones which are expected to be met along the way (for 2020, 2025 and 2030). At these points progress will be assessed and, if necessary the targets may be adjusted. To anyone unfamiliar with the current pandemic and with the multi-factorial complexities of this disease, these goals may not seem so ambitious given that the world is giving itself a full 20 years in which to achieve them. But with TB as we know things tend to happen extremely slowly, and a brief review of these first two goals in the light of some of the achievements of the last 25 years may help to illustrate this.

The new goal for reducing TB deaths has involved a fundamental shift of emphasis from the previous goal that was set in 2006 for 2015. This original goal was to halve the ***rate*** of deaths (i.e. the numbers of deaths per 100,000 population) from a baseline set at the estimated rate for 1990.[323] The new goal, meanwhile, looks to reduce by 95% the ***absolute numbers*** of deaths from a baseline in 2015 which has yet to be set.

---

[323] And this goal had already been revised from an earlier target of halving the rate of deaths from a 2000 baseline by 2010.

Currently it is being promoted that this earlier goal for 2015 may well be met – but, as we know, this is being done disingenuously. If HIV/TB deaths are included the fact is that this target will definitely ***not*** be being met by 2015 and it will be being missed by a significant margin. Meanwhile in terms of 'absolute numbers' of TB deaths (which is how the new target is to be measured), the current annual death total is today not very different to what it was estimated to be in 1990. Deaths initially consistently ***rose*** for most years after 1990, and (according to the WHO's own figures from its 2012 annual report) have only recently begun to fall at all. Because of the growth of the global population, however, the rates 'per 100,000 population' were proportionately reducing even while the absolute numbers were increasing. So it has to be accepted that a 95% numerical reduction in TB deaths is an extraordinarily ambitious target.

The second target, a 90% reduction in incidence rates of disease, presents a similar concern. These rates also rose globally after 1990, peaking around 2006, following which they began to decline very slowly (thus meeting that nondescript Millennium Development Goal of "halting and beginning to reverse the incidence of tuberculosis by 2015"). Today, 21 years into a global emergency, these rates are reducing at 2% a year. And at this current rate the new target that has been set for 2035 won't be met until the year 2180, 145 years behind schedule.

It will be realised that some serious game-changing is needed if these new targets are to be taken seriously (and they certainly should be). The resolution itself offers some carefully considered ideas as to what these need to be, and we will look at some of them shortly. But, the resolution also reveals a couple of examples of what might be viewed as aberrations from reality.

It states, for example, that the current WHO-co-ordinated global efforts to control tuberculosis (as led by its member states and as supported by its technical and financial partners) have produced "remarkable results". The idea that the recent story of TB control has achieved anything that might be described as "remarkable" is, by any account, a misrepresentation of the facts.

So how are these new targets being proposed to be achieved? The Resolution identifies three pillars to support the plan itself: one of "integrated patient-centred care and prevention"; another of "bold policies and supportive systems", and the third of "intensified research and innovation".

These pillars are themselves composed of what might be best envisaged as individual reinforcement rods – amounting to component sub-strategies, some of which are specifically identified within the text as being essential for the goals of the plan to be met. In the discussion that follows, where these sub-strategies were clearly identified within the text as being essential the relevant original words will appear in bold type.

One of the goals is to increase the reduction in incidence of disease from 2% to 10% per year. This is judged to be "ambitious yet feasible". It is projected as being possible, however, on the basis of the fastest reductions in rates of national disease ever documented. These are identified as being those "which occurred in the context of universal access to health care and rapid socioeconomic development in Western Europe and North America during the second half of the past century". Modelling this target of incidence reduction in this way renders it incredibly optimistic for the regions of the world most affected by TB today. Whilst the whole world at the time referred to may have been recovering from the devastations of a world war, Western Europe and North America were enjoying a prolonged period of enormous economic growth along with unprecedented affluence and stability. But that was not all. Incidence rates of TB certainly did dramatically decline in these regions, exactly as suggested. They did so, however, following a century of slower decline that had already reduced the disease in these regions to levels at which the disease could be attacked by the new drugs and by concerted campaigns of active case finding. Neither is remotely possible yet in those regions where the disease is now out of control.

The plan also chooses to gloss over something else of critical importance - that today's new drugs will not be able to be rolled out in anything like the scale in which the new drugs were distributed out in the 1950s and 60s in Western Europe and North America – not just because of lack of resource but also because of a fear of new resistances if they are in any way mismanaged. Furthermore the fundamental DOTS strategy that is not intended to be altered doesn't rely on active case finding at all – the realities of limited resource dictated from the outset that it relies on waiting for the patients to come for treatment. Continuing with such passive case finding can never allow the sort of reductions that are being hoped for.

The plan also depends upon tuberculosis care and prevention continuing to benefit from what it describes as "general economic growth". This is something that can hardly be relied upon given so many global uncertainties. It is also a statement that can be questioned by reviewing the situation in one of the disease's most dangerous hotspots, in southern

Africa, where the disease casts a shadow over several economies including the one which drives the wider region.

South Africa is definitely from economic growth – it is after all one of the five BRICS economies. But it has also been suggested that it has more of its citizens today earning less than a dollar a day than did under apartheid. Even its general growth, however, is at risk of being crippled by its TB epidemic, particularly because the nation has such high rates of MDR- and XDR-TB. Incidence rates of TB are the second highest in the world (100 times higher than the 2035 incidence target) and still rising, while experts are stating that drug-resistance is now out of control.

There are many factors that have had impact on these numbers – but the one relating to funding is as relevant as any given that this is another of those steel reinforcements for one of the three main pillars. The global budgets for the 2035 targets are still in development. Most of them will be irrelevant to South Africa given that it funds most of its national TB programme itself. The fact is, however, that these global budgets will prove to be both wayward and worthless if they are prepared without paying adequate heed to the South African experiences. This is because the plan also dictates that they should adequately allow for the cost of meeting one of the other implicit targets – that of "providing universal access to services for drug-resistant tuberculosis".

Universal access to treatment is rightfully another of the reinforcing steel supports to the three main pillars. Universal health coverage is defined by the plan as "the situation where all people are able to use the quality health services that they need and do not suffer financial hardship paying for them", and it qualifies this by adding that this provision is "**fundamental**" for effective tuberculosis care and prevention. It also states that providing this "will require a rapid scale up of laboratory services and programmatic management". It will also require a roll-out of second line drugs which has proved impossible to implement anywhere at any sort of scale in the last 20 years since when it was first proposed to be the only feasible option to address MDR-TB.

Diagnostics and drugs for DR-TB come at considerable cost, and providing both is being currently attempted in South Africa. According to the country's minister of health (who also happens to be the elected president of the Stop TB Partnership) despite notified drug-resistant TB comprising only a 40th of South Africa's total TB case burden the management of the DR-TB programme in the country in 2011 consumed a third of its total national TB budget. It should be added that the rates of untreated drug-resistant disease means that the real DR-TB component that needs to be met is far more than a 40th, so the true requisite budget to meet this will be much more than a third of the whole as well. Drug-resistant TB is proportionately so much more costly to treat than the straightforward drug-susceptible variety, but the nearest that the plan comes to properly addressing this financial anomaly is by stating that "funding requirements are likely to increase in the immediate post-2015 period". This must surely be an understatement. Currently funding budgets for 2015 project that 20% of the total is going to be allocated for the treatment of MDR-TB. This percentage will have to be increased substantially if the goal of universal access is to be met. This is not associated with a new goal: it was one that was made by the Assembly in 2005, and yet it still hasn't really been begun to be properly addressed.

The plan also says that the "capacity to diagnose drug-resistant tuberculosis is limited in most places where it is sorely needed". This remains a principal part of the most essential paradox of the pandemic – that almost everything that is needed to contain the disease is in far too short supply where it is most needed. The plan then notes that "only a fraction of the estimated cases of multidrug-resistant tuberculosis receive a laboratory test to confirm their disease". No-one would argue with this either, but it also states that an "adequate capacity to diagnose all cases of drug-resistant tuberculosis is **essential** to make further progress in global tuberculosis care and control". Anyone with a handle on tuberculosis realities must wonder exactly how such an "essential" part of the plan is going to be achieved as well as who is going to pay for it, particularly because the plan correctly recognises that "in most low- and middle-income countries, the currently available resources are inadequate or sufficient only for modestly ambitious plans". The plan does not go any further into this, but it should be remembered that the drug-susceptibility testing that can properly conform with the Plan's ambitions is no one-size-fits-all process. It involves both testing for first line drugs for MDR-TB and for second line drugs for XDR-TB. The capacity for testing for the former is still deficient even in high-burden MDR-TB countries where the need is recognised to be greatest, but testing for the latter is almost non-existent in most countries while rates of XDR-TB are measured as rising faster than rates of MDR-TB.

The current gaps in funding the global response to the pandemic are estimated to be around US$2 billion per year for programme implementation and around US$1.4 billion per year for research. These shortfalls are only so far computed for the current plan, however – one which is intended to address the pandemic up until 2015. This was one with far more limited ambitions than the new one. Resourcing what will be needed in order to tool up for this post-2015 plan is going to reveal shortfalls of an entirely different magnitude, and the plan itself offers no real explanations as to how these further funding gaps are going to addressed beyond vaguely accepting that they are "likely" to occur.

Meanwhile, the world is also short of approaching four million health workers. The unfortunate fact is that many of the more acute shortages also happen to occur where TB burdens are the highest, something which is hardly coincidental. This factor as much as any other should have been creating discomfort in the minds of some of the ministerial representatives of those WHO member states as they unanimously endorsed their new Plan. They must have been wondering how its implementation is going to be properly managed back on their home turfs.

In fact the plan is explicit on this: "National governments have to provide the overall stewardship to keep tuberculosis elimination high on the development agenda through political commitment, investments and oversight, while making rapid progress towards universal health coverage and social protection." While this remains an inevitable part of solving the problem of TB, it also remains as big a challenge as any. Again, the recent deteriorating story of the disease in South Africa (where almost all funding for its programme is 'in-house') is hardly encouraging in this respect. Whilst South Africa is a middle-income country, it is the low-income ones which must remain the most vulnerable.

The plan is hardly enlightening on how this challenge might be overcome either. It suggests that "co-ordinated efforts" will be required to mobilize the additional resources required to fund such truly ambitious national strategic plans, ones which will include "a progressive increase in domestic funding". Can such increases seriously be achieved by a low-income country if a middle-income one like South Africa can't make it work?

But the plan counts on something even more ambitious still. It boldly states that "effective tuberculosis prevention **will require** actions resulting in poverty reduction, improved nutrition, and better living and working conditions". It lists other requirements as well, but it is worth reminding ourselves that it was exactly these four factors that accounted for those historic reductions of disease in industrialised Europe and North America – that allowed for the subsequent rapid reductions in incidence in the second half of the 20th century that the plan has been modelled on. What appears not to have been allowed for, however, is that these same preliminary factors (reduced poverty, improved nutrition, and better living conditions) had actually been incrementally falling into place in Europe and North

America over an entire century between 1870 and 1970. For the current plan to succeed, however, they appear to be required to develop in as little as a decade.

No-one can argue that these are valid and timely ideas, not just because these same factors remain at the core of the continuing pandemic, but also because not addressing them leaves such a stain on our collective humanity. But can such wider strategies possibly be as rapidly mobilised as is apparently being imagined? The accountability for addressing this part of the plan, at least according to its authors, "will rest not only with health ministries, but also other ministries including finance, labour, social welfare, housing, mining and agriculture. Eliciting actions from across diverse ministries will require commitment and stewardship from the highest levels of government." As such, the plan begins to look to require a change in how our world is being managed. It is beginning to look like the plan will depend not just on the interventions of the WHO, but also the G7, the UN and the World Bank as well.

In one further instance it's not even certain that the plan really recognises what some of the realities are because a further steel re-inforcement rod for one of its three pillars demands the development not just of new vaccines, but of very special ones. Everyone in the field agrees that a more effective new vaccine is needed - the fundamental problem has been that developing one is so challenging. Vaccinating against any disease which, even without mutation, confers no degree of long-lasting immunity in those whom it infects creates enormous challenges for the developers. But the plan raises the stakes for this challenge: it unequivocally states that "a post-exposure vaccine that prevents the disease in latently infected individuals will be **essential** to eliminating tuberculosis in the foreseeable future". While the Plan's authors might see this special type of vaccine as being an 'essential', many other experts might consider it to be an impossibility. A post-exposure vaccine that can stop a recent infection like rabies or tetanus developing is one thing, but a vaccine that might be intended to prevent re-activation of latent tuberculosis long after an initial infection is viewed by most as a pipedream, or at best something that is many years down the road. The plan, however, insists that this dream should be realised by 2025. If this happens it will constitute perhaps the most dramatic medical achievement of our age.

There also seems to be one important component that is entirely missing in the three principal targets that the plan sets: there are no percentage target reductions set for rates of drug-resistant disease. Since the wider drug-susceptible pandemic is now reducing whilst the drug-resistant component is doing the opposite, making no fundamental attempt at monitoring this as a principal part of the new plan seems to be ignoring something important – not least because the achievements so far in this respect have been the least remarkable of all in the attempts to contain the pandemic. Pretty much all of the targets so far set to reduce DR-TB are being missed by a mile.

Drug-resistance will still be monitored, of course. The data collected just won't become part of any tick-box for disease reduction.

Some targets for MDR-TB targets for 2015 have shown little or no progress; only one seems remotely close to being met; and one (the rate of successful treatment for MDR-TB) even shows a significant reversal from the baseline target. There is not a single trend that is visible relating to drug-resistant disease that gives cause for encouragement.

The original plan for 2015 which was made in 2006 was itself revised in 2010, midway during its programme period in order to accommodate some of the emerging complexities. The original target for 2015 to reduce the rates of MDR-TB by 74%, for instance, was modified to just "reduce the global burden of drug-resistant TB". As far as most experts are concerned, even this won't be achieved. So will this new plan have to be so drastically revised midway as well? Almost certainly it will.

Meanwhile, who should be taking responsibility for the implementation of the plan and also for its success or failure? On this there is little clarity. The WHO certainly takes responsibility for developing the Plan, for providing the requisite technical advice for its implementation and for collating the numbers. They also have the challenging responsibility of stimulating the massive research initiatives which are now needed. The governments themselves have adopted the plan by endorsing it and so they also have the responsibility of implementing it. Whether the governments of those counties that are being most affected can do that much to ramp up their efforts remains the biggest question of all.

What needs to happen?

"TUBERCULOSIS IS NOT, AS DICKENS BELIEVED, A DISEASE THAT 'MEDICINE NEVER CURED, WEALTH NEVER WARDED OFF.' IT IS THE CONSEQUENCE OF GROSS DEFECTS IN SOCIAL ORGANIZATION, AND OF ERRORS IN INDIVIDUAL BEHAVIOUR. MAN CAN ERADICATE IT WITHOUT VACCINES AND WITHOUT DRUGS BY INTEGRATING BIOLOGICAL WISDOM INTO SOCIAL TECHNOLOGY, INTO THE MANAGEMENT OF EVERYDAY LIFE."

René and Jean Dubos (1952)[324]

"Dramatic changes" have been identified as being needed to have a chance of eliminating this disease whether by 2035, 2050 or by any time soon. One of these would, as the new strategy suggests, almost certainly be a post-exposure vaccine. Another is a reduction in rates of global poverty which the new plan requires as well. A list follows, almost all of which may be necessary if this goal of eradication is really to be finally achieved. They come in no particular order of importance, particularly since many are interdependent on each other:

Proper active surveillance in every country
Fast (cheaper) diagnostics which discriminate resistance
New faster acting (cheap) drugs
New fast and effective treatment of LTBI
Reliable assay indicating likelihood of LTBI developing TB
Active case finding
Reductions in poverty
Massively improved medical infrastructures
Better supplies and suppliers of reliable drugs
Extra donor funding for treatments
Extra funding at national levels
Extra funding for research
Significant reduction in rates of HIV infection
An effective vaccine (post-exposure if possible)
Proper control of bovine TB
Comprehensive management of private health providers

---

[324] "The White Plague: Tuberculosis, Man, and Society", Little, Brown, and Company, Rutgers University Press (1952), page 37.

Perhaps the most important factor of all might be an awakening to the idea that, certainly as far as the pharmaceutical battle against TB is concerned, we have not one single pandemic on our hands but several, each of which may need dealing with separately, possibly with divergent solutions to each. We have discussed this previously, but the list bears repeating because the issue may be such a fundamentally important one. The wider pandemic will need to be picked off piece by piece with different but (if at all possible) complementary strategies developed for each:

- TB (drug-susceptible "simple and straight forward")
- Polydrug-resistant TB (coming in several forms itself)
- TB with HIV
- Drug-resistant TB with HIV
- Bovine TB
- Bovine TB with HIV
- Multiple-strain TB
- Latent tuberculosis

The most important thing, however, must be to start getting the most accurate figures possible from which to build more coherent strategies.

It's easy to believe that the cause of the collapse of the epidemics in the post-industrialised nations was the discovery of the drugs, but – as massively important as their discoveries were – they were preceded by a sequence of other events that had each made a significant difference to the rates of disease, and which collectively made the job that much more possible when the drugs appeared. It's worth considering whether the story would have turned out in any way the same if the drugs had appeared earlier in the sequence. It may well not have. The post-industrialised world may just have been incredibly lucky with the way events panned out.

The rough sequence was as follows: patient isolation in sanatoria, improved living and working conditions, better nutrition, a partially effective vaccine, milk pasteurisation, discovery of drugs, and finally (with rates in real decline) active case finding.

If we want to really see the disease eradicated in our era, we have to attack at it at its source, and today, with the power of the science available to us, this might yet prove to be possible. But to stand a chance of doing this the world needs to properly wake up to the problem

With its endorsement of its new 2015-2035 plan the World Health Assembly and the WHO have embraced the word "ambitious" – using it as the fundamental adjective to describe its aspirations for the next 20 years. There can be no doubt that the plan is an ambitious one – in fact, it's so ambitious that it's difficult to believe that it was ever unanimously adopted by those who are now faced with the task of implementing it. We might even wonder whether its aims might have been drafted a little more realistically in the hope that they might be more easily achieved. But then, given what's known about what's happening with TB today and what didn't happen in the last 21 years, we must also realise that the luxury of being able to adopt more realistic strategies has been squandered by ambivalence, apathy and indecision.

There's no choice left now but to develop ambitious plans, so the WHO should be congratulated and the Assembly should be praised for having had the courage to endorse it. But are they really expecting those first waymarkers in 2020 to be met? The trick isn't in agreeing to the strategy because that's so terrifyingly easy – it's going to be in gearing up what's needed up, and in not allowing those targets to slip. It's not going to be easy: there exists a very strong possibility that the targets may have already started slipping before the plan has even been properly developed. Everything possible now needs to be done to prevent this happening.

So what sort of things might be done right now to avoid this?

There might be a few things that can be done by all of us. Just like the plan itself, however, the actions required will need to be both bold and ambitious.

One thing relates to the level of popular activism that is now needed both to promote the necessary global awareness and to demand more accountability for the management of the disease from those who have accepted the responsibilities of seeing it off. Both have been in far too short supply so far.

More often that not, whenever the words 'activism' and 'TB' are used in the same sentence they are also linked with 'HIV'. Sometimes this is because today's HIV activists are being reported to be involving themselves in promoting awareness of TB; but sometimes the link is more negatively made – comparing the limited successes of TB activism to the extraordinary achievements of HIV activists in the last 20 years.

There is something of real significance here because HIV activism went through two quite different phases of activity during this period. Today it is largely based on collaborative engagement and involvement with those managing health care both globally and nationally. Broadly speaking, everyone finds themselves on the same side; but that wasn't the way it was initially. As far as public awareness of HIV is concerned, the public relations dam that needed to be broken to enable treatment to be rolled out was breeched 15 years ago. But it was certainly not the 'engaged' style of activism that is employed today that first broke it – it was a confrontational one.

It's worth looking back 20-odd years – to review what did break that HIV dam and then consider its possible relevance for TB today. It might be much better to adapt those tactics than use the more collaborative 'down-stream' activism for tuberculosis that the HIV activists now use.

Around 20 years ago both public awareness of HIV and general attitudes towards it were vastly different to how they are today. A primetime news report from the late 1980s was suggesting that 50% of Americans wanted anyone infected with HIV to be quarantined, and 15% even wanted them tattooed so that they could more easily be identified. This was the world of fear and hostility that those early HIV activists had to confront.

The activists' initial approaches to this challenge were far from being engaged, collaborative or polite. They were, instead, deliberately conrontational. In 1990, they brought the parliamentary heartland of London, to a complete standstill by staging a mass die-in outside the offices of the Department of Social Security. Demonstrators stretched themselves out on the streets complete with fake headstones. In the USA, with more and more victims of the disease dying, things were being taken further still. These symbolic representations of HIV deaths in the die-ins were stepped up into protests which uncompromisingly involved the dead themselves – in the scattering of the ashes of victims on the lawn of the White House, and, in one instance, in a public funeral with a dead body being carried through the streets in a coffin to a park where the casket was opened for the final ceremony.

What was fuelling this uncompromising campaign was the energy and know-how of a gay rights movement that already had bitter experience of fighting discrimination against it – some of which was still legal. The campaign was being fought by its own major stake-holders which is something that has yet to happen with TB. Stepping into line behind them came a stream of celebrities, joining the campaign as the momentum gathered.

The contrast between this and today's style of activism for TB is profound. On the 21st May 2014, Phumeza Tisile, a former XDR-TB patient from South Africa (and one of the lucky few who survive), presented MSF's "Test Me, Treat Me" Drug-Resistant TB Manifesto to Mario Raviglione and so also to the 67th World Health Assembly in Geneva. MSF's important manifesto (which itself too quietly challenged the "Find me, Treat me" strapline which had been announced by the WHO for World TB Day two months earlier) had been launched online at the same time. The number of signatures on the global petition that Phumeza presented was just 53,000. If this doesn't tell us something about the general disinterest in this disease (and a loss of faith in progress against it by its stakeholders), then nothing will. MSF is probably the loudest voice in the world of TB activism today and it also carries enormous credibility as an NGO. The organisation has been conducting a campaign for wider access to medicines for 15 years. If this organisation can only raise 53,000 signatures for such a petition in a time period in which at least four times as many people will have died from the disease, then something has to be in need of change. Maybe a PR agency in New York could be enticed to take the baton off MSF for a year *pro bono* – to do the sort of work that the pharmaceutical industry might employ them to do in an opposite direction.

We can review MSF's delivery of its manifesto and compare it with the style of those early HIV activists and their shock-tactics. It's unlikely that they have would have ever considered presenting their manifesto in the hands of the articulate, healthy-looking and engaging Phumeza, for instance. Why would they consider presenting a one-in-five XDR-TB survivor story to the world when they would have been intending to wake it up to the collective demise of the other four who failed to make it? Using Phumeza as a patients' representative offers us a good example of the current 'engaged' style of activism: it remains too orchestrated by the management rather than the stake holders themselves. Those HIV activists would probably have sent someone whom the existing treatment ***wasn't*** helping – someone who had in fact been failed by the Assembly and its members whose very aims and objectives dictate that this disease should have been as good as eradicated decades ago. They would have sent someone, perhaps, who was wasting away in the final stage of the disease, presented her as an iconic representative for perhaps as many as two million others each year (because they would also have been taking the opportunity to challenge that official estimated figure of 1.3 million deaths saying that without proper surveillance all such estimates are questionable). They might even have handed out a mask to every delegate to help dramatise the event that little bit more. Of course, they would never have been allowed to do this. They would never have even been allowed into the Assembly if they had publicised these sorts of intentions, so they would have had to gatecrash it in some fashion. But this would have underlined the point they were making, and proved that such confrontational activism is what's really needed to shake an institution like the WHO and the Assembly into the action that's required. As extraordinary an organization as MSF is, and as outspoken as it often is as well, it still reluctant to really rock the establishment's boat.

Early on in the HIV campaign there was a particularly potent strapline that the activists employed. It was that "Silence = Death". Today this makes little sense for HIV, but such an uncompromising slogan is one that TB activists could certainly do worse than consider. There were other slogans as well including "Action = Life", and "Ignorance = Fear". All could be equally well adopted or adapted by TB activists, but, far more importantly, so could that original primal energy that shifted that initial public fear of HIV and the inertia of medical response. It's quite possible that those early activists conducted the most successful political campaign in recent history. It's also a fact that almost all of them are now dead. The development of ARV drugs that now mean that people living with HIV can expect to live normal lives arrived a little too late for them: but they arrived in bulk and at reducing costs on a timescale that has not been seen in any other area of medicine.

Those with the more powerful voices for HIV today simply no longer live under the same sort of storm cloud of disease. Those who are now living with a drug-resistant strain of tuberculosis do, however, and a louder voice needs to be found for them if they cannot find it for themselves. 'Die-ins' had their day for HIV and so have effectively died out. But something like them may well be what is needed to wake the world up to TB. Not 'die-ins', perhaps, but how about 'cough-ins' instead? Something really needs to be done quickly to focus the attention of the world's media (and also the G8 or G7) on what is probably the public health issue of our age and on the plight of the millions at risk and dying of TB. In fact this is exactly what the ambitious challenges set by the World Health Assembly now demand of all of us.

There is also the World Health Organisation – an institution which is well known for its inertia – ccused as it is by some of "knowing everything and doing nothing". It may have been the WHO which originally drafted this Plan, but it has passed the principal responsibilities on to others for its implementation The least it should be doing now is using some of its considerable muscle to help out.

The WHO does have the power to pass normative international legislation. Perhaps now is the moment for it to step up and demonstrate the leadership that is demanded of it, and there is at least one piece of international legislation that it could seriously consider in this respect. It's one that might genuinely help support the strained human resource that is going to be required to implement the ambitious targets it has set.

Each year a steady stream of health workers who have trained and qualified in middle- and low-income countries take up new appointments in higher-income countries. This phenomenon doesn't happen by accident: the wealthier countries, guided by increasingly selectively controlled immigration policies, recruit the most talented they can find. A 2013 Canadian study estimated that as much as US$2 billion of human investment in health worker training had been lost by just nine African countries all of which have heavy burdens of TB. Meanwhile the existing human resource that is in place in many high incidence countries is on their knees.

Such a phenomenon can no longer be morally tolerated as a feature of our globalised world. Such recruitment policies should be recognised and condemned as indefensible, particularly so in the light of the TB emergency. It should not only be shown up as such, however – it should also be legislated against and the WHO has the powers to do this. It would not be difficult: appropriate ceilings could be determined openly and equitably so that the usual blocking by the wealthier nations or by the G8 is not allowed to stymie or stall the negotiations. Such a piece of international legislation would be a benchmark moment that would demonstrate the will for change within the WHO which must exist but which is still largely invisible. Such a ceiling would set legal limits on the amount of health worker traffic allowed to travel northwards in any given year. The richer countries would still almost certainly scrape off the cream, but at least they would not continue to steal the milk as well.

Then we can also look to the patients and the health workers who are struggling to help them recover. Both are frequently identified as suffering from low morale, and both are also frequently blamed for the rise of drug-resistant disease. Both most definitely need to be better supported and more properly motivated, and far more imagination could be applied to this. When resources are poor, demotivated patients or practitioners amount to disaster. While we wait for the proper response to the necessary call-to-arms for funding for the plan and for governments to get their acts together, a far more intense focus could be made on the disease itself. It should encourage all concerned that the highest possible standards of care need to be maintained and at the same time assure those involved that, this time at least, the cavalry is really going to make it in time.

Luis Figo, the legendary Portuguese ex-footballer, is also the Stop TB Partnership's 'Goodwill Ambassador'. His face remains less visible in the Partnership's campaigns than it might, however. His is not the only well-known footballer's face that might help the cause – Figo is, after all, just one in a long line of European *Ballon d'Or* Footballers-of-the-Year. An 11-strong team of them should be recruited to help the cause under Figo's captaincy. Some of these winners are legends who are probably as well known in many TB endemic countries as they are in their own, and some of their faces are also instantly recognisable. They are the perfect poster boys for a campaign – Zinedine Zidane, Ronaldo, Ronaldinho, Andriy Schevchenko, Kaká, Cristiano Ronaldo, Messi, George Weah, Michel Platini, and Ruud Gullit. They would make up a serious team (the greatest of all, Pelé, might even help from their subs bench perhaps, given that he has an honorary awarded the '*Ballon d'Or*' award himself). Each one could help out by lending their face to an economically effective and creatively designed poster campaign intending to encourage TB patients to stick to their treatment for the 'whole match', or to help 'score the goal against TB'. Some could be photographed wearing masks, some might merely point their finger at the camera and smile encouragingly – all could help improve and repair patients' self-images whilst also helping to reduce the stigma of infection that still so persistently survives. They could be helping health workers' collective credibility in the process. A series of eye-catching posters could be displayed in every patient waiting area in every out-patient clinic in every TB-endemic country in a matter of weeks. Similar exhortative posters could encourage health workers to keep their patients on target. Who knows, could one photo-shoot lead to even more active involvement by one or more of these individuals in a campaign that is so desperately needed?

Iconic women could also be asked to join the campaign. Would Oprah Winfrey help out? Might Michelle Obama lend her face to such a campaign, or Serena Williams - or even the busy Angelina Jolie? Orchestrating such a simple campaign should not be a huge test of resourcefulness but still seems to remain beyond the authorities.

The WHO has another far tougher task ahead of it, however, which is that of stimulating active interest amongst the research community in the development of the new and faster drugs, as well as in the missing point-of-care diagnostics and the elusive new vaccines. The industry has proved itself so far to be reluctant partners in this enterprise. This doesn't mean, though, that such attitudes should continue to be accepted without active challenge.

It's not just TB patients, of course – it's the whole enterprise of biomedicine that is at risk of being held to ransom by what some have called 'medico-capitalism', at least by its excesses. The WHO is far from untainted by its own inevitable association with this multinational conglomerate, and as such is sometimes seen to suffer from conflicts of interest between its own aims and the commercial objectives of those corporate giants that compose 'big pharma'. The WHO, by designing its new Plan, might have set itself up for its own Damascene conversion, one when it can demonstrate whose interests it really serves and on whose side it is on. Dr Aaron Motsoaledi, the Minister of Health for South Africa, is perhaps the man of the moment in this respect because he is also now the elected president of the WHO's Stop TB Partnership. What marks him out from many within the organization is his public criticism of the pharmaceutical industry's stranglehold on the intellectual property rights which price millions out of accessing appropriate medical care. This places him at the heart of the new plan given that it demands the rights of "access for all" to all TB drugs and diagnostics. He hasn't minced his words on the subject, having called the industry's responses to his own government's attempts to free up access to cheaper generic medicines "genocidal".

So will the WHO be prepared to get behind the movement that is being promoted by Dr Motsoaledi, or will the doctor become more muted in his more international role? Has it got the courage to stand by the convictions that are implicit in its own Plan: that research ***must*** be developed, that diagnostics ***must*** be scaled up rapidly, that vaccines ***must*** be developed. It must because these are all imperative parts of the Plan: it has no choice. These are moral imperatives which far outweigh the commercial ones that the industry itself might want to maintain. The sort of profits that underpin the activities of the pharmaceutical industry are going to ***have to*** be either contained or side-stepped if the hopes of millions are to be met as the plan intends. A public movement now needs to be set in motion to force this to happen because it won't happen otherwise. And such a movement should threaten to shame either the WHO or the industry it is so close to (or both) if the targets look like they are not going to be met. The industry should realise that it is only going to survive if it accepts that not every new drug today needs to be a gold mine for its shareholders.

Dr Motsoaledi himself might also relate to a sideways reference to gold mines given that he is so fond of calling TB the "snake of Africa" with its head in his country's mining industry. Statistics certainly support his view with epidemiologists suggesting that a third of the region's epidemic and a ninth of the entire global pandemic has its head in those mines. Motsoaledi's own solution to the problem is also simple: if you want to kill a snake you need to stamp on its head.

So some stamping needs to begin around this issue as well, and it also needs to be done quickly. The WHO officially pronounced TB as a global emergency in 1993; it also happened to be the year when the scourge of apartheid began to be dismantled in South Africa. It could have been the year in which the country's mines were nationalized and the conditions within them begun to be improved because this is what the ANC had been promising its supporters. Once in power, however, they bowed to the irresistible pressures of wealthier nations which threatened to withdraw investment if the new government nationalised the mines as it had promised. As a result the conditions in South African mines today may be worse than ever, because autopsies suggest that the number of cases of TB has been increasing significantly during the ANC's 21-year watch. The South African mining industry, to put it bluntly, remains a public health scandal all of its own.

Back home with a copy of the new plan in his hand, Dr Motsoaledi should certainly be finding his negotiating position with his colleagues in the ANC cabinet strengthened. The plan, after all, demanded engagement from all departments of government, not just of health ministries. Effectively, they have all now been directed by the World Health Assembly to get to grips with their mining industry. So what could be done to help this particular cause, because it will be rapidly resisted by another massively profitable multinational industry?

Well perhaps a similar global campaign could be developed as was waged against the indiscriminate killing or farming of animals for their fur, or like the one that was developed against the immoral profit from 'blood diamonds' which were both legally and illegally being exported from troubled countries in Central and West Africa at huge human cost. It would need to be a punchy public campaign demanding much better working conditions in the mines, and shuoldn't just be taking place on the streets of South Africa but also on the streets in the European and North American capitals where these mining conglomerates have their headquarters. The public face of this poster campaign could be one that considers the true human cost of a gold or platinum wedding ring as opposed to the simple financial one. A photo of a ring on a beautiful hand with an inset face of a miner alongside, perhaps, accompanied by a slogan such as: "Did your lover cough up ***that*** much for your wedding ring? Because he did ..."

There is much that must be done now. The plan states that "continuing progress beyond 2015 will require intensified actions above and beyond tuberculosis programmes within and outside the health sector". Such simple initiatives as described above constitute just a few intensified areas of action but others will certainly be needed. There will be many more than can be creatively devised and initiated to get the plan kickstarted even before 2015 begins – because it looks like this is what needs to happen RIGHT NOW if anyone has any serious intention that this new plan is going to succeed.

Neglect, Indifference or Denial?

"THE CHALLENGE.. IS NOT OURS ALONE. IT IS ALSO FOR GOVERNMENTS, INTERNATIONAL GOVERNMENT INSTITUTIONS, THE PHARMACEUTICAL INDUSTRY AND OTHER NGO'S TO CONFRONT THIS INJUSTICE. WHAT WE AS A CIVIL SOCIETY MOVEMENT DEMAND IS CHANGE, NOT CHARITY."

Dr James Orbinski (1999)[325]

Archbishop Desmond Tutu talks a lot about *ubuntu*. He says that it is about looking beyond ourselves – and, in so doing, that we become more fully human. He describes *ubuntu* as a pervasive traditional African philosophy which emphasises our common humanity rather than our individualities – in other words it emphasises our interconnectedness with and interdependence on our fellow human beings.

Such an idea isn't in any way exclusive to Africa. All the major religions share such a philosophy.

In 1965, for instance, Dr Martin Luther King, similarly identified that:

> "All mankind is tied together; all life is interrelated, and we are all caught in an inescapable network of mutuality, tied in a single garment of destiny. Whatever affects one directly, affects all indirectly."

Today, in our complex era of globalisation, it is probable that such "networks of mutuality" are potentially more active than they have ever been – but sections of humanity remain as remote from each other as ever as well.

In Malawi they frame their *ubuntu* in a structure that is strikingly reminiscent of Descartes's famous aphorism but with a twist, suggesting a more existential and humane philosophy. Instead of "I think therefore I am," they simply say that, "I am because you are." Put another way perhaps, "If you are sick, then I must be sick too."

---

[325] President of MSF's International Council in his acceptance speech on behalf of MSF for the Nobel Peace prize in 1999.

Such ideas are neither foreign nor new to European traditions. In around 310 AD, Lactantius, an early Christian bishop living in North Africa, proclaimed on the subject of social justice:

> "The whole point of justice consists precisely in our providing for others through humanity what we provide for our families through affection."

This sounds like a fundamental statement of human rights, but Arundhati Roy has been identifying recent subtle shifts within such universal principles. She now differentiates two divergent notions of equality in social justice depending on whether the principle is being applied to rich or poor. Almost unconsciously, she suggests, we have allowed ourselves to become accustomed to thinking of 'justice' as being more for the rich and 'human rights' being more for the poor. This is far from fantasy in the field of public health given the two-speed model with a high standard being demanded by the developed world, and a lower one being palmed off on the developing one.

Roy suggests that any resistance movement which fights injustice should be challenging what this really means – as well as disputing what is meant by 'development'. If either amounts to no more than taking the "ugly edge off imperialism" (in Roy's words) or in superficially restoring that spoilt but "otherwise beautiful view" (in Biko's), with the poor staying poor while the rich get ever richer, then human rights NGOs are failing in their job. And Roy suspects that many of them are no more than "modern day missionaries" who passively sustain an iniquitous and unsustainable status quo on behalf of and empire of exploitation and inequality. Could the WHO even be included in such a categorisation? She touches on this:

> "Increasingly human rights violations are being portrayed as the unfortunate, almost accidental fallout of an otherwise acceptable political and economic system – as though they're a small problem that can be mopped up with a little extra attention from some NGOs."

Has the paucity of attention towards redressing the tuberculosis situation not amounted to exactly such a violation of human rights? Has it been no more than "an accidental fallout" of a political and economic system, because if so then we should face up to the fact that this system is far from being acceptable?

There are certainly some who would agree with this analysis. There are also questions that arise from the previous pages which need better explanations.

Exactly how did the ball of eradicating TB get so dreadfully dropped just when it looked like it was being carried into the end zone? How did the world's most lethal infectious disease ever get relegated to becoming a 'neglected' one? How exactly has mankind's oldest bacteriological foe been allowed to become an 'emergent' disease? How were some treatments, ones which are known to promote drug-resistance, ever approved as acceptable treatments in high incidence environments? How has the plight of children, who continue to suffer so much from this disease, been so comprehensively ignored? How did death rates from this disease, rates which would be considered unacceptable in North America and Western Europe at a hundredth of the rate that they are occurring in half of the world, become a part and parcel of normality for almost half of humanity? And how is it that barely half-a-percent of those with MDR-tuberculosis begin treatment that is considered the standard of care in the U.S. or Western Europe?

Is it simply because the poor really don't matter? Or worse, that, in Arundhati Roy's words, "chinks, negroes, dinks, gooks and wogs don't qualify as real people. Perhaps our deaths don't qualify as real deaths". One of the many poignant ironies of TB is its having been previously called the "white plague" in the 18th and 19th centuries. It certainly can't be called that today being as it is taking such a heavy toll on the black, the brown and the yellow. Even in the affluent USA, the rate of TB among native-born populations is reported to be eight times higher in non-Hispanic blacks than in non-Hispanic whites.

In 1952 the Dubos' book on tuberculosis, entitled "The White Plague", identified the danger of focusing efforts intended to solve health problems solely through prescribing medicine:

> "Some 50 years ago men of vision and of good will, physician and laymen, realized that tuberculosis could be conquered only by broadening the scope of conventional medical philosophy. Their efforts culminated in the educational program that enlisted the general public as an understanding and creative participant in the war against contagion. There is needed today a reawakening of the pioneering spirit that brought about first the sanitary revolution, and later the anti-tuberculosis campaigns."

And 70 years before René and Jules Dubos, Robert Koch was saying much the same thing:

> "It is the over-crowded dwellings of the poor that we have to regard as the real breeding places of consumption; it is out of them that the disease

> always crops up; and it is to the abolition of these conditions that we must first and foremost direct our attention if we wish to attack the evil at its root and wage war against it with effective weapons."

Bill Gates has said that, as far as he is concerned, the purpose of public health is to promote social justice, and that this includes eradicating disease. His focus has so far been mainly on malaria, HIV, and polio, but it has also been on tuberculosis. Based on the evidence available, however, it's fair to suggest that the existing global public health programmes associated with TB have been spectacularly unsuccessful using Bill Gates's definition.

Gates's viewpoint is supported by others in relation to tuberculosis:

> "Social justice is arguably the foundational animating principle of public health action. Social justice concerns direct attention to the upstream causes of TB and the broader social determinants of health. Global poverty fuels TB. In order to create communities that work towards health for all and therefore contribute to human beings flourishing in the long run, the social determinants of health must be addressed on an equal footing with medical approaches. The onus is on the global community to change perceptions and create conditions where, through solidarity, we are united in addressing a grave threat to human health. This means addressing social determinants as an explicit goal of TB control strategies. Some of the reasons for poor adherence and loss-to-follow up involve the competing priorities faced by poor populations: the need to earn money on a daily basis, duties towards family members, substance misuse as a coping strategy for impoverishment. Overcoming these problems requires a level of social support that is rarely available in an overburdened and understaffed health system."[326]

In Uganda the best that can currently be managed as far as DOTS is concerned is to enrol friends or family to act as quasi-health workers, and even that can frequently not be managed. In South Africa they use 'carers', semi-trained members of the local community who are paid a pittance to visit each registered patient each day and ensure that they take their drugs. These are effectively the front-line foot soldiers of the battle against TB in Africa – people who are unpaid or barely paid, untrained or barely trained, and unprotected or barely protected against infection in every situation outside of hospitals. They are nearly all women, and many are extraordinary in the level of their dedication to their communities. More than a few inevitably succumb themselves to the disease. Each day these women and

[326] Upshur R et al. - "Apocalypse or redemption: responding to extensively drug-resistant tuberculosis", the Bulletin of the World Health Organization, 87 (2009) 481-83.

men are exposing themselves to risks of developing disease – and, if they do, it may be a deadly resistant strain and might also then infect their children.

This isn't a fanciful risk. A study in South Africa measured incidence rates of MDR-TB hospitalization among South African health care workers and found it to be four times higher than in non-health care workers, and seven times higher in cases of XDR-TB.[327] Another study revealed that 3% of all XDR-TB patients were health workers.[328]

These health workers are the key people whom the WHO, its epidemiologists and its expert doctors, are depending upon to stall a medical apocalypse while researchers strive to catch up. This potential apocalypse envisaged by Ross Upshur and his colleagues is becoming less and less imaginary. It might not just wreak humanitarian and economic devastation in much of Africa and South Asia. Given the globalised world in which we live and the nature of the disease itself, it could yet threaten other regions as well.

A report from Sewri TB Hospital in Mumbai, India, tells a particularly shocking story. Since 2005, more than 70 workers in there have contracted TB, and 42 of them have died. At least 12 of the 70 had MDR-TB, and some were reported to have been stricken with TB as many as three times in ten years. After a brief period allowed by their employer for treatment (which is not even provided for them free of charge by their hospital employer), they have to resume work, working in the very same wards – something which unsurprisingly makes them all the more vulnerable to contracting TB again.

---

[327] O'Donnell MR et al. - "High incidence of hospital admissions with multidrug-resistant and extensively drug-resistant tuberculosis among South African health care workers", Annals of Internal Medicine. 2010153; 8 (2010) 516-22.

[328] Jarland J et al. - "Extensively drug-resistant tuberculosis (XDR-TB) among health care workers in South Africa", The European Journal of Tropical Medicine and International Health. 15; 10 (2010) 1179–84.

Journalist Maitra Porecha, in a report coinciding with World TB day 2013 entitled "Sick treating the sick at Sewri's TB Hospital", wrote about one such hapless hospital employee:

> "Amjuri is an extensively drug-resistant (XDR-TB) patient. Such patients are advised complete rest but Amjuri is compelled to do his daily duties including sweeping, disposing garbage, washing infection-laden clothes from the ward, all because he has exhausted his three-years' worth of sick leave. 'The head clerk instructed me that I will not be entitled to any more leave. In spite of being an XDR-TB patient I am compelled to work. I have spent more than Rs3 lakhs [300,000 rupees or US$5,000] for my treatment. I have to continue working to support my family.' "[329]

Sewri is not just any hospital: it is Asia's largest tuberculosis unit with 1,000 beds and as many as ten people dying from TB in its wards every day. Its high death rate is attributed partly to the fact that, despite the size of the hospital and its being dedicated to TB, it has had no facility on site for culture testing, and so (almost unbelievably) samples have to be outsourced for diagnosis.

Can all this be true? Shouldn't we be outraged if it is?

As Solomon Benatar has identified:

> "The problem of tuberculosis illustrates the paradox of how advances in scientific knowledge and in the ability to cure individual patients have not been accompanied by global public health gains. This is not the result of lack of knowledge but an example of lack of wisdom in the application of knowledge and a failure to appreciate the complex social and economic aspects of health and disease."[330]

From one particular perspective, the current pandemic of TB amounts to not one, but three elephants snoring away in the living room of modern medicine.

The first and largest elephant (still taking up an astonishing amount of room) is that of drug-susceptible TB, which was so neglected that it turned into a global emergency in the developing world while the most

---

[329] http://www.dnaindia.com/mumbai/1814991/report-sick-treating-the-sick-at-sewri-s-tb-hospital.

[330] Benatar S, - "Respiratory health in a globalizing world", American Journal of Respiratory Critical Care in Medicine, 163 (2001) 1064–7.

extraordinary medical advances have been being made and promoted elsewhere.

The second elephant is smaller, though growing fast – that of MDR-TB. It is still relatively ignored to the extent that it has been allowed to reach elephant-puberty before being recognised as the threat that it is. Meanwhile, it has entered a destructive phase of pubescent delinquency.

The third is the second elephant's younger sibling – XDR-TB. Currently it is still largely obscured, hiding behind his MDR brother. It looks for now to remain that way, effectively unrecognised in exactly the same way that MDR-TB was. Meanwhile it promises to be far more dangerous when it enters its teenage years.

There seems to be an appalling incongruity in all of this – that much of the current effort and expenditure that is being ramped up to confront this disease is almost certain to be of more potential benefit to protect those in the parts of the world where such innovation is least needed and where the disease is least active. This is the case only because these are the environments where more complex intervention can be appropriately and properly managed. Meanwhile, those living in the places where the fruits of such effort and expenditure might be most helpful have the benefit neither of the medical resource nor political resolve to mobilise any sort of orthodox response.

But there are further incongruities which are equally uncomfortable and extensive contained within this anomaly: the existing drugs that are known to be able to confront the disease are still not available where the disease is most widespread; the diagnostics that are needed for them to be properly used aren't present in these same places; even the surveillance systems are absent where they are needed. If lessons were ever needed in how ***not*** to manage a public health programme, they must surely be present in abundance in the recent story of TB.

So where did things go so terribly wrong?

Was it that the plight of the developing world got ignored when the rates of TB began to wither in the industrialised West? This must be part of the story.

Or was it more recently, when the true risks of drug-resistant disease began to emerge but when there was little done to develop an appropriate strategic response to what was already a very real threat? This certainly is part of the story as well.

But is this story also tangled up in the wider web of our modern world as the gap between rich and poor has stretched beyond comprehension? There can be no question that this is part of the problem as well.

And can this situation actually be salvaged? In an epidemiological sense, the answer to this is "yes" – either as the disease mutates into a less virulent state as the crest of the wave of the current epidemic breaks (as it inevitably will in the end), or as human ingenuity and invention manages somehow to shunt our species out of this particular risk zone.

But it seems fairer to review the answers to this question by considering them, not in terms of the larger global epidemiological picture, but rather from the perspective of those most affected by the problem, because this presents us with yet another incongruity, one which is perhaps the most disturbing of all.

The strapline of the Stop TB Partnership that was used for two years (2012 and 2013) was a call to arms to "Stop TB in my lifetime" The phrase was intended to endorse the idea that the target of eradicating TB by 2050 was still achievable, and at the same time to excite and engage the public with this idea. It was surely a positive idea to promote. It may at first seem an innocently positive turn of phrase, but it is also a revealing one in terms of what it tells us in its subtext.

The year 2050 is 36 years away, so under 'normal' circumstance the idea that stopping TB might be possible within a normal lifespan (of three-score-and-ten or more these days for the majority of us) might not seem in any way controversial. But in some parts of the world a lifetime amounts to something quite different. In Swaziland, for instance, the country with the highest rates of TB on the planet, the average life expectancy for a baby born tomorrow predicts that it may well not be alive by 2035 and is actually statistically unlikely to be so still by 2050. Unfortunately as well, many of these truncated lives will be prematurely ended by this very disease. So this makes quite a few lifetimes that are unlikely to count in this equation of life and death.

This catchy phrase should have affronted those who remain at such at risk from the disease, the same people who most need the help of the Stop TB Partnership. Their lives are not just those which are at most active risk from TB today, but they also stand as the vanguard for the millions at risk of being slaughtered by the disease year-on-year. This particular choice of strapline on the part of the Partnership suggests that TB ***even now*** isn't being properly seen from the perspective of the 95% of those who die from it, but is more consistently being viewed from the perspective of the 68% who are currently untouched by it and want to stay that way. This is the uninfected and affluent majority of us who are lucky enough not to be latently infected but still are conscious of some level of possible risk from the disease. This majority includes me, and – sure – I'd like to see it eradicated in my lifetime.

If this cruel conclusion is true, then ***still*** the lessons that TB is intent on teaching us are not being learnt, and meanwhile the suffering that is experienced in learning these lessons ironically remain almost exclusively the painful privilege of the poor.

"Stop TB in my lifetime" may have amounted to an innocently positive turn of phrase in 2012 when it first appeared, but for it to have been resurrected in 2013 suggests an institutional blind-spot as much as it might reveal an irony.

This might seem an unfair or even an extreme assessment, but an equally revelatory comment was made at the same time by Dr Chan, the Director General of the WHO. She suggested that XDR-TB "could take the world back to the pre-antibiotic era". It was a genuine statement that was similarly intended to wake the world up to the dangers of this disease as it develops ever more extensive resistance to the existing drugs. But, her statement reveals exactly the same anomaly of perspective as the Stop TB Partnership's strapline did: for the vast majority of those infected not just with XDR-TB, but also with MDR-TB, this pre-antibiotic era never went away in the first place. It effectively exists for them because those out-of-patent second line antibiotics have been and still are unavailable – exactly as they were to all in that pre-antibiotic era that Dr Chan and the rest of us so fear.

So what should be done specifically for those who are most at the mercy of this disease?

Carole Mitnick of Partners in Health suggests that we will need to:

> "… subvert a tension that has plagued TB control efforts – that is, between providing the best treatment possible to all those who need it and a perceived need to protect against emerging resistance."

By this she means that a more ethically acceptable balance needs to be struck between supplying treatment to those who need it and minimising the risk of spreading drug-resistance to the rest of us by treatment mismanagement. Such a prospect may not be comfortable for the more cautious in global health governance who feel that it is preferable to see lives sacrificed than see the disease spin out of control. TB policy, Mitnick correctly identifies, "has typically favoured caution against [engendering] resistance which has meant restricting access to the most effective treatments".

To reinforce her point she compares TB treatment to the treatment for HIV: since treatment for the latter became affordable, the balance has mostly been on the side of providing treatment to as many as possible largely because of the strength of HIV advocacy campaigning. One has to wonder, in light of this, whether the issue has really been all about the price of drugs all along – and therefore about mismanagement. If the prices could have been brought down as they were with HIV drugs would it have made the difference? What a price will have been paid in lives if this turns out to have been the truth.

Medécins sans Frontières puts an actual figure on how much the price of some of the HIV drugs were reduced even when manufactured by generic manufacturers while they are technically still under patent:

> "Competition among generic producers was instrumental in bringing down the price of the first generation of ARVs, and is one of the key reasons treatment could be scaled up to millions of people. Today, first-line ART is available for just under US$100 per person per year, which is a 99% decrease from 2000, when treatments still under patent were priced at more than $10,000 per person per year."

Perhaps the evidence on some of the previous pages suggests another tension which needs subverting as well: the tension between being forced into "doing something stupid"[331] and common sense.

An obvious example of this is the statement in the 2012 WHO report relating to the "recurring and important question ... [as to] whether the number of MDR-TB cases is increasing, decreasing or stable". The WHO's assessment was that the progress of surveillance of drug-resistance has been "unfortunately … not yet sufficient to provide a definitive assessment of

[331] Richard Coker.

trends in MDR-TB globally or regionally". This was an astonishing conclusion to be drawing. It smacked of ambivalence, ambiguity or even something worse. The 2013 report unfortunately took the same stance twice: "The estimate of MDR-TB is similar to the previous estimate"; and the rates of MDR-TB are "essentially unchanged". Meanwhile every sign and almost every expert tells us that the tide of DR disease is rising, and has been doing so for years – as does simple common logic. In another part of the 2012 report it even confirmed this stating that, "enrolments in the high MDR-TB burden countries nearly doubled between 2009 and 2011 as a result of ***steady annual increases in 12 of the countries***." The 2013 Global Tuberculosis Report contained a similar contradictory confirmatory statement, that "increases were reported by a total of 17 high MDR-TB burden countries and all WHO regions with the exception of the region of the Americas". Or are we seriously being asked to accept that these increases are occurring only in the number of cases that are being detected?

In 2007 the WHO reported 289,000 new MDR-TB cases; in 2013 they reported 650,000. The number of XDR-TB cases reported worldwide increased by 52% just between 2011 and 2012. In 2008, two years after the Tugela Ferry incident, the number of countries which had seen at least one XDR case was pegged by the WHO at 49 countries and territories; by 2012 this had risen to 92. Are these trends enough to "provide a definite assessment" of a significant surge in a slow burning disease? One would surely have thought so.

Not much common sense is needed to tell us exactly why the trend is as it is, and yet there still seem to be efforts being made to play the scale of the problem down. If this is so, then Dr Mitnick is right – some subversion is most definitely needed.

It's very difficult to be optimistic about the situation. To illustrate this further I can recount a private conversation with an expert at a meeting of the All-Party Parliamentary Group on Malaria and Neglected Tropical Diseases (APPMG) in Westminster, London.

This group is run by three Members of Parliament, one from each of the major parties. There are other politicians involved in its wings as well, however, one of whom is an elderly third Baronet of the British realm from the House of Lords – whom I found myself sitting next to during the meeting.

There were four invited speakers. One was from Save the Children, one from the WHO, one from the International Council of Nurses, and one from the Gates Foundation Malaria Consortium. The quality of presentations was mixed, and the content was in most cases so obvious that I wondered how much time, energy and money must be getting wasted by such highly qualified people gathering to hear the same old stuff.

It was the picture regarding TB, however, that I was interested in. The one that was presented began by being painted in what I felt was a quite muted fashion, with the female speaker homing in on how much the issue of stigma gets in the way of progress. She then developed her theme a little, identifying the striking contrast between the estimated figure of those newly infected with MDR-TB worldwide and the actual number receiving treatment. She then went on to describe how both DOTS and DOTS-Plus treatment regimens were invariably being hailed as successful whilst the statistics suggested that neither are being well enough implemented. After her relatively gentle start, she seemed prepared to provoke a little.

As soon as she'd finished, the Third Baronet sitting next to me stuck up his hand and asked what the situation currently was regarding new TB vaccines. Someone else answered on the speaker's behalf – suggesting that there were two in the pipeline on separate trials but that neither were anticipated to be completed before 2019. The speaker herself then responded by adding that, "Our best hope is a new vaccine."

This made me sit up, but I confess to not having felt confident enough to challenge her statement in the wider meeting. In retrospect, I'm pleased that I didn't because instead I challenged her discretely after the presentation had ended – and got a much franker answer to my question than she would have ever made to the wider gathering.

The question which I asked her was this: "You said that you thought that the best hope is for a new vaccine, but for those already latently infected with the disease – 80% of Africans according to WHO figures, and 32% of the global population – this surely presents no hope at all... so what really is the hope for them? And what does this mean, considering that many of them may be carrying drug-resistant strains?"

"We need new drugs," she said immediately, something which is indisputable. But what she said next still rings in my ears. "But frankly," she said, "our best hope is simply that they die quickly."

She was referring to the DR-TB cases, of course, and where there are high rates of co-infection with HIV there's also a far better chance that they might die quicker than might otherwise be expected. Such a frank observation made privately, in contrast to the more official response she made minutes earlier, seems to exemplify the two opposing narratives on the subject. One wishes to wake the world up to a problem it knows little or nothing about, and the other worries about what expectations might arise if such an awareness is stoked up by the very organisations that have so little with which to respond to it.

Her observation, as shocking as it may sound coming from an experienced health worker, is entirely logical. I have to confess to thinking something even more dreadful after a conversation with a TB sister in a health centre in Kampala in 2009, hearing the problems she faced with her drug failures. "I just have to leave them to die," she put it because she had no treatment for them. I realised that literally taking them out to the back of the centre and shooting them, much as the Nazis did in Poland and Russia whenever they encountered cases of potentially infectious tuberculosis, would be the logical best step from the perspective of the community since doing so would serve to protect it from their dangerous infection. So the idea that quick deaths for those with drug-resistant disease might be the best hope for everyone concerned (apart from the patient) should not have been so shocking for me to hear. But hearing someone of this calibre and experience express such an opinion did indeed shock m, and it must say something about the true immensity of the problem that is confronting Africa and elsewhere and the lack of available response.

From time to time people seriously ask whether supporting the survival of more people in societies already imperilled by precarious economies, by wars, natural disasters or by shaky social structures can possibly be, in the bigger picture, a good thing. Apart from the fact that such suggestions are both ethically and morally offensive, they are also, under normal circumstances, ill-informed and illogical. All evidence suggests that when populations are freed from the scourge of infectious disease they flourish, and their rates of population growth tend to fall rather than rise further, particularly so if there is accompanying social stability. The question, therefore, is not whether we should make proper effort to save such lives; it is rather why we aren't doing more to promote health and education in such populations so that they become capable of managing their affairs without our interference? When a vulnerable country like Swaziland is branded by the UN as being undevelopable or economically non-viable because of its burden of disease, something radical needs to be done about it, not only to help such a tiny country get back on its feet, but also to prevent others going down the same path.

Over 20 years ago, as executive secretary of the International Union against Tuberculosis, Dr Annik Rouillon proposed the idea of the 'adoption' of one highly vulnerable low-income country by a specific more affluent one as a way of helping it get on top of its TB problem. Perhaps her inspiration was an idea of its time (one that may then have had real potential given that it was made when rates of drug-resistance were still diminutive). Certainly it would be much harder to sell the idea today with the problem being that much more entrenched and developed. Raising living standards alongside bringing down the burden of disease is similarly seen to take too long and to be just too daunting a task, but that doesn't mean that it shouldn't be something that should be very seriously considered by creative and determined minds open to radical ideas.

It's beyond debate that the authorities whom we have entrusted to globally protect us from the ravages of disease have a huge problem on their hands, but it is one that is happening on all of our watches, not just theirs. So far it has proved to be a problem from which many millions have been unable to hide, whilst other millions have managed by virtue of time and place to do so quite successfully. The fact that those millions who have managed to hide from it have been the wealthier and better provided for, whilst the disease has been continuing to feed on the poor has been both the true tragedy and the stumbling block.

The authorities find themselves now struggling to ramp up commercial interest in combating the disease and sparking public interest without causing panic. But do they really want to ramp up public awareness at all? Can they develop new treatments that can be used where they are needed? Can they increase funding when the world is in recession? Can they get away with recruiting a private sector to help dig them out of their hole, when the private sector helped to dump them in it in the first place? Can they make the sort of decisions that are required if progress really is to be made in relation to a developing threat of untreatable disease that is looking to be very dangerous indeed?

The opinions of experts leave little room for debate on this. Keshavjee and Farmer have identified that:

> "Despite the enormity of the threat, investments to contain the epidemic and to cure infected patients have been halting and meagre when compared,

> for example, with those made to address the acquired immunodeficiency syndrome (AIDS) pandemic."[332]

Dr Lucica Ditiu of the Stop TB Partnership describes the fact that so many people are still dying of a curable disease as being "shameful" – and she calls the current investment in R&D "pathetic".

A host of 24 other experts headed by Professor Alimuddin Zumla of University College London have asked:

> "Why, despite nearly 20 years of WHO-promoted activity and more than 12 years of MDR tuberculosis – specific activity, has the country response to the drug-resistant tuberculosis epidemic been so ineffectual?"

And they go so far as to warn that, as things stand:

> "The cost of treatment ... could bankrupt health care financing in tuberculosis-endemic areas."[333]

They summarise this as an "ominous situation". Not everyone shares these views, however. Another UK expert, Professor Tim McHugh, also of University College London, sounds a more cautionary note:

> "I do worry when people stand up at conferences and talk about MDR-TB and say it's a big disaster and the whole world is going to collapse. It's not that severe yet."

It may be significant that Professor McHugh is the leader of a team that is testing one of the two more advanced candidate new TB drugs, and so he may feel it politically expedient to sound more positive for fear of frightening off potential funders – because he doesn't sound entirely complacent on the subject stating:

> "The big anxiety is that if we don't act now, it will easily run away from us."

---

[332] Salmaan Keshavje, and Paul E. Farmer - "Tuberculosis, Drug-resistance, and the History of Modern Medicine", New England Journal of Medicine, 367 (2012) 931-36.

[333] Zumla A et al. - "Drug-Resistant Tuberculosis—Current dilemmas, unanswered questions, challenges, and priority needs", Journal of Infectious Diseases, 205 (suppl 2) (2012) 228-40.

This idea, at least, everyone seems agreed upon. Keshavjee and Farmer again:

> "Advocacy for scaling up MDR tuberculosis treatment has been inadequate and must increase – exponentially."

They are also dismissive of what has been achieved so far:

> "The pace of scale-up of MDR tuberculosis treatment has been abysmal. We have failed to apply relevant lessons, and our approaches are outdated."[334]

Parts of clinical medicine today are dominated by what are referred to as 'algorithms' – essentially these amount to predictive equations which are composed of elements of certain or near-certain knowledge which predict probable outcomes in otherwise complex conditions.

So here are a few basic algorithms concerning DR-TB:

> **Poor infrastructure + availability of first line drugs => expected MDR-TB**
>
> **Poor infrastructure + availability of second line drugs => expected XDR-TB**
>
> **Poor infrastructure + no second line drugs but with migrant workers returning home after exposure to infection in countries where they are available => XDR-TB**

The Partnerships, the Global Plans, the initiatives – all were too slow to pick up on MDR-TB and still seem inclined to avoid the disquieting probabilities inherent within these algorithms. Now, however, perhaps 20 years later than should have ever been the case almost all the experts are agreeing that MDR-TB is out there and won't be fixed by DOTS. But so also is XDR-TB. So where is the plan to cope with XDR-TB?[335] Do we

---

334 Salmaan Keshavjee, and Paul E. Farmer - "Picking up the pace – scale-up of MDR-tuberculosis treatment programs", New England Journal of Medicine, 363 (2010)1781-84.

335 There actually is a plan, but it remains vague. The "WHO Eight-Point Plan and Additional Considerations" include:

have to wait another 20 years for further awareness to drip-feed into global health policies while vulnerable people continue to suffer and die from our oldest of enemies?

The Global Emergency was announced in 1993. It related solely to tuberculosis – no drug-resistant component was allowed for and the strategies and targets for the following decade reflected this. It took more than ten years to see the epidemic peak, and 15 to see any clear decline emerge, but even that was only with susceptible disease.

We know that the bow-wave of drug-resistance moves invisibly in the deeps of the pool of latent disease. It progresses silently and is at any moment possibly as much as 15 years ahead of what is visible on the surface of the sea of active disease. So, on this basis, we should consider another logical algorithm based both on this phenomenon and on the timescales of the current global emergency if we wish to call the world to arms to confront this drug-resistant pandemic:

> **10 years (from experience) + 15 years (drug-resistant 'pipeline' factor) => 25 years until any expected peak of the drug-resistant pandemic.**

Should we be forecasting that drug-resistance migh still be rising in 2039 even if we start to properly address it from today? Would this be a more realistic strategy than suggesting the possibility that the rates of this disease are currently "essentially unchanged" or that this disease can be "eradicated" by 2050 or "ended" by 2035? It would certainly seem not just

---

- Strengthening quality of basic TB and HIV/AIDS control
- Scaling up programmatic management of MDR-TB and XDR-TB
- Strengthening laboratory services
- Expanding MDR-TB and XDR-TB surveillance
- Developing and implementing infection control measures
- Strengthening advocacy, communication and social mobilization
- Pursuing resource mobilization at all levels
- Promoting research and development of new tools

It was also devised in 2007 and has barely begun being visibly implemented. See:
http://www.who.int/tb/challenges/xdr/xdr_mdr_factsheet_2007_en.pdf?ua=1

more sensible to be planning around such possibilities but also more ethical:

> "Drug-resistant TB is not the result of catastrophic natural forces such as earthquakes, tsunamis and hurricanes. It is not caused by malign human intent, as are terrorism and war, nor is it fostered by our dysfunctional relationship with the animal kingdom as are severe acute respiratory syndrome (SARS) and avian influenza. The locus of risk and control is entirely within the human domain. Our response to the emergence of drug-resistant TB is profoundly ethical as it raises issues of how justice and human rights are realized in our collective response to a disease. It also underscores how the global community responds to its most disadvantaged members."[336]

Mark Dybul of the Global Fund believes that we are now at a "tipping point", with the disease either going one way or the other. Mario Raviglione sees it much the same way as well..

> "The momentum to break this disease is in real danger. We are now at a crossroads between TB elimination within our lifetime, and millions more TB deaths."[337]

The final words, however, go, rather than to an expert on this disease, to a poet whose words reflect the intentions that lie behind this publication, being as it is intended to raise a set of -

"... QUESTIONS THAT HAVE NO RIGHT
TO GO AWAY."

David Whyte (2007)[338]

---

[336] Upshur R et al. - "Apocalypse or redemption: responding to extensively drug-resistant tuberculosis", the Bulletin of the World Health Organization, 87 (2009) 481-83.

[337] Mario Raviglione's comment accompanying the 2012 Global Tuberculosis Report.

[338] From the poem "Sometimes" in 'Everything is waiting for you' published by Many Rivers Press.

Appendix 1 – TB timeline

1882 – Robert Koch identifies the TB bacillus

1882 – Sputum test is developed

1890 – Koch announces discovery of tuberculin

1908 – Bacille-Calmette-Guérin (BCG vaccine) invented

1943 – Streptomycin isolated

1948 – British Medical Research Council conducts first large scale medical trial with Streptomycin

1950s & 1960s – several more drugs developed

1966 – Rifampicin discovered

*

1985 – first MDR-TB case

1991 – "Is Africa lost?" – The Lancet

1993 – WHO declares TB a global emergency

1993 – DOTS recommended

"early 1990s" – New York MDR-TB costs US$1 billion

1994 – Global Project set up to monitor drug-resistance

1996 – PIH identifies shortcomings of DOTS in Peru

1997 – first XDR-TB case

1998 – DOTS-Plus is introduced

2000 – Global Plan for 2001-2005 announced

|

2000 – Green Light Committee created to provide quality assured second line drugs

|

2005 – WHA resolution: all patients to have "universal standard 0f healthcare"

|

2005 – Global Plan 2006-2015 announced

|

2006 – outbreak of XDR-TB in KwazaZulu-Natal, South Africa

|

By 2009 – Just 0.5% of all patients with MDR-TB being treated?

|

2009 – first TDR-TB case

|

2010 -GeneXpert approved by the WHO

|

2010 – Revised Global Plan 2011-2015 announced

|

2010 – WHO report 1.5 million DR-TB deaths 2000-2009

|

2012 – Bedaquiline approved as new drug for TB by FDA

|

2014 – Global Plan 2015-2035 announced

*

2015 – completion point of 2011-2015 plan

*

2035 – completion point of post-2015 plan

Appendix 2 – National Incidence Rates

The following national rates are based on the World Health Organization's (WHO) most recently available three years (2008, 2009 and 2010) of estimated incidence (all forms of TB) per 100,000 population.[339] The three year moving average is now being used to try to allow for recognisably unstable rates in some jurisdictions. The estimated TB rates (including both new and re-treatment) are now being used, rather than the previous country/territory reported incidence rates, as these are thought to adjust for under-reporting of cases in some jurisdictions and are therefore more indicative of the current risk of being infected by residence or prolonged travel in the particular country or territory. These rates were effective as of June 2011 and it is expected that they will continue to be reviewed in this format.

Estimated burden of TB disease by country: 3 year average incidence rate per 100,000 population: 2008, 2009 and 2010

Afghanistan	189	Liberia	288
Albania	15	Libyan Arab Jamahiriya	40
Algeria	88	Lithuania	70
American Samoa	7	Luxembourg	9
Andorra	8	Madagascar	261
Angola	298	Malawi	245
Anguilla	21	Malaysia	83
Antigua and Barbuda	4	Maldives	39
Argentina	28	Mali	64
Armenia	73	Malta	12
Aruba	0	Marshall Islands	471
Australia	6	Mauritania	330
Austria	7	Mauritius	22
Azerbaijan	110	Mexico	17
Bahamas	14	Micronesia	212

339 World Health Organization - "Global tuberculosis control: surveillance, planning, financing: WHO report 2011", Geneva: World Health Organization, 2011.

Bahrain	29	Monaco	0
Bangladesh	225	Mongolia	223
Barbados	2	Montenegro	21
Belarus	71	Montserrat	10
Belgium	9	Morocco	92
Belize	40	Mozambique	539
Benin	93	Myanmar	388
Bermuda	3	Namibia	693
Bhutan	158	Nauru	49
Bolivia	140	Nepal	163
Bonaire, St Eustatius & Saba	0	Netherlands	7
Bosnia and Herzegovina	50	Netherlands Antilles	27
Botswana	548	New Caledonia	23
Brazil	45	New Zealand	8
Br Virgin Islands	10	Nicaragua	44
Brunei Darussalam	66	Niger	181
Brunei Darussalam	66	Niger	181
Bulgaria	41	Nigeria	136
Burkina Faso	59	Niue	10
Burundi	138	Northern Mariana Islands	72
Cambodia	442	Norway	6
Cameroon	182	Oman	14
Canada	5	Pakistan	231
Cape Verde	148	Palau	115
Cayman Islands	6	Panama	48
Central African Republic	327	Papua New Guinea	303
Chad	283	Paraguay	47
Chile	19	Peru	113
China	80	Philippines	280
China, Hong Kong SAR	86	Poland	23
China, Macao SAR	74	Portugal	29

Colombia	35	Puerto Rico	2
Comoros	39	Qatar	43
Congo	382	Republic of Korea	95
Cook Islands	8	Republic of Moldova	178
Costa Rica	14	Romania	125
Côte d'Ivoire	148	Russian Federation	106
Croatia	23	Rwanda	115
Cuba	9	Saint Kitts and Nevis	7
Curasao	1	Saint Lucia	8
Cyprus	4	St Vincent & the Grenadines	24
Czech Republic	8	Samoa	12
D.P.R of Korea	345	San Marino	0
D.R of the Congo	327	Sao Tome and Principe	98
Denmark	6	Saudi Arabia	18
Djibouti	620	Senegal	282
Dominica	13	Serbia	23
Dominican Republic	70	Serbia & Montenegro	0
Ecuador	68	Seychelles	31
Egypt	19	Sierra Leone	645
El Salvador	30	Singapore	36
Equatorial Guinea	126	Sint Maarten (Dutch part)	3
Eritrea	99	Slovakia	10
Estonia	30	Slovenia	11
Ethiopia	266	Solomon Islands	115
Fiji	23	Somalia	285
Finland	8	South Africa	971
France	10	Spain	17
French Polynesia	21	Sri Lanka	66
Gabon	502	Sudan	119
Gambia	268	Suriname	135

Georgia	107	Swaziland	1257
Germany	5	Sweden	6
Ghana	92	Switzerland	7
Greece	5	Syrian Arab Republic	21
Grenada	4	Tajikistan	204
Guam	63	Thailand	137
Guatemala	62	Macedonia	23
Guinea	318	Timor-Leste	498
Guinea-Bissau	229	Togo	446
Guyana	112	Tokelau	0
Haiti	238	Tonga	18
Honduras	58	Trinidad and Tobago	22
Hungary	15	Tunisia	24
Iceland	5	Turkey	29
India	190	Turkmenistan	67
Indonesia	189	Turks and Caicos Islands	22
Iran	19	Tuvalu	247
Iraq	64	Uganda	226
Ireland	9	Ukraine	101
Israel	5	United Arab Emirates	3
Italy	5	United Kingdom of GB	13
Jamaica	7	United Republic of Tanzania	183
Japan	22	United States of America	4
Jordan	6	Uruguay	22
Kazakhstan	163	US Virgin Islands	0
Kenya	314	Uzbekistan	128
Kiribati	409	Vanuatu	72
Kuwait	40	Venezuela	33
Kyrgyzstan	159	Viet Nam	200
Lao People' D. Republic	89	Wallis and Futuna Islands	53
Latvia	45	West Bank and Gaza Strip	5

Lebanon	15	Yemen	54
Lesotho	634	Zambia	481
		Zimbabwe	672

Appendix 3 – Some Alternatives

"WE HAVE TO BE READY TO BE THINKING OF NEW THINGS WITH TUBERCULOSIS BECAUSE WHAT WE'VE BEEN DOING SO FAR HASN'T WORKED OUT."

Dr Lee Reichmann[340]

Immunotherapies

If a microbe causes disease in its host it does so because of two factors – one is because of the pathogenic nature of the microbe, and the other is because of the susceptibility of the host itself. The conventional modern treatment of TB relies on attacking the microbe using active pharmaceutical agents - indeed most of the current research for new treatment relies on the same principle. As such the crucial susceptibility, or otherwise, of the host remains a relatively ignored phenomenon. It would therefore seem logical to look at this significant intrinsic factor in the disease's progression more carefully. At first glance, modulating the susceptibility of the host in ways which might resist the disease would seem to be a rather captivating idea. As ever, however, with TB things just aren't as simple as might be wished.

There is a strong probability that a small percentage of humans inherit the capacity to clear an initial TB infection simply with the strength of their own innate immune system. It's difficult to be more specific than this. Data collected in the early twentieth century from skin testing children who were most probably already exposed to TB suggests the possibility that as many as one in five may have had this capacity since around 80% of children tested in the UK by TST were showing positive signs of exposure. The 20% who weren't either hadn't been exposed to the disease at all or were showing no TST response because the disease had been cleared by an innate response which would show no subsequent antigenic evidence of occurrence. Similar studies in Canada in indigenous children suggested a higher 92% positive TST result, suggesting that this natural resistance might even be influenced by prolonged ethnic exposure to particular strains of

[340] Lung specialist at New Jersey Medical School National TB Center.

disease – the native Canadians being more susceptible to strains imported from Europe.

Whatever might be the case, we can at least assume that the immune systems of at least some of those 20% of British children were, in the sense that they could see off a TB infection at first base, naturally resistant to the disease.

The next step in disease progression is the latent infection. At this point the disease is walled off with the classic stalemate developed, remaining that way for perpetuity in 85-95% of LTBI cases. This stalemate is achieved, as we have already seen, as a result of a specific activation of the acquired immune system.

The disease, however, can break out at any time from this stalemate – re-activating into either subclinical disease or one that is fully active and lethal. The levels of symptoms will indicate which this might be, but with sub-clinical disease it will be extremely hard to spot except with good radiography.

A further range of sub-categories of disease occurs within this re-activated disease category, however: these include pulmonary and extra-pulmonary, sputum-positive and sputum-negative, culture-positive and culture-negative, drug-susceptible and drug-resistant. Each of these may involve and require a differentially discrete response by specific component parts of the immune system for the host to in any way adequately respond to it. As such, it can be immediately appreciated that a modulation of the immune host response might well not be a simple affair.

There are still very persuasive reasons not to give up on the idea however.

One is because ramping up the immune response so that it is more effective might shorten duration of treatment, and shortening treatment regimens is one of the major goals of the current research into the new drug combinations. Longer treatment regimens not only contribute to higher rates of non-completion, but they also leave what is left of the patient's host response significantly diminished, leaving him or her wide open to subsequent relapse or re-infection, or even to other opportunistic infections.

A second reason relates to the possibility of improving cure rates in both MDR- and XDR-TB cases. If the host resources can be mobilized in a way which might work in concert with the weaker more toxic drugs, it just might help tip the balance more often in favour of the host rather than the pathogenic guest. As such a more holistic TB treatment (one that works from two directions at once) could reduce this overall immune impairment, shorten the length of treatment, and even attenuate toxicities. When considering these together immunotherapy would certainly seem to promise an important potential step in a positive direction. And if it were able to be rolled out in any scale at all it might even help dam down the drug-resistant pandemic since the bacillus's opportunity to mutate (at least much of the time) is thought to be probably proportional to the extent of its exposure to therapeutic agents.

Some interesting research in this field has been completed in the last fifteen years. The results have been mixed, sometimes even the opposite of what was expected, and on occasions they are even contradictory. The overall picture, however, is an encouraging one. As our understanding of the human immune response deepens (often as a result of new discoveries in cancer research which has been more heavily focused on immunotherapy) new possibilities emerge – and they will almost certainly continue to do so.

The conclusion so far, however, tends to suggest that such interventions need to be very carefully timed, equally carefully monitored and will, at least at first, probably be very expensive.

The first part of the disease that we can be unpack a little in this respect is the phenomenon of latent infection. A rather more sophisticated model of exactly how the invading bacilli provoke a host immune response which paradoxically helps to protect them from further assault by the host's adaptive immune cells has been recently proposed. It is suggested to involve the release of bone marrow-derived 'mesenchymal stem cells' (MSCs). These stem cells are believed to somehow get 'recruited' into the granuloma where they are triggered to release a limited amount of nitric oxide. The bacilli then respond to this toxicity in their immediate environment by slowing down their metabolism.[341] In this way the immediate prospects for the bugs are effectively stymied unless or until this situation changes but, in the process, they are to some degree also protected because the effect of this chemical attack by the MSCs is also believed to decrease the bacilli's susceptibility to Isoniazid, the treatment of choice for LTBI. So, as understandings continue to develop, some sort of carefully measured infusion of autologous MSCs might just offer a novel

[341] Raghuvanshi S et al. – "*Mycobacterium Tuberculosis* evades host immunity by recruiting mesenchymal stem cells", Proceeds of the National Academy of Sciences USA, 107 (2010) 21653-68.

way of treating LTBI and might even permanently stall re-activation. As yet such an approach remains theoretical but, given the fundamental importance of getting to grips with latent disease, at least it suggests enticing possibilities, particularly so if the treatment were effective irrespective of drug-resistance.

The second part of the disease involves the subsequent re-activation of these bacilli – a condition which necessarily provokes an entirely different host immune response. It also necessitates a different immunotherapeutic response as well. Before considering this, however, there is one further potential complication to consider – which is that these two conditions may not even exist separately from each other, and this may have consequences for treatment that are still not entirely understood.

A simple understanding the development of re-activation allows us to believe that the two conditions are at least theoretically discrete – that effectively the granulomatous phase ends as the re-activated disease develops. Of course this need not necessarily be the case. Something, as yet undiscovered, causes the granulomas to burst open as the bacilli re-activate, but do they all do this? They may not do because 5% of relapse cases are believed to occur even after completion of optimal treatment. Is this because of a residue of surviving unsterilized granuloma which would have not been eradicated during first line treatment of the re-activated disease? It certainly remains a possibility, so just as in the same way that TB drugs are used in different ways for each state of TB disease, the component host immune responses may need to cope quite differently as well – even possibly simultaneously.

Be that as it may, we have already discussed the actions of the adaptive immune response to TB in an earlier section. We have seen that the elimination of *M. tuberculosis* infection depends on the success of a complex flexible interaction between the infected macrophages and the T lymphocytes – existing either as 'Th1 clones' which are characterized by the production of interferon gamma (IFN-γ) and Interleukin 12 (IL-12), or as 'Th2 clones' which are differently characterized by the production of interleukin 4 (IL-4). Overall, the cytokines IL-12, IFN-γ and TNF are now widely agreed to be critical in the control of any re-activated *M. tuberculosis* infection.

As a result the administering of these cytokines has been attempted *in vitro*, in animals or in small human studies in anticipation of their having some level of significant effect on disease progression and outcome. The results have so far been mixed and have largely only led to further complexities.

The method of administration certainly appears to be important (with aerosolysed methods seeming to be more effective than administration by injection), but there appear to be even more important factors relating to both dosage and timing to maximise effect and minimise adverse reactions. Getting either wrong looks likely to create an excessive inflammatory response and might even lead to an exhaustion of the immune response which could be catastrophic for an already weakened patient.

Two distinct methods intended to modulate the immune response to TB have been developed so far. One is to stimulate the immune response by augmenting what are believed to be deficiencies in specific cytokines, most specifically IL-12 and IFN-γ. The other is to dampen another part of the immune response, specifically related to TNF levels, something which is believed to improve the access of the TB drugs and the pathogen's susceptibility to them. Treatments which have been attempted for this second approach have used high dosage prednisolone, thalidomide and ethanercept.

Whilst there have been some positive results reported, complications have also been recorded. There also remain some uncertainties concerning possible interactions between the current combination therapies and each of these immunotherapies. The field is technically still a very challenging one, and is likely to remain so for some time to come unless an enormous effort is put into it. To date it is a field of study that remains almost completely ignored in the global strategies for future research; the possibilities that exist within it, however, mean that it is an important one to be pursued if at all possible.

Phage Therapy

Phage therapy, or perhaps more correctly, a therapy which uses bacteriophages to destroy pathogenic bacteria, has an interesting history – and it is one which actively overlaps on parts of the history of tuberculosis that we reviewed earlier.

A British bacteriologist called Frederick Twort first identified bacteriophages in 1915. Two years later, the self-taught French-Canadian medical maverick Felix d'Hérelle stumbled across them himself, quite independently, at the Pasteur Institute in Paris. Both had noticed the same phenomena - clear spots appearing on culture broths that were known to be otherwise teaming with bacteria. What both had witnessed were tiny killing fields within the cultures in which one bacterium was in the process of killing another using bacteriophages. It was d'Hérelle, however, who identified the microscopic marvel as some new type of parasite and realised its possibilities, writing, "In a flash I had understood what caused my clear spots was in fact an invisible microbe...a virus parasitic on bacteria." He then called what he saw 'bacteriophages', deriving the term from two Greek words meaning 'bacteria devouring'.

Bacteriophages are indeed viruses, far tinier than bacteria and slightly tadpole-shaped. They are among the simplest organisms on the planet, no more than a millionth of an inch in size and are only visible with an electron microscope. One millilitre of water can contain up to a trillion of them. They can thrive anywhere that bacteria exist – particularly favouring raw sewage, but also occurring in more open water and in human beings – in fact they occur to some degree practically everywhere. Sewage effluents, though, have been one of the most favoured places for their collection by phage researchers.

These phages get down to their work by first settling on the surface of a bacterium 'tail down', secreting enzymes to soften up the bacterial cell wall and then injecting their deadly DNA into the bacillus. Once 'infected' the bacterium finds itself helplessly playing host to the virus, with the invader replicating itself 100–150 times in as little as ten minutes before exploding out of the bacterium, causing its death. A single phage can thus produce tens of thousands of offspring in an hour. Other phages reproduce in a slightly more moderate fashion by becoming a part of the bacterium's genome, so that when the bacterium reproduces, so does the phage. In other cases still, the phage's DNA simply binds to the bacterial DNA, with the phage becoming a virtual tenant in the outer cytoplasm of the germ. In either of these latter cases, sooner or later the phage DNA or the actual phages themselves confer the infected bacteria with an involuntary capacity to kill other bacteria.

D'Hérelle, in partnership with microbiologist George Eliava, went on to set up an institute in Tbilisi, the capital of Georgia, in order to continue the specialist study of this phenomenon. There they harvested phages from the nearby Kura River for culture and further examination. D'Hérelle himself left the institute during the Stalinist era whilst Eliava stayed behind and ended up being executed. But the 'Eliava Institute of Bacteriophage Microbiology and Virology' flourished and still exists today. By the late 1930s it was churning out phages in quantity, and some major U.S. pharmaceutical companies including Eli Lilly, ER Squibb and Abbott had also got involved in their development as well, each manufacturing their own particular phage preparations.

Then, in 1934, a poorly designed study found that treatment with systemic phages showed mixed results, concluding that host body fluids strongly inhibited and destroyed most bacteriophages before they could reach target tissue and so interest in the treatment in the West began to wane.

The advent of sulfa drugs and antibiotics in the 1940s pretty much finished phage therapy off completely, effectively relegating both phage therapy and theory to the backseat in all Western countries. While phages were now being seen to frequently and inexplicably fail, antibiotics, at least at first, appeared to be completely fail-safe. Doctors preferred them as well not just because they were so relatively easy to use, but also because they also often killed a broad spectrum of bacterial infections. And t they weren't seen to pose the sorts of risk that introducing living organisms into a patient might do.

In wartime Russia, however, there was no real knowledge of the Western advances in antibiotic production and phage therapy was still being successfully used at some scale on infections including on both wartime gangrene and dysentery. And as a result Soviet research into phage therapy continued after the war was over. Russian researchers continued to develop and refine their treatments, and also to publish the results of their research but, due to the scientific barriers created by the Cold War, their research was rarely if ever translated and so, bafflingly, it failed to be shared across the world.

Antibiotics, meanwhile, became the mainstay of TB treatment directly as a result of soil biologist Selman Waksman's original research. Waksman had correctly realised that there was something in the soil that was able to kill tuberculosis and he then figured that it must be other bacteria. His early research had effectively proved. When Albert Schatz finally isolated the tuberculosis-killing streptomycin from an actinomyces cultured in a well-manured soil both scientists thought that that their case was comprehensively proven. They completely ignored the possibility that mycobacteriophages, known to exist in the soil, might have also been causing at least some the *M. Tuberculosis* deaths that they had previously witnessed in certain soils.

In fact they may well have considered this possibility since another of the early drug pioneers, the extraordinary Rene Dubos, had actually published a study in 1943 on phage treatment, the very same year that they discovered Streptomycin.[342] Dubos's paper had confronted some of those earlier concerns which had arisen from the faulty 1934 study which had quetioned phage therapy's safety and efficacy. He showed that there was actually no real problem in the phages reaching and safely destroying pathogenic bacteria, demonstrating that this was even the case when done in the brain. The phages multiplied and remained at substantial levels in the blood, and they did so only as long as there were sensitive bacteria in which they could reproduce. There had quite clearly been problems with some of the earlier research: some of the preparations had almost certainly been contaminated, and also many of the early researchers hadn't sufficiently realised how highly specific each phage type might be for a given bacteria species or even for a strain of a species - something which might have accounted for the reports of lack of effect

It had also been Dubos who had laid the groundwork for all of the antibiotic research that was going on at the time of the discovery of Streptomycin and well after. He had done this with his discovery of gramicidin in 1939. It was actually as a result of this single discovery that, in spite of Dubos's 1943 paper which thus appeared as no more than a sideline, all attention had become focused on antibiotic development.

Interest in phage therapy was regenerated for a short while in the West in the mid-1980s but it was the burgeoning frequency of antibiotic-resistant bacterial infections that prompted the more recent surge of interest in the

---

[342] Dubos RJ, Straus JH - "Multiplication of bacteriophages in vivo and its protective effect against an experimental infection with Shigella Dysenteriae", Journal of Experimental Medicine, 78; 3 (1943) 161–8.

West. The question that was beginning to be asked was whether phage therapy might now be 'resurrected' to respond to the unresolved problems of antibiotic resistance that were being recognised to challenge large parts of modern medicine.

In fact bacteria have also been seen to quite naturally develop resistance to their specific bacteriophages just as they do to antibiotic drugs. The phages themselves, however, have the natural capacity to adapt in turn in order to keep hunting down their prey bacteria, matching them, if they possibly can, mutation for mutation. This is something that has been described by Alexander Sulakvelidze, a former Georgian lab director at the Eliava Institute, as being a "biological arms race". If this is indeed consistently the case, then, the trick would appear to be simply to spot the successful mutations in the phage and then continue to culture and exploit them.

Phages also offer other significant advantages over antibiotics. They are target-specific, so leaving the myriad benevolent bacteria which lives in symbiosis with their human hosts completely untouched. This leaves the treated patient far less open to opportunistic infections by other pathogens whilst under treatment and also far less likely to suffer side effects. Because phages can replicate *in vivo* after administration, a small initial dosage is also all that is needed for it to be effective.

It's not all good news, however. Some specific phages can actually make the bacteria they infect even more lethal to the host than they were originally. This happens, for example, when certain phages infect the bacteria that cause cholera, scarlet fever, and diphtheria. The phages' high bacterial strain specificities also almost mean that different phage 'cocktails' would be needed for the treatment of the same infection or disease if the bacterial components of such diseases differ only slightly from region to region or even from person to person. Such cocktails would necessitate the development of 'phage banks' which would contain many different phages, and these banks in turn would need to be regularly updated with new phages. This would be challenging enough, but the need for such phage banks would also necessitate individual regulatory testing of each newly developed phage for treatment safety in humans. This single factor makes the whole enterprise far more complex and expensive. It must certainly challenge the prospect for any future large-scale production or roll-out given the existing technologies. But that is not all, unfortunately, because individual patents for each new phage will inevitably be being sought and will almost certainly prove complicated with companies competing in efforts to maintain exclusive rights on their best phage 'inventions'.

Nevertheless a handful of companies are in the process of developing their own 'phage catalogues' which intend to sequence the genetic code of a select few of the almost infinitely large number of species of bacteria-killing viruses found in nature. Some have opted to use only naturally occurring species, whilst others are attempting to use genetic engineering to help them overcome bacterial resistances (and quite probably make their patenting much easier). Human trials have yet to begin, but they might well do so soon.

Meanwhile, back in Tbilisi bacteriophages never really fell out of fashion at all. They've been in continuous use in humans for 70 years with intermittent reports of miraculous results.[343] Claims are now being made that they are effective for a range of clinical pathogens that have developed resistance to antibiotics, amongst them staphylococcus, enterococcus, streptococcus, salmonella and shigella. Tuberculosis has yet to appear on any list, however.

Theoretically, however, the possibilities have been being explored, not least because it's been known for at least 30 years that *M. tuberculosis* is vulnerable to certain specific phages. In fact an innovative and specific hypothetical approach has even been proposed based on the results of some other TB-specific research.[344] This 'hypothesis' is this – that the mycobacteriophage TM4, when 'parentally' injected into a diseased patient whilst within the cells of another benign mycobacterium which is also susceptible to it, might thus susbequently destroy drug-resistant tuberculosis mycobacteria as it encounters them. The idea was developed from results of a research study originally published in the Journal of Infectious Diseases, itself designed and developed on particular foundational ideas.

Back in 1981, a Czech study had shown that such 'parenterally' injected mycobacteriophages (this time bacteriophage DS-6A) could destroy *M. tuberculosis* in guinea pigs.[345] The results suggested that the results were approximately as effective as Isoniazid. Since then other phages have been

[343] Phage therapy, in fact, has yet to be approved for human use in any country except for Russia and Georgia.

[344] Lawrence Broxmeyer - "Bacteriophages: antibacterials with a future?" Medical Hypotheses, 62 (2004) 889–893.

[345] Sula L - "Therapy of experimental tuberculosis in Guinea Pigs with mycobacterial phages DS-6A, GR21T, MY-327", Czech Medicine, 4; 4 (1981)209–14.

shown to attack TB, and meanwhile the concept of 'shuttle plasmid delivery systems' have been developed. The term 'shuttle phasmid' (or 'shuttle vector') describes phages that can replicate in, not one, but in two different host species. The clever trick is that they can harmelessly exist in a non-pathogenic and non-disease-causing form in one strain or species of bacteria whilst at the same time having the capacity to multiply as a potentially lethal agent when they encounter the other pathogenic strain. This idea suggests that a bacteria that is known to be non-pathogenic to man, but which still has the capacity to generate specific phages that are known to kill other virulent pathogens already in the body, might be quite deliberately injected into a diseased patient with the bacteriophage tucked harmlessly away inside the non-pathogenic bacteria and then eradicate the virulent disease when it encounters its bacteria. The harmless bacteria will all the while have been protecting and nurturing the viral phages that are deadly to the pathogen before finally delivering its payload. It remains a truly compelling idea. The general process involved is known as 'lysogeny', a term which describes how one colony of bacteria can kill another by means of its phage weaponry without itself being harmed. Lawrence Broxmeyer, the author of the hypothesis, has poetically described the act of cunningly injecting a harmless phage-laden bacterium into a diseased organism as being like "a veritable Trojan horse to conquer heretofore incurable disease": all the while a hidden host of phages (the deadly "Greek soldiers") stay quiet inside the harmless Trojan bacteria waiting to break out.

The original study that the hypothesis is based upon had selected *M. smegmatis* as the best candidate for its trojan horse both because of its general gene sequence and because its chromosomal organization is very similar to that of the closely related streptomyces – the same bacteria which Schatz had worked with whilst isoloating streptomycin. *M. smegmatis* is also used in other research work on mycobacteria both because it is so fast-growing and also because it is non-pathogenic to humans and therefore much safer to work with. One further factor is that, despite being fast-growing, it still shares those unusual lipid cell-wall properties of *M. tuberculosis*. It is an interesting organism: first identified in 1884, *M. smegmatis* is most abundantly found in the secretions that collect under the prepuce of the foreskin of the penis or of the clitoris, and is more commonly referred to as 'smegma'.

The phage that was selected for the study, meanwhile, was the TM4 mycobacteriophage. This is a phage which might be described as being 'broad spectrum' in phage terms since it can equally infect both fast- (*M. smegmatis*) and slow- (*M. tuberculosis*) growing mycobacteria. The study had intrigingly suggested that, when properly introduced via the non-virulent *M. smegmatis*, this TM4 phage had a killing rate for virulent TB that was far in excess of modern day antibiotics.[346] Of further significant interest was the finding that neither *M. smegmatis* nor TM4 alone was able, in and of itself, to kill the virulent mycobacteria, and yet they so efficiently did so in combination.

The potentials from this study are enormous if it is clinically reproducible since the technique could then be applied to treat otherwise untreatable drug-resistant strains of TB. As presented, however, the idea was claimed to be 'proof of concept' only, with further animal and toxicity studies required before human trials might begin to be attempted. There are, as identified above, still clear difficulties in researching this extraordinary field however.

The final words on this topic go to Lawrence Broxmeyer, the author of the hypothesis, since they so sadly reflect mankind's ongoing struggle with its ancient enemy:

> "Mycobacteria were chosen because they have created a vast reservoir of disease on earth, the last chapter of which has yet to be written.
>
> "And unfortunately we are a major host."

[346] Broxmeyer L et al. - "Killing of Mycobacterium avium and Mycobacterium tuberculosis by a mycobacteriophage delivered by a nonvirulent mycobacterium: a model for phage therapy of intracellular bacterial pathogens", Journal of Infectious Diseases, 186; 8 (2002).

Moxibustion – the 'Moon at the Window'?

"THE MOON AT THE WINDOW –
AT LEAST THE THIEF
LEFT THAT BEHIND."

Ryōkan Taigu (1758-1831)[347]

Direct 'small-cone' moxibustion (or 'moxa') is a treatment which involves burning tiny pieces of a dried and refined herb (mugwort) on the skin. It produces a tiny instantaneous 'pinch' of heat. The therapy is a part of the larger canon of East Asian medicine which originated in China and it is closely associated with acupuncture. In many parts of East Asia this treatment used to be carried out in a very aggressive way, creating both blisters and sometimes suppurative scarring by using sizeable bean-sized 'cones' of moxa. The treatment was particularly refined in Japan, however, resulting in a much more delicate treatment using only tiny 'half-rice-grain-sized' pieces of the herb. Despite these being so small and weighing just 1mg, it is still customary to refer to these these 'cones'.

The Japanese refinement of the technique has resulted in a more adaptable, appropriate and safe treatment, especially for immuno-compromised patients.

It has been confirmed by a series of scientific Japanese studies published over several decades that this treatment promotes an immune response. There is a quantity of documentary and historical accounts from earlier periods of it having been used to treat TB. The earliest documentary Chinese evidence comes from as long ago as the 6th AD[348] with more

[347] Ryōkan Taigu was an eccentric Japanese Zen Buddhist monk who lived much of his life as a hermit. In Japanese, this quotation in its original Japanese exists as a poem in *haiku* format.

[348] "The Moxibustion Method for Consumptive Disease", written by a Tang dynasty physician called Cui Zhidi but was subsequently lost from posterity. While still extant, however, it was frequently quoted and referred to in several centuries.

evidence from the Ming Dynasty in the 17th century, although all of these used aggressive blistering treatment with claims of complete cure.[349]

There is only one piece of scientific evidence for the use of moxa to treat TB. It was a study the results of which were published in Japan in 1929. They described the treatment being used on animals, conducted by a physician who also elsewhere documented his own successful use of the treatment on his human patients. The doctor's name was Shimetaro Hara.

Doctor Hara (1883-1991) started his medical career in 1901 and began doing medical research in 1924. He was already fascinated by the actions of moxibustion, using the treatment on both himself and his patients. Intrigued by the responses he was finding (and he was already claiming that his treatment was curing TB if done over a long term) he conducted his research into its effects on guinea pigs, deevloping a series of experiments on five groups of guinea pigs, deliberately infecting them all with the TB bacillus.

The first group was treated with moxa for a month before their infection and with treatment continuing after it. The second group had their moxa started three weeks after their infection. The third group had moxa started ten weeks after infection. A fourth group received moxa for a month before their infection but then had their moxa treatment discontinued. A fifth group was the control, with no moxa therapy at all. All the moxa treatments consisted of three 1mg cones on nine points which he described as being "under the waist", with the frequency and dosage reduced if there were any observable signs of overdosage which he judged mainly from signs of fur loss.

The first group did the best; the second group did nearly as well; the third group did not do so well but still compared favourably to the control group; and the fourth group survived an average two months longer than the control group.

His results amazed him and caused him to write: "Disease is not cured by someone else outside but through regenerative powers within." The treatment as far as he saw it would certainly be describable in today's terms as being an immunotherapy. He went on to specifically advocate the use of

[349] The Ming dynasty was a golden period for China in many fields including medicine. Several famous medical texts including the famous "Great Compendium of Acupuncture and Moxibustion" repeatedly recommended moxa for the treatment of TB, promising reliable results if applied correctly.

moxa for the treatment of TB, which was a common killer disease in 1930s Japan. By 1933 Hara was describing moxa as a "peoples" medicine, the only resort for those Japanese living in poverty who were deprived of access to any decent form of health care.

Japan in the 1930s was a very different country to the one which we know today. The vast majority of its population was rural and poor. TB was a common disease which particularly decimated this stratum of society. There are many fascinating similarities between then and now in terms of whom it most devastatingly affects – people with low incomes, low levels of literacy, poor living conditions, little access to affordable or effective health care, living on a poor diet and with constitutionally weakened immune systems.

Hara entitled a chapter of his subsequent 1933 book on moxa[350] "the Proletariat's War". In it he identified that more lives were being lost to TB in Japan each year than were being lost in the ongoing Sino-Japanese war. As importantly, he stressed the social consequences of the disease – that, not only did it affect the person who was infected (who was generally poor), but also both infected and affected the rest of the family. "For a family with no savings", he wrote, "the first page of a tragedy immediately opens to them."

One question still needs answering before his claims can be taken seriously, however. Was the treatment really as effective as his documentary evidence suggested? It was in order to answer this question that the author, along with friend and colleague Jenny Craig, co-founded the Moxafrica charity in 2008.

There are other well-known Japanese reports of moxibustion specialists who claimed to be treating TB effectively with moxa from this time. As the possibilities began to materialise for us, however, it was Hara's treatments which began to interest us more and more. There were four reasons for this. Firstly he was a medical doctor and his approach was therefore largely scientific. Secondly his protocols were designed to be simple and were intended to be done at home by the patients themselves and their relatives with the anatomical locations for the treatment easily mastered with little needed in the way of instruction. Thirdly, they were extremely light in terms of dosage in terms of both size and numbers of cones, and therefore represent the most appropriate and safest approach. In fact his treatment involved the daily application of the tiny moxa cones in the smallest

[350] Shimetaro Hara, "Moxibustion, Therapy effective for all Diseases" (Old Japanese) out of print but currently in translation into Englush (1933).

possible doses in order to create a cumulative effect. Fourth, his reports come with some interesting (apparently rigorous) scientific research, despite the fact that some of his explanations of the mechanisms of response appear today to be a little outdated.

Although his research only used animal subjects, his results remain persuasive. Dependent upon dosage he reported that the treatment aided recovery from TB. We had to accept that his claims may have been overstated and also recognised that his research was only done on animals, but his accounts of his human patients' responses provided us with incentive enough to look more carefully at the Japanese literature and particularly his reports.

For general health maintenance he simply advocated daily moxa on St36 (a bilateral acupuncture point on the leg) using seven tiny moxa cones at each location. "This is all you have to do and something great will happen" he wrote. He had gone on on to form the "Great Japan National Health Alliance". On joining, its members had to swear to carry on self-administering moxa for health promotion for the remainder of their life. Hara himself lived to the grand old age of 108. For the last couple of months of his life he was himself officially the oldest living male in Japan.

His claims of efficacy concerned not just TB, but a wide range of other diseases as well and for these he advocated the bilateral leg points together with his own eight "loin points". These were eight points which he located by applying simple geometry from anatomical landmarks on the patient's lower back. It was these same eight points along along with the two points on the leg that he advocated as being effective for TB. It's unclear to us today as to exactly how he chose their locations since they are not classic acupuncture points, but he described them as being both logical and convenient, hidden from sight, and more pleasant in terms of heat perception than any other points on the body.

He was also fairly certain that some of moxa's effects could be obtained from applying moxa almost anywhere on the body, but he considered that this was only a part of the matter. He was quite certain that the anatomical locations were important.

Be that as it may, we found no more recent repetition of his experiments. Since the advent of TB drugs, there has been no apparent interest at all in Japan in investigating moxa's effects on tuberculosis. Those who were conducting the treatment have since died, their knowledge along with them, and the disease has been adequately controlled by drugs so no incentive exists.

Doctor Hara, however, also investigated the wider effects of moxa on the immune system, particularly monitoring White Blood Cell counts, and there is plenty of more recent information on this subject which casts the treatment in better light for us today. In fact there exists a record of Japanese research into the immunological and serological effects of moxibustion which spans over 80 years right up till today. More recently the focus of the research has been on its effects on tumour growth. In addition, since the advent of HIV/AIDS a far deeper appreciation of the complexities of the immune system has developed than that which was ever understood by Doctor Hara in the 1930s.

The story which emerged for us from this more recent research is not conclusive although it remained persuasive enough for it still to be encouraging. Problems arose particularly from the fact that the published research used widely differing approaches in terms of cone sizes, cone numbers and in the points that were used. It also, more often than not, employed various small mammals for subjects, with different papers asking differing questions from differing treatment approaches.

Not unexpectedly, perhaps,quite widespread variations in immune response have been reported. What was of primary importance to us, however, was that immune responses were indeed being confirmed. In this regard these papers endorsed what was reported to us by every experienced moxibustion practitioner we encountered or contacted based on their clinical experience: that moxa cumulatively strengthens a patient's constitution if it has been weakened by chronic disease.

Seen as a whole, this provided (and still provides) an irresistible argument for us as to why this treatment might be re-examined in the light of the current pandemic – particularly in the developing world. We wanted to find out if it might improve tendencies in recovery, reduce morbidity and mortality, be in any way effective in the treatment of drug-resistant strains, and even help improve prognoses in cases of co-infection with HIV/AIDS. From the outset we could see that the treatment had enormous possibilities for the treatment of TB where resources are poor, but most particularly in Africa if it was applicable in cases of co-infection.

1. First and foremost it is extremely easy to administer. Generally it can be self-administered by the patient, who can be taught how to do the treatment in less than an hour. We have also

subsequently proved that we can teach health workers enough about the treatment in two days for them to be confident in both introducing their patients to the treatment and teaching them how to safely administer it themselves.

2. Furthermore, it is cheap. US$10 will buy enough moxa for a year's supply for the average patient.

3. The treatment itself and the technology required to refine the dried leaf of the plant are both traditional and cannot be patented. This means that no organisation or institution can monopolise any part of the treatment.

4. It also seems to be safe, even with immune compromised patients. Three pilot studies have reported this, and now a clinical trial in Uganda appears to be confirming these earlier findings.

5. It is also a potentially sustainable treatment. Moxa can be easily made from several strains of Artemisia, all of which are found in the temperate zones of the northern hemisphere. We have conducted growth trials of four of these strains on farms in the Western Cape of South Africa (which has a Mediterranean climate), and found that two grow well there. We have yet to establish whether or not they can be cultivated at all in tropical parts of Africa.

6. Everything about the treatment is low-tech and therefore particularly appropriate for rural Africa. Neither does it require electricity. The refining process from leaf to 'moxa floss', in fact, can be achieved with little more than a stone pestle and mortar and a kitchen sieve.

7. No sophisticated diagnostics are required for its application and it need not even be disease-specific for it to be usefully administered. The results from three pilot studies lead us to strongly suspect that the treatment, if applied properly, will not harm, and will probably help, anyone who is suffering from either TB or from TB-like symptoms.

8. Because the treatment works by apparently promoting immune response there are no issues likely to arise relating to drug-resistance or drug interactions.

9. Based on theoretical extrapolation of the immune response, we would suggest that the treatment could even be used prophylactically. It is quite possible that this might stall or prevent the re-activation of a latent infection. It might even help prevent re-infection after drug treatment In some instances it might prevent primary infection from a close-contact infectious case, although much more research would be needed in order to confirm all of this.

10. Finally, we would tentatively suggest that, if drugs are simply unavailable (which we know to be often an unfortunate reality in rural situations) the treatment might prevent worsening of symptoms, reduce infectivity and even promote recovery. We have no evidence to support this idea from our own investigations to date since they have all been conducted adjunctively to first line TB drugs. A theoretical case for this can still be made, however, from the Japanese documentary evidence from the 1930s – from the decade before the first TB drugs were developed and when many recoveries were being reported. This could be an important asset if there are cases of drug-resistant TB in a community which has no access to second line drugs as is becoming increasingly common.

Our initial primary research involved a pilot study in Uganda to establish how African patients and health workers might experience such a culturally foreign traditional treatment. The study ran for a year during which we gathered as much anecdotal evidence as possible concerning patient response. The reports from both patients and health workers were generally very positive, with no reports of adverse effects and a couple of quite dramatic recoveries reported. The picture we were given by the staff involved was that all those who persisted with the daily treatment reported benefits. We also received consistent reports of reduced side effects from the drugs if patients used the treatment. We came to realise that this might be of potential importance if it could be capitalised upon to help patients complete their challenging drug treatment. Last of all we saw no noticeable differences in responses between patients co-infected with HIV and patients infected only with TB.

We then repeated the process in South Africa. We were already well aware that South Africa is the furnace for tuberculosis in Africa, with rates of both disease and drug-resistance that are much higher than further north. We wanted to see how the treatment might be received by what would most probably be a far more challenging group of patients. We conducted two pilots - one in Nyanga (a Cape Town township) and the other in Robertson, a rural town about 200 miles further east with high rates of TB amongst its vineyard workforce. And we received almost exactly the same anecdotal reports, again including a couple of dramatic unexpected recoveries.

In summary, the following observations were made:

No adverse effects of moxa were reported.

Most patients reported unpleasant side effects developing after the start of their TB drug therapy. These were less marked or absent if moxa was used at the same time.

After starting moxa, most patients reported improved appetite, weight gain, reduced joint pains, reduced peripheral neuropathy and a general increase in strength and energy.

In patients who began using moxa some time after starting their TB drugs, there was a reduction in side effects which began sometimes only one or two weeks after starting moxa.

Some patients stopped using moxa when they began to feel better, but some symptoms then returned. They were then encouraged to resume their daily moxa treament, and the symptoms soon reduced accordingly. This served to convince them of the benefits, and many patients wanted to continue using moxa after they had finished their drug course and had been discharged.

Patients co-infected with HIV reported similar improvements with moxa to those having only TB.

Clinic staff suspected that the patients receiving moxa treatment were recovering from TB faster than those on TB drugs alone.

The results of these pilot studies attracted the attention of Makerere University's School of Health Sciences and we were invited to give a presentation about the progress that we had made. As a result of this, we began collaboratively designing a Phase II Randomised Control Trial to test the treatment's use as an adjunctive treatment in a properly controlled scientific study. The study was to be managed by the University, by Professor Paul Waako, with the charity is funding it.

The trial has been comprehensively analysing the response of 180 newly diagnosed patients, with regular sputum tests, full blood counts (which include CD4 and CD8 counts), radiological assessments and quality of life scores (using the Karnofsky scoring method). Currently the study is in its second half, but the preliminary data at half way stage is showing up some exciting preliminary data.

The data so far available is from the first 90 patients and remains preliminary but has revealed serological evidence of an immune response in the CD8 counts in the moxa patients which has not occurred in the patients who are only using TB drugs. The study has also revealed a significantly better bacteriological clearance in the more infectious cases in the moxa group (defined as '++' and '+++' by sputum smear microscopy). If the final analyses confirm this finding there might be an important recommendation that might be made: it could be recommended that all more infectious cases might be considered as being able to potentially benefit from adjunctive moxa therapy in order to improve their recovery rates. It might also suggest that wider use of the treatment on such patients might help reduce the pool of active infection in a community by improving conversion rates in these most infectious cases. Delayed sputum conversion or reduced rates of decline of infectious sputum content during the first month are recognised as reasonable indicators of increased risk of later relapse – there might even be an implication from this as well.

The study is also demonstrating significantly reduced side effects from the TB drugs group. This relates specifically to much fewer reported incidences of arthralgia symproms, which has most probably been caused by Rifampicin or Pyrazinamide. Arthralgia (referred to by both patients and health workers simply as "joint pain") was quite easily the most readily side effect reported in all three pilot studies as well, and they had also reported improvements with moxa therapy. It is our opinion that patients particularly report this side-effect because of the challenges they face when using latrines, squatting over small holes in the floor with painful knees. We consider this to be a likely cause that some patients default on treatment once they feel that their symptoms have cleared. Ameliorating this side effect alone could, we suspect, potentially improve compliance and treatment completion.

We have seen no evidence as yet to support our earlier hypothesis that daily moxa treatment might increase CD4 count in HIV patients, although the preliminary data has yet to be cleansed to properly analyse this factor. Approximately 30% of the enrolled patients are also HIV-positive so offer

an important window into how useful this treatment might be in co-infected cases.
We also have no idea at all about drug-resistant cases. All cases that are confirmed resistant by the GeneXpert device have had to be withdrawn[351] or excluded from the study. Such patients, of course are exactly the ones who might possibly benefit the most from the treatment if it is finally demonstrated to be of benefit.

Pyrazinamide is also frequently used in second line treatment if appropriate, so the same benefits relating to side effects might occur for patients on treatment for MDR- and even XDR-TB treatment. Fluoroquinolones are also identified as frequently causing side effects which include arthralgia. As a result, there would seem to be good reason to develop further investigations using adjunctive moxa on MDR-TB patients, monitoring both their bacteriological conversion rates and their side effects, treatment completion sand rates of cure.

Theoretically (at least if the Japanese claims from the 1930s are to be believed and the evidence of the immunological effects of moxibustion allowed any credit), it should make little and possibly no difference to the suggested efficacies of moxa therapy whether a particular strain of TB is either resistant or susceptible to drug treatment. It should only matter how virulent the strain is and how susceptible the patient is to it. What this suggests is that a higher dosed moxa treatment might be assessed for XDR-TB patients or even MDR-TB patients who are otherwise functionally untreatable because of drug availabilities.

The dosage that was used in the Ugandan RCT was deliberately minimal. This was for several reasons. The reports from the pilots suggested that, when used adjunctively to first line drugs, only minimal treatment would be needed for measurable effect. Maximising patient compliance to the treatment was also seen as being vital to the quality of any final data, and a more complex protocol which could not be self-administered by the patient was seen to present a risk of a much higher drop-out rate.

Under normal circumstances only 5-10% of those infected by the bacillus go on to develop active infectious TB. We feel that we can reasonably suggest that the use of moxa in Japan in the 1930s might have sufficiently stimulated the host responses of some of these statistically prone 5-10% to

---

[351] Access to GeneXpert became available some months after the trial was begun.

have enabled the disease to be re-confined to a state of non-infectious latency. Whether it actually ever 'cured' the disease remains an unknown. But then, under the WHO's current definitions of cure in bacteriologically confirmed cases of disease, the same doubt still exists symptoms subside and there would be no further bacteriological evidence of existence of disease. In this sense, nothing has changed since the 1930s.

Those Japanese practitioners, however, never had to consider the problems of co-infection with HIV/AIDS, and so the idea that moxa might today help fight TB in Africa (or India, or in any resource-poor environment) can still only really be mooted on a theoretical model which considers only half of the current syndemic without good new clinical data.

We also remain unsure as to exactly how the treatment works (if it does). We are now more confident that there is an immune response from the heat stimulation, but we also believe that there may be a secondary chemical response from tiny amounts of one of the chemicals in the moxa being absorbed into the skin.[352]

The most important question of all, however, remains: could this simple treatment possibly make a real difference in a general context where resources are poor, but also particularly when and where the disease is functionally untreatable?

We started with a blank slate. That slate is little by little being filled in, and what it tells us so far is that it might do.

---

[352] This chemical is borneol. See Merlin Young – "The Moon over Matsushima – Insights into Moxa and Mugwort", Godiva Books (2012).

Index